RADIOGRAPHIC PATHOLOGY FOR TECHNOLOGISTS

Sixth Edition

NINA KOWALCZYK, PHD, RT(R)(QM)(CT), FASRT
Assistant Professor
Radiologic Sciences and Therapy
The School of Health and Rehabilitation Sciences
The Ohio State University
Columbus, Ohio

ELSEVIER

ELSEVIER
MOSBY

3251 Riverport Lane
Maryland Heights, MO 63043

Notices

Library of Congress Control Number 2007932477
Kowalczyk, Nina, author.
    Radiographic pathology for technologists / Nina Kowalczyk. – Sixth edition.
        p. ; cm.
    Includes bibliographical references and index.
    ISBN 978-0-323-08902-9 (pbk. : alk. paper)
    I. Title.
    [DNLM: 1. Radiography–methods.   2. Pathology–methods.   WN 200]
    RC78
    616.07–dc23

                                                    2013021567

Executive Content Strategist: Sonya Seigafuse
Content Development Specialist: Amy Whittier
Publishing Services Manager: Catherine Jackson
Production Editor: Sara Alsup
Design Direction: Paula Catalano

Working together
to grow libraries in
developing countries

www.elsevier.com • www.bookaid.org

Printed in China

Last digit it the print number: 9 8 7 6 5 4 3 2 1

Kevin D. Evans, PhD, RT(R)(M)(BD), RDMS, RVS, FSDMS
Associate Professor/Director
Radiologic Sciences and Therapy
The School of Health and Rehabilitation Sciences
The Ohio State University
Columbus, Ohio

Tricia Leggett, DHEd, RT(R)(QM)
Assistant Professor and Radiologic Technology Clinical Coordinator
Assessment Coordinator
Zane State College
Zanesville, Ohio

Jonathan Mazal, MS, RT(R)(MR), RRA
MRI Technologist
National Institutes of Health
Bethesda, Maryland
*Contributing in his personal capacity

Beth McCarthy, BS, RT(R)(CV)
Research Coordinator
Cardiovascular Medicine
The Ross Heart Hospital at The Ohio State University Wexner Medical Center
Columbus, Ohio

Deanna Butcher, MA, RT(R)
Program Director
St. Cloud Hospital School of Diagnostic
    Imaging
St. Cloud, Minnesota

Robert J. Comello, MS, RT(R)(CDT)
Radiologic Science Program
Midwestern State University
Wichita Falls, Texas

Gail Faig, BS, RT(R)(CV)(CT)
Clinical Coordinator
Shore Medical Center
Somers Point, New Jersey

Kelli Haynes, MSRS, RT(R)
Program Director
Northwestern State University
Shreveport, Louisiana

Deborah R. Leighty, MEd, RT(R)(BD)
Clinical Coordinator, Radiography Program
Hillsborough Community College
Tampa, Florida

Marcia Moore, BS, RT(R)(CT)
Instructor
St. Luke's College
Sioux City, Iowa

Jeannean Rollins, MRC, BSRT(R)(CV)
Associate Professor, Medical Imaging and
    Radiation Sciences Department
Arkansas State University
Jonesboro, Arkansas

**Melissa Hale Smith, BSRT(R)(MR)(CT),
    CNMT**
Instructor, Magnetic Resonance Imaging
    Program
Forsyth Technical Community College
Winston-Salem, North Carolina

Staci Smith, RT(R), MHA
Program Director
Holy Cross Hospital School of Radiologic
    Technology
Silver Spring, Maryland

Timothy Whittaker, MS, RT(R)(CT)(QM)
Associate Professor of Radiology
Hazard Community and Technical College
Hazard, Kentucky

The sixth edition of *Radiographic Pathology for Technologists* has been thoroughly updated and revised to offer students and medical imaging professionals information on the pathologic appearance of common diseases in a variety of diagnostic imaging modalities. It also presents basic information on the pathologic process, signs and symptoms, diagnosis, and prognosis of the various diseases.

The sixth edition includes the latest information concerning recent advances in genetic mapping, biomarkers, and up-to-date imaging modalities used in daily practice. The authors have attempted to present this material in a succinct, but reasonably complete, fashion to meet the needs of professionals in various imaging specialties. With each new edition, the authors have also expanded the scope of the material covered in the text to provide the reader with a broader base of knowledge.

NEW TO THIS EDITION

- The chapter order and arrangement have been changed to accommodate the general revision of existing material.
- Over 50 new illustrations have been added to complement new, updated, or expanded material.
- Human genetic technology information has been expanded, and altered cell biology has been added to Chapter 1.
- Genetic marker and information regarding biomarkers have been added throughout the text.
- The most recent American College of Radiology Appropriateness Criteria has been incorporated throughout the text.
- Several new terms have been added to the glossary, and other definitions have been expanded or updated.

LEARNING ENHANCEMENTS

- Each chapter begins with an outline, followed by key terms and learning objectives.
- Chapter content is followed by a summary table, general discussion questions, and multiple-choice review questions, all of which can be used by the reader to assess acquired knowledge or by the instructor to stimulate discussion.
- Bold print has been used to focus the reader's attention on the key terms in each chapter, which are defined in the glossary at the end of the book along with other relevant terms.

USING THE BOOK

The presentation of the sixth edition presumes that the reader has some background in human anatomy and physiology, imaging procedures, and medical and imaging terminology. The reader may build on this knowledge by assimilating information presented in this text.

To facilitate a working knowledge of the principles of radiologic pathology, study materials presented in the sixth edition remain sophisticated enough to be true to the complexity of the subject, yet simple and concise enough to permit comprehension by all readers. For student radiographers, sonographers, radiation therapists, and nuclear medicine technologists, this text is best used in conjunction with formal instruction from a qualified instructor. The practicing imaging professional may use this book as a self-teaching instrument to broaden and reinforce existing knowledge of the subject matter and also as a means to acquaint himself or herself with changing concepts and new material. The book can serve as a resource for continuing education because it provides an extensive range of information.

ANCILLARIES

Evolve Resources

Evolve is an interactive learning environment designed to work in coordination with *Radiographic Pathology for Technologists*. Included on the Evolve website are a test bank in Exam View containing approximately 400 questions, an electronic images collection consisting of images from the textbook, and a PowerPoint presentation. Instructors may use Evolve to provide an Internet-based course component that reinforces and expands the concepts presented in class. Evolve may be used to publish the class syllabus, outlines, and lecture notes; set up "virtual office hours" and e-mail communication; share important dates and information through the online class calendar; and encourage student participation through chat rooms and discussion boards. Evolve also allows instructors to post examinations and manage their grade books online. For more information, visit http://evolve.elsevier.com/Kowalczyk/pathology/ or contact an Elsevier sales representative.

ACKNOWLEDGMENTS

Over twenty years ago, two young and fairly naïve radiography educators collaborated to undertake the task of developing a pathology textbook for radiography students. At that time, only one small textbook was commercially available and little did we know that the text-book we conceived and created would result in five subsequent editions spanning almost 25 years! As I began to revise this sixth edition, I was amazed at the changes that have occurred over the past 20 years relative to understanding pathologic processes. Great strides have been made in genetic mapping and the identification of biomarkers that allow the advent of personalized medicine. Although this is a complex area of study, basic information has been added to the sixth edition of this text because it is crucial for all radiation science professionals to have an understanding of the impact of genomics in current medical practice.

In 1986, working together, JD Mace and Nina Kowalczyk combined their course materials, added information by researching outside pathology sources, and began the task of contacting publishers with the concept of creating a comprehensive textbook to meet this need. Although both authors worked on developing the content for review, JD Mace assumed the lead role in contacting and communicating with various publishers to bring the work to fruition. JD's initiative and dedication to this project led to the first edition of *Radiographic Pathology for Technologists*, which was published in 1988. JD Mace played a major role in the development of the concept for this textbook, its format, and all administrative tasks associated with this project. JD also continued to be a major contributor to the following three editions of *Radiographic Pathology for Technologists*. However, shortly after the first edition was published, his professional career path led him away from education to radiology and healthcare administration. JD remained committed to the role of lead author for subsequent editions, but over the years his professional focus led him further away from clinical practice and education. Although his role was limited in the fifth edition, the textbook would never have been created if not for the lead role he assumed in the late 1980s. JD Mace is a true professional and has given much to the field of radiologic technology. I am sorry that he is no longer a co-author in this current edition, but thankful he is a true friend for life. His foresight and contributions are greatly missed.

I certainly could not have completed the sixth edition of this text without a great team of people who wanted it to be successful and to accomplish its primary mission. I would like to thank my son, Nick, for his support; my students, past and present, for their inspiration; and my colleagues for their encouragement. I also want to thank the editorial team at Elsevier who worked diligently to keep me on track throughout the revision process.

The images in this book come from a variety of fine organizations that are to be thanked for graciously allowing us to use their material. They include the American College of Radiology, as well as The Ohio State University Wexner Medical Center, Riverside Methodist Hospitals, and Nationwide Children's Hospital—all located in Columbus, Ohio.

Nina Kowalczyk

Introduction to Pathology

Incidence
Infection
Inflammatory
Invasion
Lesion
Leukemia
Lymphatic spread
Lymphoma
Malignant neoplasm
Manifestations
Metabolism
Metaplasia
Metastatic spread
Morbidity rate
Morphology
Mortality rate

Neoplastic
Nosocomial
Pathogenesis
Physical mapping
Prevalence
Prognosis
Sarcoma
Seeding
Sequelae
Sign
Single-nucleotide polymorphisms
Symptom
Syndrome
Traumatic
Virulence

Pathology is the study of disease. Many types of disease exist, and, in general, many conditions can be readily demonstrated by imaging studies. Additionally, image-guided interventional procedures and therapeutic protocols are often utilized in the management of disease. Therefore, it is critical for radiologic professionals to have a thorough understanding of basic pathologic processes. This foundation begins with a working knowledge of common pathologic terms, an understanding of impact of disease and prevention on U.S. health care expenditures, and the role of genetics in the development and individualized treatment of different pathologic processes. It is also important to understand the role of the Centers for Disease Control and Prevention (CDC) in terms of tracking, monitoring, and reporting trends in health and aging. This information is captured and reported by the National Center for Health Statistics (NCHS).

This chapter serves as a brief introduction to terms associated with pathology, recent health trends, and a review of cellular biology and genetics.

PATHOLOGIC TERMS

Any abnormal disturbance of the function or structure of the human body as a result of some type of injury is called a **disease**. After injury, **pathogenesis** occurs. *Pathogenesis* refers to the sequence of events producing cellular changes that ultimately lead to observable changes known as **manifestations**. These manifestations may be displayed in a variety of fashions. A **symptom** refers to the patient's perception of the disease. Symptoms are subjective, and only the patient can identify these manifestations. For example, a headache is considered a symptom. A **sign** is an objective manifestation that is detected by the physician during examination. Fever, swelling, and skin rash are all considered signs. A group of signs and symptoms that characterizes a specific abnormal disturbance is a **syndrome**. For example, respiratory distress syndrome is a common disorder in premature infants. However, some disease processes, especially in the early stages, do not produce symptoms and are termed **asymptomatic**.

Etiology is the study of the cause of a disease. Common agents that cause diseases include viruses, bacteria, trauma, heat, chemical agents, and poor nutrition. At the molecular level, a genetic abnormality of a single protein may also serve as the etiologic basis for some diseases. Proper infection control practices are important in a health care environment to prevent hospital-acquired **nosocomial** disease. Staphylococcal infection that follows hip replacement surgery is an example of a nosocomial disease, that is, one acquired from the environment. The cause of the disease, in this case, could be poor infection-control practices. **Iatrogenic** reactions are adverse responses to medical treatment itself (e.g., a collapsed lung that occurs in response to a complication that arises during arterial line placement). If no causative factor can be identified, a disease is termed **idiopathic.**

The length of time over which the disease is displayed may vary. **Acute** diseases usually have a quick onset and last for a short period, whereas **chronic** diseases may manifest more slowly and last for a very long time. An example of an acute disease is pneumonia, and multiple sclerosis is considered a chronic condition. An acute illness may be followed by lasting effects termed **sequelae**—for example, a stroke, or cerebrovascular accident, resulting in long-term neurologic deficits. Similarly, chronic illnesses often manifest in acute episodes, for example, an individual diagnosed with diabetes mellitus experiencing hypoglycemia or hyperglycemia.

Two additional terms refer to the identification and outcome of a disease. A **diagnosis** is the identification of a disease an individual is believed to have, and the predicted course and outcome of the disease is called a **prognosis.**

The structure of cells or tissue is termed **morphology.** Pathologic conditions may cause morphologic changes that alter normal body tissues in a variety of ways. Sometimes, the disease process is destructive, decreasing the normal density of a tissue. This occurs when tissue composition is altered by a decrease in the atomic number of the tissue or the compactness of the cells or by changes in tissue thickness, for example, atrophy from limited use. Such disease processes are radiographically classified as *subtractive, lytic,* or *destructive* and require a decrease in the exposure technique. Conversely, some pathologic conditions cause an increase in the normal density of a tissue, resulting in a higher atomic number or increased compactness of cells. These are classified as *additive* or *sclerotic* disease processes and require an increase in

the exposure technique. It is important for the radiographer to know common pathologic conditions that require an alteration of the exposure technique so that high-quality radiographs can be obtained to assist in the diagnosis and treatment of the disease.

Government agencies compile statistics annually with regard to the incidence, or rate of occurrence, of disease. **Epidemiology** is the investigation of disease in large groups. Health care epidemiology is grounded in the belief that the distributions of health states (good health, disease, disability, and death) are not random within a population and are influenced by multiple factors, including biologic, social, and environmental factors. Health care epidemiologists conduct research primarily by working with medical statistics, data associations, and large cohort studies. The **prevalence** of a given disease refers to the number of cases found in a given population. The **incidence** of disease refers to the number of new cases found in a given period. Diseases of high prevalence in an area where a given causative organism is commonly found are said to be *endemic* to that area. For example, histoplasmosis is a fungal disease of the respiratory system endemic to the Ohio and Mississippi River valleys. It is not uncommon to see a relatively high prevalence of this disease in these areas. Its appearance in great numbers in the western United States, however, could represent an epidemic.

MONITORING DISEASE TRENDS

Over the past century, life expectancy in the United States has continued to increase. The majority of children born at the beginning of the twenty-first century are expected to live well into their eighth decade (Fig. 1-1). Over the past 100 years, the principal causes of death have shifted from acute infections to chronic diseases. These changes have occurred as a result of biomedical and pharmaceutical advances, public health initiatives, and social changes over the past century (Fig. 1-2). But experts disagree about the trend of increased life expectancy

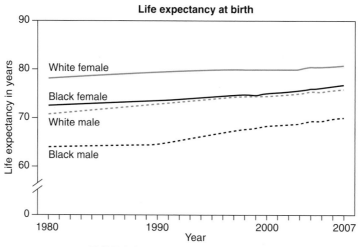

FIGURE 1-1 Life expectancy at birth.

continuing into the twenty-first century. Some believe that increased knowledge of disease etiology and continued development of medical technology in combination with screening, early intervention, and treatment of disease could have positive results. However, many experts express concern about the quality of life of older adults. In other words, the possibility of older adults spending their added years in declining health and lingering illness, instead of being active and productive, is a concern.

The **mortality rate** is the average number of deaths caused by a particular disease in a population. Death certificates are collected by each state, forwarded to the NCHS, and subsequently processed and published as information on mortality statistics and trends. The NCHS and the U.S. Department of Health and Human Services (USDHHS) monitor and report mortality rates in terms of leading causes of death according to gender, race, age, and specific causes of death such as heart disease or malignant neoplasia. Trends in these mortality patterns are identified by age, gender, and ethnic origin and tracked to help identify necessary interventions. For instance, the age-adjusted death rate for heart diseases has steadily decreased for both women and men in the United States. This trend demonstrates a 30% to 40% decline over the past 20 years resulting, in part, from health education and changes in lifestyle behaviors. Because mortality information is gathered from death certificates, changes in the descriptions and coding of "cause of death" and the amount of information forwarded to the NCHS may alter these statistics. For instance, changes in the way deaths were recorded and ranked in terms of the leading causes of death occurred between 1998 and 1999. Since 1999, mortality data and cause-of-death statistics have been gathered and classified according to the *Tenth Revision, International Classification of Diseases* (ICD-10), and in 2007 additional ICD-10 codes were added to clarify the underlying causes of death.

Chronic diseases continue to be the leading causes of death in the United States for adults age 45 years and older. Heart diseases and malignant neoplasia remained the top two causes of deaths in 2007 for both males and females, responsible collectively for 48.6% of all deaths. The third, fourth, and fifth top causes of death in 2007 were stroke, chronic lower respiratory diseases, and accidents, respectively. Alzheimer disease continues to increase and was ranked as the sixth leading cause of death in 2007. Emphasis has been placed on reducing the deaths

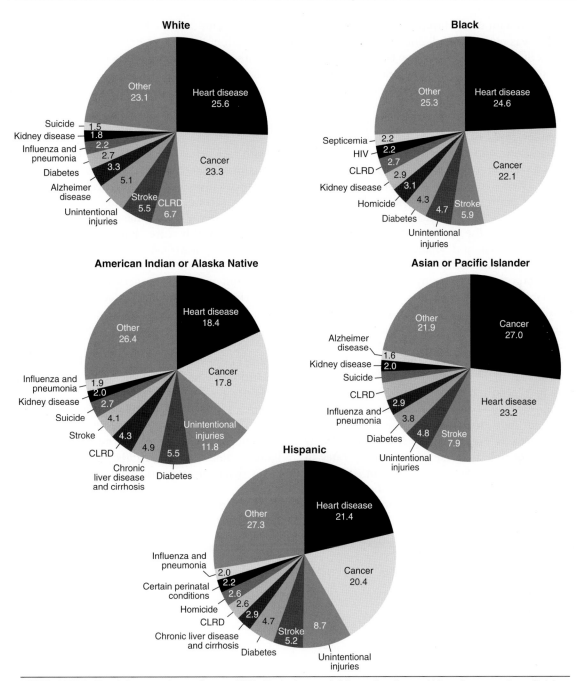

NOTES: CLRD is Chronic lower respiratory diseases; HIV is Human Immunodeficiency virus disease. Values show percentage of total deaths. ICD–10 code J09 (Influenza due to avian influenza virus) was added to the influenza and pneumonia category in 2007; no deaths occurred from this cause in 2007.)
SOURCE: CDC/NCHS, National Vital Statistics System, Mortality.

FIGURE 1-2 National Vital Statistics Report of the 10 leading causes of death by race and ethnicity: United States, 2007.

associated with these chronic diseases, and slight decline was noted through 2007. The decrease in deaths due to heart disease may be clearly attributed to advances in the prevention and treatment of cardiac disease. An increased understanding of the genetics of cancer is certainly responsible for better screening and individualized treatment for many types of neoplastic disease. Advances in diagnostic and therapeutic radiologic procedures have also played a role in the reduction of deaths associated with these chronic diseases.

As the mortality rate for heart disease and cancer have declined, increases have been noted in Alzheimer disease and diabetes mellitus. Among children and young adults (age 1–44 years), injury remains the leading cause of death.

Mortality rates from any specific cause may fluctuate from year to year, so trends are monitored over a 3-year period. These data are used to evaluate the health status of U.S. citizens and identify segments of the population at greatest risk from specific diseases and injuries. Current data are available on the NCHS Web site and may be accessed at www.cdc.gov/.

The incidence of sickness sufficient to interfere with an individual's normal daily routine is referred to as the **morbidity rate**. The CDC is also responsible for trending morbidity rates in the United States. States must submit death certificates to the NCHS, making it fairly easy to obtain accurate data about the mortality rate of a specific population. It is more difficult to obtain accurate data about the morbidity rate. This information comes primarily from physicians and other health care workers reporting morbidity statistics and information to the various governmental and private agencies.

Health Care Resources

Health care delivery in the United States has two fundamental and diverse functions, with one area focused on healthy lifestyle for prevention and the second area focusing on restoration of health after a disease has occurred. Improvements in health care interventions such as technology, electronic communications, and pharmaceuticals have greatly contributed to a shift from inpatient services to outpatient services (Fig. 1-3). Ambulatory care centers range from hospital outpatient and emergency departments to physicians' offices. In response to this shift, emphasis has been placed on increasing the number of physician generalists, including family practitioners, internal medicine physicians, and pediatricians. Inpatient admissions and hospital length of stay have remained fairly consistent over the past 10 years; however, emergency department visits have continued to steadily increase since the late 1990s, with many emergency departments reporting admissions exceeding their capacity (Fig. 1-4).

The rate of growth in U.S. health expenditures is staggering. In 2010, U.S. health spending

FIGURE 1-3 Number of outpatient hospital visits per 1000 persons during 1988 to 2008.

FIGURE 1-4 Percent of hospitals reporting emergency department capacity issues by type of hospital, 2010.

accounted for 17.3% of the gross domestic product, a larger share than in any other major industrialized country, with U.S. health care expenditures totaling $2.6 trillion (Table 1-1). The average annual health spending increase from 2010 through 2020 is projected to outpace average annual growth in the overall economy by 4.7%. The major sources of funding for health care include Medicare, funded by the federal government for older adults and disabled individuals; Medicaid, funded by federal and state governments for the poor; and privately funded health care plans. However, the Centers for Medicare and Medicaid Services (CMS) project that private insurance and out-of-pocket spending on health care will almost double to a rate of 4.8% in 2013. Estimates from the CDC National Health Interview Survey for 2010 indicated that approximately 16% of the U.S. population was uninsured at the time of the interview (Fig. 1-5). For those under the age of 18 years, the percentage of the uninsured has continued to decline since 1997 as a result of governmental legislation with regard to Medicaid and other government insurance for children. The diagnosis and treatment of cancer and other chronic diseases consume enormous financial and other resources in health care. Therefore, emphasis on wellness and disease prevention must continue to reduce these costs. Studies have shown that it is much more cost-effective to provide preventive care than to wait until a disease has progressed.

TABLE 1-1	National Health Expenditures,[1] 1980–2019[2]
Year	**Expenditures (Billions)**
1980	$253
1990	$714
2000	$1353
2001	$1469
2002	$1602
2003	$1735
2004	$1855
2005	$1983
2006	$2113
2007	$2239
2008	$2339
2009	$2472
2010	$2570
2011	$2703
2012	$2850
2013	$3025
2014	$3225
2015	$3442
2016	$3684
2017	$3936
2018	$4204
2019	$4483

[1]Years 2009–2019 are projections.

[2]CMS completed a benchmark revision in 2006, introducing changes in methods, definitions, and source data that are applied to the entire time series (back to 1960). For more information on this revision, see http://www.cms.hhs.gov.

From Centers for Medicare & Medicaid Services, Office of the Actuary. Data released February 4, 2010.

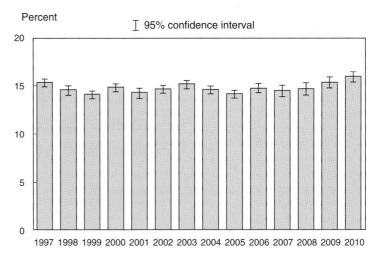

FIGURE 1-5 Percentage of persons of all ages without health insurance coverage, United States, 1997–2010.

HUMAN GENETIC TECHNOLOGY

The Human Genome Project was a 13-year (1990–2003) project coordinated by the U.S. Department of Energy and the National Institutes of Health. The goals of the project were to identify the 30,000 genes in the human deoxyribonucleic acid (DNA); to determine the sequences of the three billion chemical base pairs that make up the human DNA; to electronically store the data; to improve tools for data analysis; and to address ethical, legal, and social issues that arose from the project.

With the exception of reproductive cells, each cell in the human body contains 22 pairs of autosomal chromosomes, 2 sex chromosomes (XX or XY), and the small chromosome found in each mitochondria within the cell. Collectively, this is known as a **genome**. The genome contains between 50,000 to 100,000 genes that are located on approximately three billion base pairs of DNA and forms the basic unit of genetics. Genetics play a significant role in the diagnosis, monitoring, and treatment of disease; thus, it is imperative that radiologic science professionals have a basic understanding of the role of genetics and genetic markers in the development and treatment of disease.

The genome project resulted in the identification of thousands of DNA sequence landmarks and the development of two types of gene maps (Fig. 1-6). **Physical maps** are used to determine the physical location of a particular gene on a specific chromosome. **Genetic maps** are used to assign the distance between the genetic markers, that is, mapping or linking DNA fragments, to a specific chromosome. Genetic linkage maps are useful in tracking inheritance of traits and diseases that are transmitted from parent to child because genetic markers that are in proximity increase the probability that the genes will be inherited together.

As more information was discovered through the Human Genome Project, researchers determined that the genome sequence was 99.9% identical for all humans, leaving only a small percentage of variation among people. However, this 0.1% variation greatly affects an individual's predisposition to certain diseases and his or her response to drugs and toxins. Researchers were able to identify common DNA pattern sequences and common patterns of genetic variations of single DNA bases termed **single-nucleotide polymorphisms** (SNPs). This led to the development of haplotype mapping, often referred to as the *Hap Map*. A **haplotype** comprises closely linked SNPs on a single chromosome, and it is a very important resource in identifying specific DNA sequences affecting disease, response to pharmaceuticals, and response to environmental factors.

Mapping genes to whole chromosomes

chromosome banding
DNA hybridization to somatic cell
   hybrids or sorted chromosomes
in situ hybridization
karyotyping

Genetic linkage mapping

Physical mapping of large DNA fragments

yeast artificial chromosome
cloning gel electrophoresis

Physical mapping of small DNA fragments

FIGURE 1-6 Mapping genes to whole chromosomes at different levels of resolution.

©1992 by BSCS & The American Medical Association.

This continued research has led to improved diagnosis of disease, earlier detection of genetic predispositions to disease, gene therapy, newborn screening, customized pharmaceutical applications, DNA fingerprinting, and DNA forensics. This serves as the basis for the current emphasis on individualized medicine, as no two patients are the same. It also has resulted in the ability to predict the development of certain diseases, thus allowing earlier intervention. Additional information about the National Human Genome Institute can be found at www.genome.gov.

ALTERED CELLULAR BIOLOGY

To protect themselves and avoid injury, cells adapt by altering the genes responsible for their function and differentiation in response to their environment. When a cell is injured and unable to maintain homeostasis, it can respond in several ways. It may adapt and recover from the injury, or it may die as a result of the injury (Fig. 1-7). Many cells adapt by altering their pattern of growth, as demonstrated in Figure 1-8. **Atrophy** is a generalized decrease in cell size. An example of atrophy is when muscle cells decrease in size after the loss of innervation and use. **Hypertrophy** is a generalized increase in cell size. If the aortic valve is diseased, then the left ventricle enlarges because of the increased muscle mass

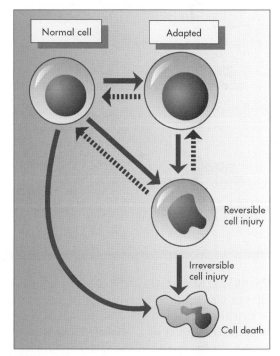

FIGURE 1-7 Cellular injury and responses of normal adapted and reversibly injured cells and cell death.

needed to pump blood into the aorta. **Hyperplasia** is an increase in the number of cells in a tissue as a result of excessive proliferation. An estrogen-secreting ovarian tumor causing endometrial epithelial cells to multiply is an example of

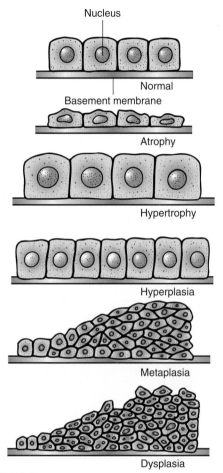

FIGURE 1-8 Adaptive alterations in simple cuboidal epithelial cells.

TABLE 1-2	Altered Cellular Biology
Cell Type	**Description**
Anaplasia	Absence of tumor cell differentiation, loss of cellular organization
Dysplasia	Abnormal changes in mature cells; also termed *atypical hyperplasia*
Metaplasia	Abnormal transformation of a specific differentiated cell into a differentiated cell of another type

DISEASE CLASSIFICATIONS

Diseases are grouped into several broad categories. Those in the same category may not necessarily be closely related, but groupings such as those discussed in the following sections tend to produce lesions that are similar in morphology—that is, their form and structure. Pathologies discussed in this text are generally grouped into the following classifications:

- Congenital and hereditary
- Inflammatory
- Degenerative
- Metabolic
- Traumatic
- Neoplastic

Congenital and Hereditary Disease

Diseases present at birth and resulting from genetic or environmental factors are termed **congenital**. It is estimated that 2% to 3% of all infants born live have one or more congenital abnormalities, although some of these may not be visible until a year or so after birth. A major category of congenital diseases is caused by abnormalities in the number and distribution of chromosomes. In somatic cells (those other than germ cells), chromosomes exist in the nucleus of each cell in pairs, with one member from the male parent and the other from the female parent. In humans, chromosomes are normally composed of 22 pairs of autosomes (those other than the sex chromosomes) and one pair of sex

hyperplasia. **Metaplasia** is the conversion of one cell type into another cell type that is not normal for that tissue (Table 1-2). The epithelial cells in the respiratory tract of a smoker undergo metaplasia as a response to the chronic irritation from the chemicals in the smoke. **Dysplasia** refers to abnormal changes of mature cells. Individual cells within a tissue vary in size, shape, and color, and they are often nonfunctional. Dysplastic adaptations are considered precancerous and are most commonly associated with neoplasms within the reproductive system and the respiratory tract.

chromosomes. Down syndrome is a congenital condition caused by an error in autosomal mitosis that leads to an extra twenty-first chromosome, so the affected individual has 47 chromosomes rather than the normal 46.

Hereditary diseases are caused by developmental disorders genetically transmitted from either parent to a child through abnormalities of individual genes in chromosomes and are derived from ancestors. For example, hemophilia is a well-known hereditary disease, in which proper blood clotting is absent. A genetic abnormality present on the sex chromosome is a sex-linked inheritance; an abnormality on one of the other 22 chromosomes is an autosomal inheritance. The inherited disease may be *dominant* (transmitted by a single gene from either parent) or *recessive* (transmitted by both parents to an offspring). Amniocentesis, a standard procedure typically guided by sonography, is used prenatally to assess the presence of certain hereditary disorders.

A congenital defect is not necessarily hereditary because it may have been acquired in utero. Intrauterine injury during a critical point in development may have been caused by maternal infections, radiation, or drugs. Abnormalities of this type occur sporadically and cannot generally be recognized before birth. However, their likelihood is greatly lessened by following proper precautions against infection, avoiding radiation (particularly during the early term of pregnancy), and avoiding drugs or agents not specifically recognized by a physician as safe for use during pregnancy.

Inflammatory Disease

An **inflammatory** disease results from the body's reaction to a localized injurious agent. Types of inflammatory diseases include infective, toxic, and allergic diseases. An infective disease results from invasion by microorganisms such as viruses, bacteria, or fungi. Viruses consist of a protein coat surrounding a genome of either ribonucleic acid (RNA) or DNA, without an organized cell structure. They are classified by the type of viral genome and are not capable of replicating outside of a living cell. Bacteria are unicellular organisms that lack an organized nucleus. They tend to colonize on environmental surfaces and are extremely adaptable, which allows them to become resistant to antibiotics over time. Fungi are microorganisms that can form complex structures containing organelles and may grow as mold or yeast. For instance, pneumonia is a type of inflammatory disease that may result from a viral, bacterial, or fungal infection. Toxic diseases are caused by poisoning by biologic substances, and allergic diseases are an overreaction of the body's own defenses.

Some diseases in this classification are considered autoimmune disorders. Under normal conditions, antibodies are formed in response to foreign antigens. In certain diseases, however, they form against and injure the patient's own tissues. These are known as **autoantibodies**, and diseases associated with them are termed **autoimmune disorders**. Rheumatoid arthritis is an example of an autoimmune disorder.

An inflammatory reaction (i.e., inflammation) is a generalized pathologic process that is nonspecific to the agent causing the injury. The body's purpose in creating an inflammatory reaction is to localize the injurious agent and prepare for subsequent repair and healing of the injured tissues. Substances released from the damaged tissues may cause both local and systemic effects (Fig. 1-9). Those effects seen local to the injury include capillary dilatation to allow fluids and leukocytes, specifically, to infiltrate into the area of damage. Cellular necrosis (death) is common in acute inflammation, and the leukocytes serve to remove dead material through phagocytosis. The characteristics of such acute inflammation include heat, redness of skin, swelling, pain, and some loss of function as the body tends to protect the injured part. If the inflammatory process is significant, systemic effects such as an elevation of body temperature become evident.

Chronic inflammation differs from the acute stage in that damage caused by an injurious agent may not necessarily result in tissue death. In fact, necrosis is relatively uncommon in cases

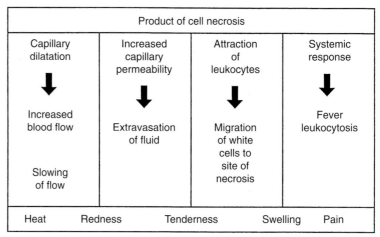

FIGURE 1-9 Local and systemic effects of cell necrosis induced by various agents.

of chronic inflammation. It differs also in the duration of the inflammation, with chronic conditions lasting for long periods, such as the presence of neuropathy resulting in an individual with chronic diabetes mellitus.

The repair of tissues damaged by an inflammatory process attempts to return the body to normal. Tissue regeneration is the process by which damaged tissues are replaced by new tissues that are essentially identical to those that have been lost. Although this is the most desirable type of repair, tissues vary in their ability to replace themselves. Damaged nerve cells, for example, are not likely to readily regenerate. Fibrous connective tissue repair is the alternative to regeneration, but it is less desirable because it leads to scarring and fibrosis. Damaged tissues are replaced by a scar and lack the structure and function of the original tissue.

Debridement (removal of dead cells and materials) is an essential component of the healing process. It may be accomplished both at the cellular level and through human intervention, as in the case of burns or removal of foreign objects such as pieces of glass. The repair process begins with the migration of adjacent cells into the injured area and replication of the cells via mitosis to fill the void in the tissue. This new growth includes capillaries, fibroblasts, collagen, and elastic fibers. Remodeling of the new tissue, the last phase in the healing process, occurs in response to normal use of the tissue. For instance, remodeling of the bone after a skeletal fracture may take months, but the results often return the injured bone to its original contour.

Infection refers to an inflammatory process caused by a disease-causing organism. Under favorable conditions, the invading pathogenic agent multiplies and causes injurious effects. Generally, localized infection is accompanied by inflammation, but inflammation may occur without infection. **Virulence** refers to the ease with which an organism can overcome body defenses. An organism with high virulence is likely to produce progressive disease in susceptible persons; one with low virulence produces disease only in highly susceptible persons under favorable conditions. A variety of factors such as the presence of dead tissue or blockage of normal body passages may predispose an individual to bacterial infection.

Degenerative Disease

Degenerative diseases are caused by deterioration of the body. Although they are usually associated with the aging process, some degenerative conditions may exist in younger patients. For instance, an individual may develop a degenerative disease following a traumatic injury, regardless of age.

The process of aging results from the gradual maturation of physiologic processes that reach a peak and then gradually fade (i.e., degenerate) to a point at which the body can no longer survive. Heredity, diet, and environmental factors are known to affect the rate of aging. Over time, the functional abilities of tissues decrease because either their cell numbers are reduced or the function of each individual cell declines, with both typically participating in pathologies resulting from aging. Atherosclerosis, osteoporosis, and osteoarthritis are three diseases commonly associated with the aging process. Each is discussed later in this text.

Metabolic Disease

Metabolism is the sum of all physical and chemical processes in the body. Diseases caused by a disturbance of the normal physiologic function of the body are classified as metabolic diseases. These include endocrine disorders such as diabetes mellitus and hyperparathyroidism and disturbances of fluid and electrolyte balance.

Endocrine glands secrete their products (hormones) into the bloodstream to regulate various metabolic functions. The major endocrine glands include the pituitary, thyroid, parathyroid, and adrenal glands; pancreatic islets; ovaries; and testes. An endocrine disorder may consist of hypersecretion, which causes an overactivity of the target organ, or hyposecretion, which results in underactivity. The clinical effects of an endocrine disturbance depend on the degree of dysfunction as well as the age and sex of the individual.

Dehydration is the most common disturbance of fluid balance. It is caused by insufficient intake of water or excessive loss of it. Electrolytes are mineral salts (most commonly sodium and potassium) that are dissolved in the body's water. They may be depleted because of vomiting, diarrhea, or use of *diuretics* (substances that promote the excretion of salt and water). Disturbance of either fluid balance or electrolyte balance upsets *homeostasis*, the body's normal internal resting state.

Traumatic Disease

Another general classification of diseases is **traumatic** diseases. These diseases may result from mechanical forces such as crushing or twisting of a body part or from the effects of ionizing radiation on the human body. In addition, disorders resulting from extreme hot or cold temperatures, for example, burns and frostbite, are also classified as traumatic.

Trauma may injure a bone, resulting in *fractures*, which are covered extensively in Chapter 12. It may also injure soft tissues. A *wound* is an injury of soft parts associated with rupture of the skin. Traumatic injuries may damage soft tissues even if the skin is not broken. Bleeding into the tissue spaces as a result of capillary rupture is known as a *bruise* or a *contusion*.

Neoplastic Disease

Neoplastic disease results in new, abnormal tissue growth. Normally, growing and maturing cells are subject to mechanisms that direct cell proliferation and cell differentiation, controlling their growth rate. *Proliferation* refers to cell division, and *differentiation* refers to the process of cellular specialization. When this control mechanism goes awry because of mutations within the chromosomes of the cell (genetic instability), an overgrowth of cells develops and results in a neoplasm. Cells are classified as either differentiated or undifferentiated, depending on the resemblance of the new cells to the original cells in the host organ or site. If the differences are small, the growth is termed *differentiated* and has a low probability for malignancy. If the cells within the neoplasm exhibit atypical characteristics, they are termed *poorly differentiated* or *undifferentiated* and have a higher probability of malignancy. Neoplastic cells are similar to normal cells in that they include both parenchymal and supporting tissues. In neoplastic disease, parenchymal cell proliferation and differentiation are altered, and since the parenchymal tissue is the functional tissue of the cell, it must receive adequate blood supply to survive. Classification of the neoplasm depends on the type of altered parenchymal cells, that is, tissue type of the tumor (Table 1-3).

Neoplasms originate from mutations within the genetic code (Box 1-1), which may silence the genes, that is, *tumor-suppressor genes*, or cause them to become overactive, that is, *oncogenes* (Fig. 1-10). This abnormal growth of cells leads to the formation of either a benign tumor or a malignant tumor (a neoplasm). A **benign neoplasm** is composed of well-differentiated cells with uncontrolled growth. Thus, a benign neoplasm remains localized and is generally noninvasive. However, a **malignant neoplasm** exhibits the loss of control of both cell proliferation and cell differentiation, which changes its functional capabilities. Malignant neoplasms grow at a faster rate compared with benign neoplasms and tend to spread and invade other tissues. Malignant neoplasms may be solid tumors confined to

a specific organ or tissue, or they may be hematologic in nature, affecting blood and lymph.

Sometimes, it is difficult to classify abnormal cells as either benign or malignant because they may exhibit characteristics of both types. Thus, the abnormal growth is graded, depending on the composition of particular cells.

The spread of malignant cancer cells resulting in a secondary tumor distant from the primary lesion is termed *metastasis*. **Metastatic spread** may occur in a variety of ways. If the cancerous cells invade the circulatory system, they may be spread via blood vessels, and this process is termed **hematogenous spread**; or they may spread via the lymphatic system, and this is termed **lymphatic spread**. The lymph node into which the primary neoplasm drains is termed the *sentinel*

FIGURE 1-10 Development of neoplastic cells.

BOX 1-1	Types of Genetic Lesions in Cancer

1. Point mutations
2. Subtle alterations (insertions, deletions)
3. Amplifications
4. Gene silencing
5. Exogenous sequences (tumor viruses)

TABLE 1-3 Nomenclature And Classification Of Benign And Malignant Tumors*

Cell or Tissue of Origin	Benign Tumor	Malignant Tumor
Tumors of Epithelial Origin		
Squamous cells	Squamous cell papilloma	Squamous cell carcinoma
Basal cells		Basal cell carcinoma
Glandular or ductal	Adenoma	Adenocarcinoma
Epithelium	Cystadenoma	Cystadenocarcinoma
Transitional cells	Transitional cell papilloma	Transitional cell carcinoma
Bile duct	Bile duct adenoma	Bile duct carcinoma (cholangiocarcinoma)
Liver duct	Hepatocellular adenoma	Hepatocellular carcinoma
Melanocytes	Nevus	Malignant melanoma
Renal epithelium	Renal tubular adenoma	Renal cell carcinoma
Skin adnexal glands		Sweat gland carcinoma
Sweat glands	Sweat gland adenoma	Sebaceous gland carcinoma
Sebaceous glands	Sebaceous gland adenoma	Seminoma (dysgerminoma)
Germ cells (testis and ovary)		Embryonal carcinoma, yolk sac carcinoma
Tumors of Mesenchymal Origin		
Hematopoietic/lymphoid tissue		
Leukocytes		Leukemias
Granular leukocytes and precursors		Granulocytic leukemia
		Myelocytic leukemia
		Myelogenous leukemia
Plasma cells		
Lymphoid		
Nongranular leukocytes and prelymphocytes		Lymphoma
Proliferating lymphocytes and monocytes		Lymphocytic leukemia
Proliferating immature precursor monocytes		Lymphoblastic leukemia
Solid tumors of lymph tissue (thymus, spleen, lymph nodes)		Lymphoma or lymphosarcoma
Neural and retinal tissue		
Nerve sheath	Neurilemoma, neurofibroma	Malignant peripheral nerve sheath tumor
Nerve cells	Gangiloneuroma	Neuroblastoma
Retinal cells (cones)		Retinoblastoma
Connective tissue		
Fibrous tissue	Fibromatosis (desmoid)	Fibrosarcoma
Fat	Lipoma	Liposarcoma
Bone	Osteoma	Osteogenic sarcoma
Cartilage	Chondroma	Chrondrosarcoma
Muscle		
Smooth muscle	Leiomyoma	Leiomyosarcoma
Striated muscle	Rhabdomyoma	Rhabdomyosarcoma
Endothelial and related tissues		
Blood vessels	Hemangioma	Angiosarcoma
		Kaposi sarcoma
Lymph vessels	Lymphangioma	Lymphangiosarcoma
Synovium		Synovial sarcoma
Mesothelium		Malignant mesothelioma
Meninges	Meningioma	Malignant meningioma
Tumors of Uncertain Origin		

*This list is intended to provide only an introduction to tumor nomenclature.

Modified from Murphy GP, et al: *American Cancer Society's textbook of clinical oncology,* ed 2, New York, 1995, American Cancer Society.

node. If the cancerous cells spread into surrounding tissue by virtue of the proximity of the areas, it is termed **invasion**. However, if the cancerous cells travel to a distant site or distant organ system, it is termed **seeding**. Certain types of cancer appear more often as metastases from other areas rather than originating in a given organ.

Lesion is a term used to describe the many types of cellular change that may occur in response to disease. Some lesions may be visible immediately; others may be detectable initially only through diagnostic means such as laboratory testing. *Cancer* is a general term often used to denote various types of malignant neoplasms. Note that the terms *cancer* and *carcinoma* are not synonymous. A **carcinoma** is one type of cancer and is derived from epithelial tissue. Adenocarcinoma of the colon is an example of a type of carcinoma. Other cancers include **sarcoma**, which arises from connective tissue (e.g., fibrosarcoma); **leukemia**, which arises from blood cells; and **lymphoma**, which arises from lymphatic cells. Both benign and malignant tumors are also named according to the tissue type of origin (see Table 1-3). In the case of a benign neoplasm, the suffix "oma" is added to the word root, for instance, *adenoma*. Malignant neoplasms are named by adding the name of the tissue type to the word root, for instance, *adenocarcinoma*. Medical imaging plays a major role in the diagnosis and staging of a variety of neoplastic diseases. The primary diagnostic and staging methods include imaging procedures such as computed tomography (CT), magnetic resonance imaging (MRI), positron emission tomography (PET), radiography, and ultrasonography; others include endoscopic procedures, identification of tumor markers in blood, clinical laboratory tests of cells and tissues, and gene profiling. Treatment modalities often include radiation therapy in combination with surgery, chemotherapy, hormone or antihormone therapy, immunotherapy using biologic response modifiers such as interferons and interleukins, and targeted drug therapies. The choice of a modality or a combination of modalities depends on many factors, including the type of cancer, its location and stage, and the treating oncologist. The goal of treatment may be curative, allowing the patient to remain free of disease for 5 years or more, or palliative, which is designed to relieve pain when a cure is not possible and to improve the quality of life.

Staging and Grading Cancer. Decisions regarding the appropriate treatment of malignant tumors and in determining prognosis and end results are guided by classifications that stage and grade the disease. Although several clinical classifications of cancer exist, the TNM (tumor–node–metastasis) system emerged in the 1950s and is now considered a recognized standard and is endorsed by the American Joint Committee on Cancer (AJCC). The AJCC is co-sponsored by several prominent health organizations, including the American Cancer Society and the American College of Radiology.

The TNM system is based on the premise that cancers of similar histology or origin are similar in their patterns of growth or extension. The "T" refers to the size of the untreated primary cancer or tumor. As the size increases, lymph node involvement (N) occurs, eventually leading to distant metastases (M). The addition of numbers to these three letters indicates the extent of malignancy and the progressive increase in size or involvement of the tumor. For example, T0 indicates that no evidence of a primary tumor exists, whereas T1, T2, T3, and T4 indicate an increasing size or extension. Lack of regional lymph node metastasis is indicated by N0, and N1, N2, and N3 indicate increasing involvement of regional lymph nodes. Finally, M0 indicates no distant metastasis, and M1 indicates the presence of distant metastasis.

Neoplastic cells are examined histologically, and these growths are graded according to their degree of differentiation based on a scale of I (well differentiated) to IV (poorly differentiated). The combination of tumor classification and grading serves as a shorthand notation for the description of the clinical extent of a given malignant tumor. It facilitates treatment planning, provides an indication of prognosis, assists in evaluating treatment results, facilitates information exchange among treatment centers, and allows unambiguous categorization of malignancies to aid in the continuing investigation of cancer.

SUMMARY

Technologic advances in the field of radiology have, without a doubt, done much to relieve human suffering, but medical imaging alone cannot provide a definitive diagnosis. Medical imaging must be used in conjunction with other diagnostic and therapeutic modalities to provide the best treatment for each specific disease process. The following chapters provide the student radiographer with a better understanding of the disease processes of the various physiologic systems. This information should help students analyze and critique each radiograph to ensure that it provides optimal information to assist physicians in their diagnosis.

REVIEW QUESTIONS

1. The prediction of the course and end of a disease and an outlook based on that prediction best define its:
   a. Diagnosis
   b. Etiology
   c. Prognosis
   d. Syndrome
2. A compression fracture of the lumbar spine that results from steroid treatments for pain reduction of arthritis would be an example of _____ disease.
   a. Degenerative
   b. Iatrogenic
   c. Idiopathic
   d. Traumatic
3. A disease such as Tay-Sachs syndrome that is transmitted genetically is termed:
   a. Congenital
   b. Hereditary
   c. Metabolic
   d. Neoplastic
4. Sickness sufficient to interfere with normal daily routines is termed:
   a. Etiology
   b. Morbidity
   c. Mortality
   d. Pathogenesis
5. Which of the following would be considered a symptom of a disease process?
   a. Bloody stool
   b. Nausea
   c. Skin rash
   d. Swelling
6. A disease that manifests slowly and is present for a long period is said to be:
   a. Acute
   b. Asymptomatic
   c. Chronic
   d. Congenital
7. Which of the following disease classifications is usually associated with the normal aging process?
   a. Congenital
   b. Degenerative
   c. Inflammatory
   d. Metabolic
8. If 4000 cases of a given disease are found in a given population, the _____ of the disease is defined.
   a. Incidence
   b. Morphology
   c. Metabolism
   d. Prevalence
9. The relative ease with which an organism can overcome normal bodily defenses refers to its:
   a. Infection
   b. Necrosis
   c. Pestilence
   d. Virulence
10. A neoplastic growth is evaluated to determine its degree of histologic differentiation. This is termed:
    a. Grading
    b. Metastasis
    c. Morphology
    d. Staging

11. Generalized increase in cell size refers to:
    a. Hypertrophy
    b. Atrophy
    c. Metaplasia
    d. Hyperplasia
12. Which of the following terms refers to abnormal changes of mature cells?
    a. Hypertrophy
    b. Dysplasia
    c. Metaplasia
    d. Hyperplasia
13. Explain the concept of neoplastic disease. Are all neoplasms cancer?
14. What is the difference between mortality and morbidity rates? How is each important to the practice of medicine and to public health agencies?
15. Differentiate between an acute illness and a chronic illness. Give two examples of each type of disease.

2

Skeletal System

LEARNING OBJECTIVES

On completion of Chapter 2, the reader should be able to do the following:

- Describe the anatomic components of the skeletal system on a macroscopic level and basic microscopic level.
- Identify and explain the criteria for assessing technical adequacy of skeletal radiographs.
- Characterize a given condition as congenital, inflammatory, arthritic, or neoplastic.
- Specify the pathogenesis, signs and symptoms, and prognosis of the skeletal pathologies cited in this chapter.
- Explain the role of various imaging modalities in the diagnosis and treatment of skeletal pathologies.

OUTLINE

KEY TERMS

Chondrosarcomas
Clubfoot
Compact bone
Craniosynostosis
Craniotubular dysplasias
Developmental dysplasia of the hip
Diaphysis
Diploë
Endochondroma
Epiphysis
Escherichia coli
Ewing sarcoma
Exostoses
Ganglion
Giant cell tumors
Gouty arthritis
Hyperostosis frontalis interna
Involucrum
Juvenile rheumatoid arthritis
Medullary canal
Metaphysis
Osteoarthritis
Osteoblastoma
Osteoblasts
Osteochondroma
Osteoclastomas
Osteoclasts

Osteogenesis imperfecta
Osteoid osteoma
Osteoma
Osteomyelitis
Osteopetrosis
Osteophytes
Osteosarcoma
Polydactyly
Pott disease
Psoriatic arthritis
Reiter syndrome
Rheumatoid arthritis
Scoliosis
Sequestrum
Simple unicameral bone cyst
Spina bifida
Spondylolisthesis
Spondylolysis
Staphylococcus aureus
Syndactyly
Tendonitis
Tenosynovitis
Trabeculae
Trabecular pattern
Transitional vertebra
Tuberculosis
Whiplash

ANATOMY AND PHYSIOLOGY

The skeletal system is composed of 206 separate bones and is responsible for body support, protection, movement, and blood cell production. It contains more than 98% of the body's total calcium and up to 75% of its total phosphorus. The system is commonly divided into the axial skeleton (Fig. 2-1), which contains 80 bones, and the appendicular skeleton (Fig. 2-2), which contains 126 bones. Bone is a type of connective tissue, but it differs from other connective tissue because of its matrix of calcium phosphate. The construction of this matrix further classifies bone tissue as either compact (dense) or cancellous (spongy) (Fig. 2-3).

The outer portion of bone is composed of **compact bone**, and the inner portion, termed the **medullary canal**, is made up of **cancellous bone**. Bone marrow is located within the medullary canal and is interspersed between the **trabeculae**. This intricate, weblike bony structure is visible on a properly exposed radiograph of the skeletal system and is often referred to as the **trabecular pattern**. The term **diploë** is specific to the cancellous bone located within the skull. The red bone marrow is responsible for the production of bone erythrocytes and leukocytes. Red bone marrow is found, in a normal adult, primarily in the bones of the trunk. At the approximate age of 20 years, the majority of the red bone marrow is

FIGURE 2-1 Axial skeleton.

FIGURE 2-3 Bone composition.

FIGURE 2-2 Appendicular skeleton.

replaced by yellow bone marrow composed mainly of fat.

Osteoblasts are the bone-forming cells that line the medullary canal and are interspersed throughout the periosteum. They are responsible for bone growth and thickening, ossification, and regeneration. **Osteoclasts** are specialized cells that break down bone to enlarge the medullary canal and allow for bone growth. This production and breakdown of bone play an important role in serum calcium and phosphorus equilibrium. Certain metabolic disease processes may alter the percentage of calcium, resulting in either hypocalcemia or hypercalcemia.

The bones of the skeletal system may also be classified according to their shape to include long, short, flat, and irregular bones. The **diaphysis** of a long bone refers to the shaft portion and is the primary site of ossification, whereas the **epiphysis** refers to the expanded end portion and is the secondary site of ossification (Fig. 2-4). The **metaphysis** refers to the growth zone between the epiphysis and the diaphysis. It is the area of

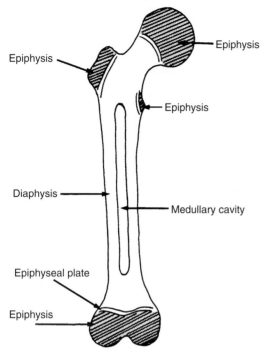

Epiphysis

Epiphysis

Epiphysis

Diaphysis

Medullary cavity

Epiphyseal plate

Epiphysis

FIGURE 2-4 Endochondral ossification.

greatest metabolic activity in a bone. A cartilaginous growth plate is located between the metaphysis and the epiphysis in the bone of a growing child. Radiographically, these growth areas appear radiolucent. As the body matures, this cartilage calcifies and is no longer radiographically visible in the adult.

The periosteum is a fibrous membrane that encloses all of the bone except the joint surfaces and is crucial to supplying blood to the underlying bone. Osteoblasts located within the periosteum increase bone thickness relative to individual activities. The more physical stress a bone is under, the more thickly the compact portion develops; therefore, it is common medical practice to allow patients with healing fractures of the hip or femur to bear weight on the injured bone, which helps shorten the healing period. Disuse atrophy occurs when a bone is not allowed to bear weight and results in significant decalcification and thinning of the bone.

The 206 bones of the body are connected to one another by one of three types of joints: (1)

Fibrous (synarthrodial) joints form firm, immovable joints such as the sutures of the skull; (2) *cartilaginous (amphiarthrodial) joints* such as those found between the vertebral bodies are slightly movable; (3) *synovial (diarthrodial) joints* such as the knee are freely movable. The ends of the bones composing a synovial joint are lined with articular cartilage and are held together by ligaments. The joint capsules are lined by a synovial membrane responsible for the secretion of synovia, a lubricating fluid containing mucin, albumin, fat, and mineral salts.

IMAGING CONSIDERATIONS

Radiography

In examining a skeletal radiograph, it is important to begin by properly orienting the image receptor and recognizing the radiographic projection. The radiographic exposure technique selected is very important in achieving a proper diagnosis. Proper technique is achieved when the soft tissues and bony structures of interest are both adequately penetrated and the trabecular pattern is visible. Any motion of the part in question impairs the visibility of the detail present.

Soft tissue areas often hold clues to the diagnosis and are examined by the interpreting physician. Any signs of muscle atrophy, soft tissue swelling, calcifications, opaque foreign bodies, or the presence of gas may indicate disease. Analysis of the configuration of the bone and its relationship to other bones serves to detect or exclude fractures, dislocations, congenital anomalies, or acquired deformities.

The interface between cortical (compact) bone and soft tissue is also important. Any periosteal new bone formation seen may be a response to trauma, tumors, or infection. Juxtaarticular erosions are often seen in cases of arthritis. Cortical resorption may be demonstrated as smudgy, irregular loss of the cortical margin. In addition, the internal bone structure is important and should be examined for abnormally altered texture, alterations in the amount of mineralization, or foci of destruction. Careful consideration of all areas mentioned assists the physician in arriving at the correct diagnosis.

Magnetic Resonance Imaging

Magnetic resonance imaging (MRI) is an important modality used in imaging of skeletal pathology, particularly in providing soft tissue detail because of its superior contrast resolution. It is considered the modality of choice for detection and staging of soft tissue tumors involving the extremities. It is also extremely useful in evaluation of joints, particularly the knee and the shoulder (Fig. 2-5). Newer imaging techniques and improved equipment allow MRI to detect a greater number of musculoskeletal subtleties with higher-resolution imaging (Fig. 2-6). Sometimes these subtleties mimic bone pain but involve soft tissues instead, which is an important distinction. Bone marrow imaging done with MRI is superior to other modalities in visualizing subtle abnormalities within the musculoskeletal system. Also, MRI may play a larger role in trauma medicine, particularly with the refinement of open-bore and short-bore technologies.

Computed Tomography

Computed tomography (CT) is an important tool in skeletal imaging because with newer technology the examination can be performed quickly and noninvasively, even in cases of trauma. CT has the ability to define the presence and extent of fractures or dislocations, to assess abnormalities in joints and associated soft tissues, and to help diagnose spinal disorders (Fig. 2-7). Cortical bone gives no signal in MRI, but CT provides ready visualization of bone details and is often used as a follow-up to conventional radiographic imaging for improved detail. Bone tumors, in particular, are now usually imaged with spiral or helical CT because of its excellent ability to display bone margins and trabecular patterns and to assess both bone and soft tissue involvement of tumors. Although CT results in greater contrast resolution compared with radiography, much of the role for imaging other related soft

FIGURE 2-5 Magnetic resonance imaging scan (short-τ inversion recovery sequences) showing a subcutaneous cyst on the scapula.

FIGURE 2-6 Magnetic resonance imaging scan (short-τ inversion recovery sequences) showing synovitis of the metacarpophalangeal and interphalangeal joints.

FIGURE 2-7 Computed tomography scan demonstrating a burst fracture of the third lumbar vertebra.

tissues has been usurped by MRI. Quantitative computed tomography (QCT) is also used in evaluating bone mass loss, especially within the vertebral bodies of the spine.

Nuclear Medicine Procedures

Nuclear medicine retains an advantage not offered by either MRI or CT in skeletal imaging: the ability to look at the entire body at one time in a convenient fashion (Fig. 2-8). It allows ready decision making as to whether any pathology shown is an old injury or a new problem, with activity indicating that the bone involved is affected by some new process. In addition, the bone scan is still the standard of care for examination of metastatic processes because it demonstrates metabolic reaction of the bone to the disease process and is more sensitive than comparative radiographic studies. This is also true in many other traumatic or inflammatory diseases of the skeletal system. However, the utilization of positron emission tomography (PET) scanning in skeletal pathologies has started to increase, particularly the use of 18F-NaF (2-deoxy-2-[18F] fluoro-D-glucose). Although primarily used in diagnosing and staging

of metastatic disease, it may be appropriate in certain individuals with back pain, to confirm child abuse (especially rib fractures) following abnormal radiographs, and for the diagnosis of osteomyelitis, trauma, inflammatory and degenerative arthritis, avascular necrosis, osteonecrosis of the mandible, condylar hyperplasia, metabolic bone disease, Paget disease, bone graft viability, complications of the prosthetic joints, and reflex sympathetic dystrophy.

CONGENITAL AND HEREDITARY DISEASES

Osteogenesis Imperfecta

Osteogenesis imperfecta (OI), sometimes referred to as *brittle bone disease,* is a quite serious and rather rare heritable or congenital disease affecting the skeletal system. OI is most commonly an autosomal dominant defect. The eight recognized types are classified as type I to type VIII, with type I being the mildest and type VIII the most severe. Prenatal testing of cultured skin fibroblasts (CSF) helps diagnose types II, III, and IV. It is caused by mutations in the two structural genes that encode the α_1- and α_2-peptides of type I collagen, the main collagen of bone, tendon, and skin. The specific mutations occur in the *COL1A1, COL1A2, CRTAP,* and *LEPRE1* genes. Thus, deficient and imperfect formation of osseous tissue, skin, sclera, inner ear, and teeth is noted in individuals with this disease. The two main clinical groups of OI are based on the age of onset and the severity of the disease. (1) *Osteogenesis imperfecta congenita* is present at birth. Infants with this disease usually have multiple fractures at birth that heal only to give way to new fractures. This results in limb deformities and dwarfism and may lead to death. (2) In *osteogenesis imperfecta tarda,* fractures might not appear for some years after birth and then generally stop once adulthood is reached (Fig. 2-9). In some cases, however, a hearing disorder persists because of otosclerosis, which is the formation of abnormal connective tissue around the auditory ossicles. Radiographic evaluation will demonstrate

FIGURE 2-8 Bone scan demonstrating metastatic disease throughout the ribs, thoracic vertebrae, and pelvis resulting from carcinoid disease.

multiple fractures in various stages of healing and a general decrease in bone mass. The bone cortex is thin and porous, and the trabeculae are thin, delicate, and widely separated.

Achondroplasia

The most common inherited disorder affecting the skeletal system is **achondroplasia**, which results in bone deformity and dwarfism. It occurs in 1 in 15,000 to 40,000 newborns. It is caused by an autosomal dominant gene (*FGFR3*) at the 4p chromosome location, and this gene does not skip generations. Individuals with this gene have about a 50% chance of transmitting it to their children. Because of a disturbance in endochondral bone formation, the cartilage located in the epiphyses of the long bones does not convert to

FIGURE **2-9** Tibia–fibula radiograph demonstrating bowed lower extremities resulting from osteogenesis imperfecta tarda. This condition was recognized shortly after the child began to walk.

attempt to lengthen the shortened limbs. This procedure was perfected by Dr. Gavriil Ilizarov and has been used for over 30 years. It consists of a corticotomy of the limb, followed by attachment of an Ilizarov fixator, which consists of two circular frames that surround the limb, wires, and rods. By using this method, bones may be made to grow at a rate of approximately 1 mm per day. Bone age radiographic studies may be used to monitor patients with growth hormone (GH) deficiency. These images are analyzed to compare the chronologic age with the radiographic bone age by using one of two methods: (1) the atlas matching method, which was established by Greulich and Pyle in the 1950s; or (2) the point scoring system of Tanner and White-house, which was developed in the 1960s. Most recently, clinical trials have involved GH injections in the treatment of children with achondroplasia. Conclusive results cannot be determined until the children in the current study reach their adult heights. Early research indicates that introduction of GH may have an adverse effect on the cardiovascular system. In addition, these patients may receive genetic and social counseling.

Osteopetrosis

Osteopetrosis and *marble bone* are terms used to characterize a variety of disorders involving an increase in bone density and defective bone contour, often referred to as *skeletal modeling*. These pathologies involve mutations at the *CLCN7* gene. The spectrum of osteopetrosis includes (1) infantile malignant *CLCN7*-related autosomal recessive osteopetrosis (ARO), which has its onset in infancy; (2) intermediate autosomal osteopetrosis (IAO), which develops in childhood; and (3) autosomal dominant osteopetrosis type II (ADOII), which occurs in late childhood or adolescence. In osteopetrosis, bones are abnormally heavy and compact but nevertheless brittle. The disorders characterizing osteopetrosis include osteoscleroses, craniotubular (affecting the cranium and tubular long bones) dysplasias, and craniotubular hyperostoses. It is important for the technologist to be aware that both the

bone in the normal manner, impairing the longitudinal growth of the bones. Thus, patients with this type of osteochondrodysplasia have a normal trunk size and shortened extremities (Fig. 2-10, *A*). In some instances, ultrasonography may be used for prenatal diagnosis of achondroplasia. An adult with achondroplasia is usually no more than 4 feet in height, with lower extremities usually less than half the normal length. Additional clinical manifestations of this disorder include extreme lumbar spine lordosis, bowed legs, a bulky forehead with midface hypoplasia (see Fig. 2-10, *B),* and a narrowing of the foramen magnum within the skull, which causes neural compression. Occasionally, orthopedic surgery may be necessary in the management of complications associated with achondroplasia. The Ilizarov procedure has also been used in an

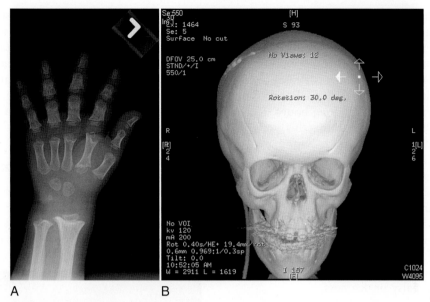

A   B

FIGURE 2-10 A, Bone age radiograph of a 3-year-old demonstrating an abnormal flared appearance of the metaphyses and shortened, broad phalanges consistent with achondroplasia. **B,** Three-dimensional reconstruction of computed tomography scan demonstrating midface hypoplasia typical of achondroplasia.

osteosclerotic and craniotubular hyperostotic disorders require an increase in exposure factors to adequately penetrate the bony anatomy because of abnormal bone density (Fig. 2-11). In some cases, adequate radiographic density may never be achieved. All bones are affected, but the most significant changes occur in the long bones of the extremities, vertebrae, pelvis, and base of the skull. Radiographs demonstrate an increase in the density and thickness of the cortex as well as an increase in the number and size of trabeculae, with a marked reduction of the marrow space.

Albers-Schönberg disease is a fairly common form of osteosclerotic osteopetrosis. This autosomal dominant, delayed, benign skeletal anomaly involves increased bone density in conjunction with fairly normal bone contour. In fact, many patients with Albers-Schönberg disease are asymptomatic, and it is often discovered after radiographing the patient for an unrelated problem. Although this is a hereditary disorder, the bone sclerosis is not radiographically visible at birth. As the individual ages, radiographic manifestations of the osteopetrosis become

FIGURE 2-11 Anteroposterior lumbar spine radiograph demonstrating uniform sclerosis of the bone associated with osteopetrosis.

visible, especially in the region of the cranium and spine; however, the general health of the individual is unimpaired.

Craniotubular dysplasias are a group of rare autosomal recessive hereditary diseases, which mainly result in abnormal or defective bone contour of the cranium and long bones. Radiographs are useful in demonstrating this alteration in contour, scleroses, and changes within the cortical bone. Craniotubular hyperostoses include a variety of fairly rare hereditary diseases, causing both an increase in bone density and abnormal bone modeling. Both of these craniotubular anomalies manifest in childhood. Although these disorders do not normally impair the individual's general health, bony overgrowth may entrap cranial nerves, resulting in some dysfunction such as facial palsy or deafness.

Hand and Foot Malformations

A variety of abnormalities of the fingers and toes may occur during fetal development but can be surgically corrected at birth. Failure of the fingers or toes to separate is called **syndactyly** and causes the physical appearance of webbed digits (Fig. 2-12). It is also associated with Apert syndrome, which is a genetic syndrome involving mutations of fibroblast growth factor receptor 2. Apert syndrome is also responsible for craniosynostosis. **Polydactyly** (Fig. 2-13) refers to the presence of extra digits, and treatment includes surgical intervention and therapy.

Clubfoot (talipes) is a congenital malformation of the foot that prevents normal weight bearing. The foot is most commonly turned inward at the ankle. This congenital malformation is more common in males than in females and may occur bilaterally. It is generally corrected by casting or splinting the foot in the correct anatomic position.

Developmental Dysplasia of the Hip

A malformation of the acetabulum often results in **developmental dysplasia of the hip** (DDH). Because the acetabulum does not form completely, the head of the femur is displaced

FIGURE 2-13 Foot radiograph demonstrating additional digits associated with familial polydactyly.

FIGURE 2-12 Hand radiograph of an infant demonstrating acrosyndactyly.

FIGURE 2-14 Frog leg lateral projection of the pelvis of an infant demonstrating congenital dislocation of the left hip.

FIGURE 2-15 Anteroposterior lumbar spine radiograph demonstrating congenital scoliosis.

superiorly and posteriorly (Fig. 2-14). Often, the ligaments and tendons responsible for proper placement of the femoral head are also affected. DDH may be unilateral or bilateral and occurs more frequently in females than in males. Other risk factors include a breech position in utero, being the first child, or low levels of amniotic fluid. DDH affects approximately 1 in 1000 births and may be associated with cerebral palsy, myelomeningocele, arthrogryposis, and Larsen syndrome. Larsen syndrome is a mutation of the *FLNB* gene affecting the production of filament B protein. Sonography may be used to diagnose this anomaly early in life through visualization of the cartilaginous structures of the hip. Conventional radiographs of the hip are often difficult to interpret in the neonate. Radiographic measurements of the anteroposterior (AP) pelvis are obtained and compared with standardized lines. This anomaly should be treated early with immobilization through casting or splinting the affected hip to allow the acetabulum to grow and form a normal joint. If left untreated, this anomaly may result in uneven limb length, hip muscle weakness, and an uneven gait.

Vertebral Anomalies

Scoliosis refers to an abnormal lateral curvature of the spine (Fig. 2-15). Structural scoliosis is associated with vertebral rotation. The lateral curves are usually convex to the right in the thoracic region and to the left in the lumbar region of the spine. Up to 80% of all structural scolioses are idiopathic, although factors such as connective tissue disease and diet have been implicated. Scoliosis does not generally become visually apparent until adolescence. It tends to affect girls more frequently than boys and may cause numerous complications, including cardiopulmonary complications, degenerative spinal arthritis, and fatigue and joint dysfunction syndromes. Nonstructural scoliosis, in which the primary issue is not vertebral rotation, usually results from unequal leg lengths or compensatory postural changes affected by chronic pain elsewhere in the body.

Radiography is important in the diagnosis and treatment of scoliosis. Initial evaluation requires initial AP or posteroanterior (PA) and lateral standing radiographs and follow-up radiographs on a fairly routine basis. Radiologists use one of several methods to measure the spine's curvature, so consistent quality from one examination to another is important. Effective radiation protection techniques are vital because of the large size of the exposure field, the young age of the patient, and the frequency of the examinations. Special attention is necessary in shielding the breasts of young female patients during radiographic examination throughout the treatment process. The PA projection should be obtained whenever possible because it significantly reduces the radiation dose to the breast area. Scoliosis may be corrected by placing the individual in a brace or body cast in patients with curves of 25 to 35 degrees. Surgical treatment with spinal fusion is prescribed for curves greater than 40 degrees.

A **transitional vertebra** is one that takes on the characteristics of both vertebrae on each side of a major division of the spine. Most frequently, such vertebrae occur at the junction between the thoracic and lumbar spine or at the junction between the lumbar spine and the sacrum. The first lumbar vertebra and the seventh cervical vertebra may have rudimentary ribs articulating with the transverse processes (Fig. 2-16). A cervical rib most commonly occurs at C7 and may exert pressure on the brachial nerve plexus or the subclavian artery, requiring surgical removal of the rib.

Spina bifida is an incomplete closure of the vertebral canal that is particularly common in the lumbosacral area (Fig. 2-17). Often, such patients have no visible abnormality or neurologic deficit, but failure of fusion of the two laminae is visible radiographically (spina bifida occulta). In more severe cases, the spinal cord or nerve root may be involved, which results in varying degrees of paralysis. Treatment of spina bifida is determined on the basis of the extent of the anomaly and requires the services of a variety of physicians.

Cranial Anomalies

The premature or early closure of any of the cranial sutures is called **craniosynostosis**. This congenital anomaly causes an overgrowth of the unfused sutures to accommodate brain growth, which alters the shape of the head (Fig. 2-18). It

FIGURE 2-16 Anteroposterior lumbar spine radiograph demonstrating bilateral lumbar ribs.

FIGURE 2-17 Abdominal radiograph of a patient with spina bifida occulta of the lower lumbar vertebrae.

FIGURE 2-18 Lateral skull radiograph demonstrating premature closure of the sagittal suture. This results in dolichocephaly and prominent convolutional markings caused by the increased intracranial pressure.

FIGURE 2-19 Abdominal radiograph of a pregnant woman carrying a fetus with anencephaly. Note the absence of the cerebral cranial bones.

is often associated with Apert syndrome, a genetic disorder that is caused by a mutation of the *FGFR2* gene on chromosome 10. Although this defect may be corrected with surgery, brain damage may occur.

Anencephaly is a congenital abnormality in which the brain and cranial vault do not form (Fig. 2-19). In most cases, only the facial bones are formed. This abnormality results in death shortly after birth and may be diagnosed before birth by ultrasonography. Anencephaly is a neural tube defect, and its cause is unknown. It is suspected that anencephaly may be caused by a combination of multiple genetic (*MTHFR* gene) and environmental factors such as deficiency of folate, diabetes mellitus, exposure to high heat in early pregnancy, or use of certain antiseizure medications during pregnancy.

INFLAMMATORY DISEASES

Osteomyelitis

Osteomyelitis is an infection of the bone and bone marrow caused by a pathogenic microorganism spread via the bloodstream (hematogenous), from an infection within a contiguous site, or through direct introduction of the microorganism (Fig. 2-20). Signs and symptoms

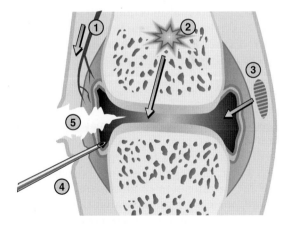

1. The hematogenous route
2. Dissemination from osteomyelitis
3. Spread from an adjacent soft tissue infection
4. Diagnostic or therapeutic measures
5. Penetrating damage by puncture or cutting

FIGURE 2-20 Routes of infection to the joint.

may include dull pain, heat in the affected area, and an intermittent low-grade fever. Generally, hematogenous osteomyelitis develops at the ends of the long bones. The distal femur, proximal tibia, humerus, and radius are most commonly affected in children and the vertebrae in adults. Infants and children are more commonly affected by acute hematogenous osteomyelitis because of increased vascularity and the rapid growth of their long bones. In addition, children often have a lowered resistance to the pathogenic organism, most commonly *Staphylococcus aureus.* Infection may be spread to the marrow space via the nutrient artery from an infection of the skin, ear, or pharynx. In infants, hematogenous osteomyelitis may also be caused by group B streptococci and *Escherichia coli.* In adults, hematogenous osteomyelitis is commonly secondary to bacteremia caused by genitourinary tract, soft tissue, or respiratory infections. As in children, *S. aureus* and streptococci are the pathogenic microorganisms primarily responsible for the infections.

Osteomyelitis resulting from contiguous infections is often associated with burns, sinus disease, periodontal infection, soft tissue infection, or skin ulcers resulting from peripheral vascular disease. Pathogenic microorganisms may also be directly introduced to bones by penetrating wounds, open fractures, fractures treated with internal fixation devices, or prosthetic replacements.

No specific bone changes may be demonstrated radiographically in the very early stage of infection. But the infection spreads rapidly, with the acute stage of osteomyelitis characterized by the formation of an abscess, leading to an inflammatory reaction within the bone that causes a rise in internal bone pressure. Osteomyelitis may be diagnosed with elevated erythrocyte sedimentation rate (ESR) or cross-reactive protein (CRP) levels; however, normal laboratory values should not exclude this diagnosis. Because of the constriction of the periosteum, blood vessels compress and thrombose, leading to bone necrosis within 24 to 48 hours. Unfortunately, not until about 10 to 14 days later is new periosteal bone repair evident radiographically to indicate the presence of the disease. Therefore, it is imperative that the condition be recognized clinically and treated with antibiotics and local drainage.

Initially, radiography may demonstrate soft tissue swelling in the area around the affected bone. MRI demonstrates waterlike signal characteristics. Follow-up radiography may be performed 10 to 14 days after medical treatment to aid in the diagnosis.

With the effective use of antibiotics, osteomyelitis seldom passes the acute stage. When it does, treatment with antibiotics in combination with surgical drainage of pus from under the periosteum often results in a complete cure of the bone lesion in a majority of cases. Chronic osteomyelitis, however, is characterized by extensive bone destruction with irregular, sclerotic reaction throughout the bone (Fig. 2-21). A **sequestrum** is dead, devascularized bone that appears very dense. An **involucrum** is a shell of new supporting bone laid down by the periosteum around the sequestrum. An accurate diagnosis is extremely important to distinguish osteomyelitis from a neoplastic bone disease.

Radiography is not a very sensitive means of diagnosing the condition because a 30% to 50% loss of bone calcium is required before the destructive changes of osteomyelitis are visible radiographically. Nuclear medicine bone scan studies and MRI are much more sensitive in detecting osteomyelitis.

Tuberculosis

Tuberculosis of the bone is a chronic inflammatory disease caused by *Mycobacterium tuberculosis.* It is usually more advanced and often left untreated for a longer period compared with pulmonary tuberculosis. It most commonly affects the hip, knee, and spine. Radiographically, the ends of the long bones display a "worm-eaten" appearance, with the disease slowly destroying the epiphyses, spreading to the articular cartilage, and, in some cases, infecting the joint space (Fig. 2-22). Tuberculosis of the spine is also

FIGURE 2-21 A, Chronic osteomyelitis demonstrated in a knee with prior fusion. An involucrum surrounded by fluid densities is seen in the middle of a large intramedullary cavity approximately 3 cm above the fusion site. **B,** The involucrum demonstrated on a sagittal magnetic resonance imaging (MRI) scan from the same patient. **C,** The sequestrum demonstrated on an axial MRI image from the same patient, appearing as very dense bone as a result of devascularization.

called **Pott disease**. Recognized in ancient times, it has been described in Egyptian mummies dating back to 3000 BC. It destroys the spine, causing softening and eventual collapse of the vertebrae, which results in paravertebral abscess formation and exerts abnormal pressure on the spinal cord.

Arthropathies

Arthropathy, a collective term used to denote disorders of the joints, includes, but is not limited to, arthritis, bursitis, tendonitis, and tenosynovitis. Joint inflammation is known as **arthritis** and may be caused by a variety of etiologic factors.

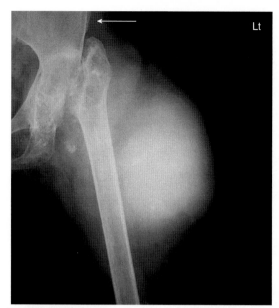

FIGURE 2-22 Hip radiograph of a 47-year-old man with extensive destruction of the femoral head and neck caused by tuberculosis of the hip with a cold abscess.

For many years, osteoarthritis was believed to be a noninflammatory type of arthritis; however, current research has indicated that all types of arthritis involve inflammation of joints. An accurate clinical history is of extreme importance because different types of arthritis are characterized by specific features. For example, it is important to identify the number of joints involved, the location of the joints involved, and the presence of any other disease process. Some types of arthritis involve several joints, but others involve only one joint. In addition, certain types of arthritis have a preference for specific joints while sparing others. Finally, some types of arthritis are associated with specific disease processes caused by a host of factors such as bacteria or autoimmune response. Arthritis may be further classified as *acute* and *chronic*; the most common forms are chronic and disabling.

Infectious Arthritis. Infectious arthritis is caused by a variety of factors including *S. aureus,* streptococci, and *Neisseria gonorrhoeae.* The infectious agents may enter the joint through a break in skin, via extension from an adjacent infection such as osteomyelitis or an infected wound, or as a result of bacteremia. Common clinical symptoms of an acute bacterial infectious arthritis are rapid onset of pain, redness, and swelling of the affected joint, often accompanied by fever. Diagnosis is generally made by analysis of blood and synovial fluid from the infected area. Infectious arthritis usually responds rapidly to antibiotic therapy. Early radiographic changes demonstrate soft tissue swelling and joint effusions, with joint space narrowing that is visible only approximately 2 weeks after the infection. Radiographs obtained during the healing stage demonstrate recalcification and sclerosis, which often result in joint ankylosis.

Psoriatic arthritis is an inflammatory arthritis associated with psoriasis of the skin and involves a rheumatoid-like destructive process that predominantly affects the distal interphalangeal (DIP) joints of hands and feet. It may cause asymmetric destruction of digits. Radiographic findings characteristic of psoriatic arthritis include bony ankylosis of the interphalangeal (IP) joints of hands and feet and resorption of the terminal tufts of the distal phalanges. A distinctive radiographic difference between psoriatic arthritis and **rheumatoid arthritis** (RA) is that in psoriatic arthritis bone density is usually preserved.

Reiter syndrome is a variant of rheumatoid arthritis occurring most commonly in young males. It has been associated with bacterial infections of the gastrointestinal (GI) and genitourinary systems by organisms such as *Chlamydia trachomatis, Shigella, Salmonella, Yersinia,* or *Campylobacter.*

The sacroiliac joints, heels (calcanei), and toes are generally affected in this syndrome, sometimes referred to as "lover's heel." Although the radiographic appearance may mimic RA, Reiter syndrome affects feet instead of hands. It is characterized by asymmetric involvement of the joints of the lower extremities, ill-defined erosions of bone with adjacent areas of proliferation, and a tendency to produce heterotrophic bone.

Nuclear medicine bone scans are helpful in diagnosing early stage Reiter syndrome in the sacroiliac joints, and the disease may be imaged before any findings are visible on a conventional radiograph. The preferred treatment is nonsteroidal antiinflammatory drugs (NSAIDs).

Rheumatoid Arthritis. RA is a chronic autoimmune disease that may fluctuate in severity. It is triggered by exposure of an immunogenetically susceptible host to an arthritogenic antigen and is characterized by chronic inflammation and overgrowth of the synovial tissues, most often in the extremities. RA develops slowly, and as synovial tissues proliferate, they progressively destroy cartilage, bone, and supporting structures. Genetic factors also are believed to predispose an individual to RA. An analysis of blood chemistry identifies the presence of an autoantibody against γ-globulin, also known as the *serologic rheumatoid factor* (RF). It usually occurs between the ages of 30 and 40 years and is three times more common in women than in men. In the United States, approximately 2.5 million adults are affected by RA. Symptoms include pain, swelling, and stiffness of the affected joint, with periods of activity or exacerbations and remissions of the disease process.

Although any joint may be involved, RA typically begins in the peripheral joints, particularly in the small bones of hands and feet and in the knee. The radiographic changes seen early in this disease are soft tissue swelling and osteoporosis of the affected bones (Fig. 2-23). As the disease progresses, cortical erosion with joint space narrowing occurs because of the overgrowth of synovial tissue into the articular spaces. This severe damage makes the joint unstable and leads to deformity caused by displacement of the bones in the joint. The late changes of this condition may be quite severe, resulting in bone and cartilage destruction and subluxation or dislocation of the involved joint (Fig. 2-24). Eventually, the joints become ankylosed (fused), which necessitates surgical intervention. Surgical procedures such as synovium excision, dislocation corrections, joint reconstructions, and prosthetic joint replacements may be performed to improve joint function (Fig. 2-25). New advancements in disease-modifying antirheumatic drugs (DMARD) such as methotrexate and

FIGURE 2-23 Hand radiograph demonstrating soft tissue joint swelling associated with early rheumatoid arthritis.

the availability of new biologic agents have enhanced the success of the management of RA. Diagnosis of RA in adults was originally based on the 1987 revised classification criteria of the American College of Radiology (ACR); however, in 2010, a new set of criteria was developed by the ACR and EULAR (European Leagues Against Rheumatism). These new criteria present a specific approach in identifying patients earlier in the disease process so that intervening treatment may begin sooner. The 2010 criteria indicating the presence of RA are as follows:

- Confirmed presence of synovitis in at least one joint
- Absence of an alternative diagnosis that better explains the synovitis
- Achievement of a total score of 6 or greater (of a possible 10) from the individual scores in the following four domains:
  - Number and site of involved joints (score range 0–5)

FIGURE 2-24 Posteroanterior **A,** and lateral **B,** hand images demonstrating advanced rheumatoid arthritis with subluxation of the first metacarpophalangeal joint.

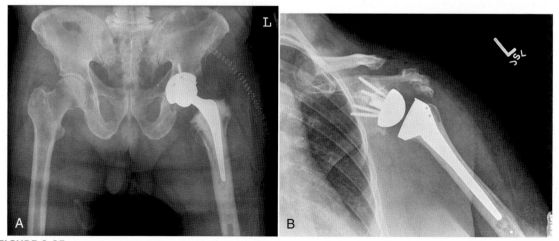

FIGURE 2-25 A, Radiograph of an anteroposterior pelvis demonstrating proper placement of a prosthetic hip replacement. **B,** Radiograph of an oblique shoulder demonstrating proper placement of a prosthetic shoulder replacement.

- Serologic abnormality (score range 0–3)
- Elevated acute-phase response (score 0–1)
- Symptom duration (2 levels, range 0–1)

Juvenile rheumatoid arthritis (JRA), also known as Still disease, affects children under age 16 years and is similar to the adult form of RA. However, differences in the pattern of involvement and prognosis do exist. Generally, fibrosis and proliferation are less than in the adult form. JRA affects nearly 100,000 children in the United States. Symptoms include pain, swelling, and stiffness of the affected joint with periods of activity or exacerbations and remissions of the disease process. The majority of children have long periods of remission without significant joint damage. The prognosis is generally good, with fewer than 20% having progressive destructive disease.

The ACR criterion for the diagnosis of JRA differs from that of adult RA. JRA is indicated if (1) the child is younger than 16 years at the onset of the disease, (2) symptoms of arthritis (swelling or effusion) are present in one or more joints for at least 6 weeks, and (3) the onset can be assigned to one of three JRA onset types: (a) pauciarticular, (b) polyarticular, and (c) systemic. Pauciarticular JRA is the most common form, and it is more common in females than in males. It affects four or fewer joints, most commonly the knee, ankle, and elbow joints. Polyarticular RA affects five or more joints, generally those in hands, feet, and weight-bearing joints. Systemic JRA is the least common form of RA in children, and it can affect many areas of the body, including joints and internal organs.

Ankylosing Spondylitis. Ankylosing spondylitis (Marie-Strümpell disease) is a progressive form of arthritis, mainly involving the spine; in this disease, joints and articulations become ankylosed, especially the sacroiliac joints. It tends to affect men between the ages of 20 and 40 years and is believed to have a genetic predisposition because it is 20 times more common in the first-degree relatives of individuals known to have this disorder. Most commonly, an individual will report low back pain of varying intensities, often nocturnal in nature and associated with morning stiffness. Other early signs and symptoms include low-grade fever, fatigue, weight loss, and anemia. Early radiographic changes demonstrate bilateral narrowing and fuzziness of the sacroiliac joints. Eventually, the sacroiliac joints become obliterated, and the condition progresses up the spine. Later radiographic changes show calcification of the bones of the spine and ossification of the vertebral ligaments. The articular cartilage is destroyed, and fibrous adhesions develop. These adhesions lead to bone fusion and calcification of the annulus fibrosis of the intervertebral disks as well as the anterior and lateral spinal ligaments. The spine becomes a rigid block of bone, giving the condition its characteristic nickname "bamboo spine" (Fig. 2-26). In addition to radiographic indications, blood serum analysis is used in the diagnosis of ankylosing spondylitis. The human leukocyte antigen B27 (HLA-B27) test may be ordered individually or as part of a group of tests that includes rheumatoid factor (RF), ESR, or CRP. It is treated with NSAIDs, cyclooxygenase 2 (COX-2) inhibitors, therapeutic exercise, and postural training.

Osteoarthritis. The most common type of arthritis is **osteoarthritis**, also known as *degenerative joint disease*. It affects men and women equally, although patients are usually asymptomatic until they are in their 50s. Osteoarthritis is a disease of cartilage and is classified as *primary* or *secondary*. Primary osteoarthritis may be inflammatory or erosive and destructive, resulting from a noninflammatory deterioration of the joint cartilage that occurs with normal wear and tear. In some cases, individuals may have a genetic predisposition for developing osteoarthritis. Secondary osteoarthritis occurs as a result of bone stress associated with trauma, congenital anomalies, or other diseases that alter the hyaline cartilage and surrounding tissue. Osteoarthritis generally affects the large, primary weight-bearing joints of the body such as the hip, where it is particularly disabling, or the knees and ankles (Fig. 2-27). Osteoarthritis may also affect the interphalangeal joints of fingers.

FIGURE 2-26 A, Lateral cervical spine radiograph depicting ankylosing spondylitis with granulation tissue beneath the anterior longitudinal ligament destroying the corners of the contiguous vertebra. **B,** Lateral lumbar spine radiograph of a 64-year-old man with ankylosing spondylitis. Note the fusion of the vertebrae into a solid block of bone.

FIGURE 2-27 Anteroposterior and oblique ankle radiographs demonstrating osteoarthritis.

Osteoarthritis of fingers, which is thought to be hereditary, affects women, especially after menopause, more than it affects men. With this condition, fingers become enlarged and often develop bony knobs termed *Heberden nodes* and *Bouchard nodes.* Osteoarthritis of the fingers is most often managed with medications, splints, and heat treatments.

In joints affected by this disease, articular cartilage degenerates and is gradually worn away, exposing underlying bone. Radiographically, this loss of articular cartilage appears as a narrowing of the joint space. An overgrowth of articular cartilage occurs on the peripheral surfaces of the joint and often calcifies, which results in **osteophytes** or bone spurs that are visible

FIGURE 2-28 Shoulder radiograph demonstrating the formation of an osteophyte at the inferior lip of the glenoid labrum caused by primary osteoarthritis.

radiographically (Fig. 2-28). In terms of radiographic diagnosis, the formation of osteophytes is indicative of osteoarthritis and helps distinguish it from other types of arthritis.

Clinically, an individual with osteoarthritis experiences pain and progressive stiffening of the affected joint. Methods of halting its gradual progression are few; it is second only to cardiovascular disease in causing long-term disability. Treatment consists of the use of medications such as NSAIDs, COX-2 inhibitors, and acetaminophen. Exercise is one of the best treatments to decrease pain, increase flexibility, and help with weight control. The use of corticosteroid injections, walking aids, rest, and heat treatment may also be incorporated in the treatment regimen. Surgery may be used to resurface or reposition bones or remove loose pieces of bone or cartilage; in cases of severe pain, surgical prosthetic joint replacement provides great relief and allows return of joint mobility.

Gouty Arthritis. **Gouty arthritis** is an inherited metabolic disorder in which excess amounts of uric acid are produced and deposited in the joint and adjacent bone. The condition occurs more frequently in men and most commonly affects the metatarsophalangeal joint of the great toe. It is characterized by acute attacks with intervals of remission. This disease may occur in patients placed on long-term diuretics, for instance, to treat congestive heart failure.

The crystallization of uric acid within the joint causes an acute inflammatory reaction. Large masses of these sodium urate crystalline deposits in joints and other sites are called *tophi*. Bone changes include erosion (Fig. 2-29) with overhanging edges. One long-term complication of gout is the formation of radiolucent kidney stones caused by increased excretion of uric acid by the kidneys. Treatment of gout consists of medications either to promote excretion of uric acid by the kidneys or to inhibit the production of uric acid within the body.

Inflammation of Associated Joint Structures. The specialized connective tissues that attach muscle to bone are called *tendons*. Tendons are enclosed in a synovial sheath. **Tendonitis** is inflammation of a tendon, and inflammation of the tendon and the sheath is a condition known as **tenosynovitis** (Fig. 2-30). Tenosynovitis may spread to the associated tendon, resulting in tendonitis. Chronic tendonitis may also cause the formation of calcium deposits in either the affected tendon or an associated sheath. Such calcium deposits that form in the shoulder joint as a result of chronic trauma often cause rotator cuff tears, which can be detected on shoulder radiographs, shoulder arthrogram studies, and MRI examinations of the shoulder (Fig. 2-31). Bursae, which are sacs lined with a synovial membrane, are found in locations where tendons pass over bony prominences. If the bursa becomes inflamed, it is called **bursitis**. Inflammation of these associated structures may be caused by acute or chronic trauma (e.g., "housemaid's knee"), acute or chronic infection, inflammatory arthritis, gout, and, rarely, infection by pyogenic or tuberculous organisms. These inflammatory conditions are characterized by pain, localized tenderness, and limited motion of the involved joint. In cases of chronic bursitis, the walls of the bursa become thickened, and calcium deposits

FIGURE 2-29 Posteroanterior **A,** and lateral, **B,** foot radiographs demonstrating erosion of the tarsal bones from gout.

FIGURE 2-30 Magnetic resonance imaging scans (A, sagittal; B, axial) of right ankle demonstrate tenosynovitis involving the posterior tibialis muscle following a strain injury.

FIGURE 2-31 Calcific tendonitis of the left shoulder resulting from rotator cuff disease. The radiograph demonstrates radiopaque calcium deposits within the shoulder joint.

FIGURE 2-32 Coronal magnetic resonance image of the wrist demonstrating a cystic lesion on the volar aspect of the wrist along the ulnar side.

may be visible radiographically within the bursa. Common areas for bursitis are the shoulder, elbow, knee (prepatellar), and greater trochanter of the hip.

Common medical treatment of bursitis and tendonitis includes NSAIDs in combination with analgesics. In severe cases, aspiration of any accumulated fluid and corticosteroid injections may be included in the treatment. Surgical intervention is necessary when tendons or bursae ossify, especially in conjunction with rotator cuff tears. A **ganglion** is a cystic swelling that develops in connection with a tendon sheath (Fig. 2-32). Ganglions commonly occur in the back part of the wrist joint, but they can occur in any joint space. Ganglion cysts are treated with simple aspiration, aspiration with corticosteroid injection, or surgical excision, if symptomatic.

VERTEBRAL COLUMN

The causes of vertebral column injuries include direct trauma, hyperextension–flexion injuries,

osteoporosis, and metastatic destruction. **Whiplash** is a broad term that encompasses soft tissue neck injuries from a variety of causes and is discussed further in Chapter 12.

Radiographic indications of spinal column injuries include the interruption of smooth, continuous lines formed by the vertebrae stacked one on another and may result from hyperextension or hyperflexion injuries (Figs. 2-33 and 2-34). *Anterospondylolisthesis* refers to the anterior slipping of the body of the vertebra (Fig. 2-35), and *retrospondylolisthesis* refers to the posterior slipping of the body of the vertebra. Anterospondylolisthesis is also known as **spondylolisthesis**. The patient with this condition may have symptoms identical to those of a herniated disk. Approximately 90% of such slippage commonly occurs at the L5-S1 junction and is best detected on a lateral projection. Conservative medical management (e.g., rest, chiropractic manipulative therapy) is the preferred choice for treatment before surgical fusion. Surgical intervention (Fig. 2-36) depends on the degree of slippage and is classified as grade I to IV, with grade I being the least severe and grade IV the most severe.

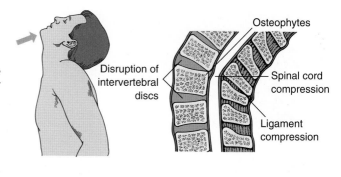

FIGURE 2-33 Hyperextension injuries of the spine. Hyperextension may result in fracture or nonfracture injuries with spinal cord damage.

FIGURE 2-34 Hyperflexion injury of the spine. Hyperflexion produces subluxation of vertebrae, which compromises the central canal and compresses spinal cord parenchyma or vascular structures.

The vertebral bodies may also lose some height, or the interspace may narrow. Perhaps the most common condition of the vertebral column is generalized back pain, typically in the lumbar area. Such back pain may not always result from bone involvement. Disk disease may cause muscle spasm with referred pain throughout the back. Finally, back pain may be secondary to referred pain from the hip. Conventional radiography is the most common imaging modality used to assess low back pain because it can demonstrate vertebral fractures and subluxation, **spondylolysis**, or erosion of vertebral bodies. However, they are of little value in the evaluation of disk pathologies.

A cleft, or breaking down, of the body of a vertebra between the superior and inferior articular processes (pars interarticularis) results in spondylolysis. Typically, this occurs in the arch of the fifth lumbar vertebra as a result of developmental or congenital anomaly rather than acute trauma. It appears radiographically as a "collar" or "broken neck" on the "Scotty dog" (Table 2-1) and is demonstrated on an oblique projection of the lumbar spine (Fig. 2-37).

In cases of disk disorders, myelography may be performed. Myelographic examination alone may visualize the nerve roots and subarachnoid space and clearly demonstrate posture-related disk anomalies. Myelography performed in combination with CT (Fig. 2-38) enables evaluation of bone detail; however, it is still an invasive procedure. MRI provides a noninvasive alternative to CT myelography. MRI demonstrates the spine in multiple planes and is unsurpassed in its ability to demonstrate the spinal cord, nerve roots, subarachnoid and epidural spaces, vertebral disks, and the paraspinal tissues (Fig. 2-39). MRI does have limitations, such as patient compliance and contraindications for performing MRI examination such as pacemakers, aneurysm clips, and so on. In cases of vertebral fracture,

FIGURE 2-35 Lateral spine radiograph demonstrating anterospondylolisthesis of the cervical spine.

TABLE 2-1	Anatomic Components of the Scotty Dog
Dog Part	**Anatomic Component**
Eye	Pedicle
Nose	Transverse process
Ear	Superior articular process
Foreleg	Inferior articular process
Neck	Pars interarticularis
Body	Lamina

FIGURE 2-36 A, Sagittal reconstruction of lumbar spine demonstrating spondylolisthesis before surgical intervention. **B,** L5-S1 lateral radiograph after surgical fusion for spondylolisthesis. **C,** Sagittal reconstruction of lumbar spine demonstrating spondylolisthesis after surgical intervention.

FIGURE 2-39 Magnetic resonance image of the lumbar spine reconstructed in a sagittal plane demonstrating the spinal cord, subarachnoid space, and intervertebral disks.

FIGURE 2-37 Oblique radiograph of the lumbar spine demonstrating spondylolysis of the fourth and fifth lumbar spines on the left side. Note the "break in the Scotty dog's neck."

CT is the modality of choice for demonstrating bone anatomy.

NEOPLASTIC DISEASES

Many varieties of bone tumors are seen in patients of all ages; however, primary bone tumors are more common in children than in adults, and metastatic bone lesions far outnumber the incidence of primary bone neoplasms in the adult. The most common benign tumors are osteoma, osteochondroma, and giant cell tumor. The primary malignant bone tumors are osteosarcoma, Ewing tumor, and multiple myeloma.

The diagnosis of a bone abnormality is often made radiographically on the basis of the patient's age, the pattern of bone destruction, the location of the tumor, and the tumor's position within the bone. In terms of age, benign tumors most often occur within the first three decades of life; a bone tumor in older adults is likely to be malignant. The pattern of bone destruction in benign lesions is expansion of bone and sharp, sclerotic margins. Malignant neoplasms often infiltrate, permeate, and destroy anatomic margins. The location of a

FIGURE 2-38 Computed tomographic myelogram demonstrating the subarachnoid space and intervertebral disks.

tumor is also important. For example, half of all osteosarcomas appear in the distal femoral or proximal tibial metaphysis. Similarly, **chondrosarcomas** tend to involve the trunk, shoulder girdle, and proximal long bones.

Alkaline phosphatase, osteonectin, osteocalcin, and collagen are used as potential bone tissue markers; however, these proteins may be difficult to distinguish if the origin is the bone matrix or from collagenous mimics, which are found in bone neoplasms. For this reason, they may not be helpful as genetic markers.

Radiographic studies contribute greatly to the diagnosis and management of patients with bone tumors. Radiographs are used to disclose the lesions and show the growth characteristics that assist in determining their benign or malignant nature. In conjunction with CT, plain radiographs identify malignant growth patterns and the proper site for biopsy. Sometimes, seemingly unrelated examinations such as a barium enema or chest radiography are ordered by the physician to rule out distant metastases.

CT plays a key role in the primary diagnosis and continued evaluation of neoplasms of the skeletal system because of its ability to produce images with excellent soft tissue and contrast resolution. Sectional images of the area of interest provide physicians with the exact location and extent of the specific tumor, allowing the surgeon to identify the optimal surgical procedure and possibly limiting the surgical resection of the affected bone as well as assisting in the postsurgical management of the disease process. CT is also commonly used to assist during bone biopsy procedures.

As mentioned earlier in this chapter, radionuclide bone scans are helpful in assessing neoplastic diseases because the bone scan reflects the metabolic reaction of bone to the neoplastic disease process. Nuclear medicine procedures may also be performed during the initial stages of treatment planning to identify possible metastatic involvement of other anatomic sites.

Because cortical bone does not produce a signal, MRI provides the unique ability to clearly demonstrate fat and bone marrow because of

their high water content. This information is helpful in differentiating between normal bone marrow and tumor tissue in the assessment of many neoplastic diseases of the skeletal system.

It is important to note that many neoplastic lesions may have similar radiographic appearances or are difficult to differentiate with imaging procedures alone. Therefore, the final diagnosis must include a biopsy of the abnormality. Some biopsies may be performed under CT, MRI, or fluoroscopic guidance, whereas others must be performed surgically to obtain sufficient tissue for analysis. Histopathologic diagnosis is required for a definitive diagnosis.

A staging system for both benign and malignant bone tumors was developed by Enneking in 1980. Arabic numerals are used for benign lesions (1, 2, 3) and Roman numerals (I, II, III) for malignant lesions. For benign lesions, three stages exist: (1) stage 1, which includes benign, inactive tumors; (2) stage 2, in which the bone tumor is benign but active; and (3) stage 3, which includes aggressive benign lesions with bone destruction, soft tissue extensions, or pathologic fractures. Malignant bone lesions need to be staged after biopsy and histologic analysis have been done. Staging for malignant skeletal lesions includes histologic grade (low G1 or high G2), local extent of tumor (intracompartmental T1 or extracompartmental T2), and presence or absence of metastatic disease. The classification examples of IA, IB, IIA, IIB, III, and so on are assigned on the basis of the tumor characteristics, lymph node involvement, metastasis, and grade of the neoplasm.

Osteochondroma (Exostosis)

The most common benign bone tumor is **osteochondroma** (Fig. 2-40), which is three times more common in men than in women. An osteochondroma arises from the growth zone between the epiphysis and diaphysis of long bones, also called *metaphysis*. Most commonly, it involves the lower femur or upper tibia and is capped by growing cartilage attached to the skeleton by a bony stalk. The cortex of an osteochondroma

FIGURE 2-40 Bilateral anteroposterior knee radiographs demonstrating osteochondroma with exostoses within the knee joint.

blends with normal bone, and the growth tends to protrude up and away from the nearest joint, most commonly the knee. **Exostoses** or excessive bone growth may appear as singular or multiple lesions and are normally diagnosed in childhood or adolescence. Multiple hereditary exostoses (MHE) indicate a hereditary disorder and usually appear at an earlier age than compared with the single-lesion osteochondroma. MHE have been linked to mutations in the following genes: *EXT1* on chromosome 8q23-q24, *EXT2* on chromosome 11p11-p12, and *EXT3* on the short arm of chromosome 19. It is theorized that the *EXT* genes also have the function of tumor suppression. In addition, MHE may transform to malignant neoplasms such as chondrosarcoma. Many times, osteochondromas are asymptomatic unless the affected long bone is traumatized, which results in a pathologic fracture of the diseased bone. An osteochondroma has an osteosclerotic or osteoblastic radiologic appearance. CT and MRI are used in initial differentiation between an osteochondroma and a malignant lesion.

Osteoma

An **osteoma** is a less frequent benign growth most commonly located in the skull. These lesions are composed of very dense, well-circumscribed, normal bone tissue that usually projects into the orbits or paranasal sinuses. They are generally slow-growing tumors of little significance unless they cause obstruction, impinge on the brain or eye, or interfere with the oral cavity. A term associated with osteoma of the skull is **hyperostosis frontalis interna**.

Endochondroma

An **enchondroma** is a slow-growing benign tumor composed of hyaline cartilage and is hypothesized to be a result of incomplete endochondral ossification. It grows in the marrow space and most commonly affects the small bones of the hands and feet of individuals between the ages of 30 and 40 years. These benign tumors do not invade surrounding tissue as they grow; however, they do expand the cortical bone, causing thinning. Radiographically, endochondromas appear as radiolucent lesions containing small, stippled calcifications (Fig. 2-41). They are well circumscribed and appear as a "bubbly" lesion of the bone. The erosion of the cortex may cause pain and swelling and increase the incidence of pathologic fractures. Multiple growths, termed *enchondromatosis* (Ollier disease), may also occur in childhood and, like multiple osteochondromas, may undergo malignant transformation with a risk of 25% to 30%. CT and MRI are useful in distinguishing endochondromas from chondrosarcomas.

Simple Unicameral Bone Cyst

A **simple unicameral bone cyst (UBC)** is a wall of fibrous tissue filled with fluid. These frequently occur in the long bones of children, most commonly in the humerus and proximal femur. Eighty percent of all simple bone cysts occur between 3 and 14 years of age and twice as often in boys as in girls. The cyst is usually first noticed when the patient reports pain, caused by increased tumor growth or as a result of a pathologic fracture.

Radiographically, UBCs appear radiolucent with well-defined margins from normal bone surrounding the lesion (Fig. 2-42). Occasionally,

FIGURE 2-41 A, Conventional shoulder radiograph in a 66-year-old man demonstrates calcification in the proximal diaphysis of the right humerus. **B,** Follow-up magnetic resonance image demonstrates an intramedullary lesion without breakthrough of the cortex, consistent with an endochondroma.

FIGURE 2-42 A, Anteroposterior (AP) projection demonstrating multiple well-circumscribed radiolucencies in the proximal humerus consistent with a simple unicameral bone cyst. **B,** AP humerus radiograph demonstrating a well-circumscribed radiolucency midshaft consistent with a simple unicameral bone cyst.

the cyst may be surrounded by a thin rim of sclerotic bone. Small cysts tend to heal and obliterate themselves; larger cysts require surgical intervention. The benign bone cyst is treated by surgical excision and packing with bone chips to obtain complete healing. Percutaneous steroid injection into the lesion is another form of treatment that was introduced in the 1970s, and it is inexpensive and has a decreased morbidity rate compared with surgical intervention.

Aneurysmal Bone Cyst

An **aneurysmal bone cyst** (ABC) is an idiopathic condition and not a true neoplasm. These cysts generally occur in the metaphysis of long bones in individuals under the age of 20 years and consist of numerous blood-filled arteriovenous communications. Vertebral lesions usually occur in the lumbar region and account for 15% to 20% of aneurysmal bone cysts. Following the Human Genome project, it has been discovered that this bone cyst is most likely caused by translocation of 17p13 and overactivity of the oncogene *USP6* (ubiquitin-specific protease). These are slow-growing lesions, and the most common symptoms are pain and swelling at the site of the cyst. This cystic growth causes a thinning of the cortex that is apparent radiographically and as a well-circumscribed lesion associated with soft tissue extension and periosteal bulging. A bone scan demonstrates peripheral uptake with a centralized decreased uptake. Angiography shows persistent accumulation of contrast media throughout the cyst. CT and MRI may also be used for imaging ABCs. CT better delineates the cyst in the vertebral column, and MRI shows fluid levels or the presence of soft tissue mass. The most common treatment of an ABC is surgical removal of the lesion and subsequent bone grafting; however, radiation therapy may be used for treatment in some areas in the vertebral region where surgical removal is difficult. Caution is used with radiation therapy because of the risk of postradiation malignancies.

Osteoid Osteoma and Osteoblastoma

Other common benign tumors of the skeletal system are **osteoid osteoma** and **osteoblastoma**. Although similar in histologic features, they differ in size, origin, and symptoms. Osteoid osteomas are less than 2 cm in dimension, whereas osteoblastomas are larger. Osteoblastomas more frequently involve the spine, and pain may not be present. Furthermore, they are not associated with a marked bone reaction or new bone production and are classified radiographically as osteolytic lesions. Osteoblastomas have a higher recurrence rate compared with osteoid osteomas and, in rare cases, may undergo malignant transformation to osteogenic sarcoma.

Osteoid osteomas occur twice as often in men as in women and almost always develop before the age of 30 years. It has been discovered that genetic markers include an elevated amount of E2 but may also include F2 alpha, 6-keto-F1 alpha, and thromboxane B2. Osteoid osteomas are most commonly found in the femur, tibia, or spine of the young adult. They arise within the cortical bone and erode underlying bone tissue, resulting in a lytic lesion called a *nidus*. The area of erosion is surrounded by a zone of dense, sclerotic bone, making the radiographic appearance of osteoid osteomas very distinctive (Fig. 2-43). The radiographic appearance of an osteoid osteoma demonstrates a well-circumscribed, small radiolucent area containing a dense center (nidus). The radiolucent area is surrounded by very dense, sclerotic bone. The nidus is composed of osteoid or newly formed bone; thus, this tumor is classified as an osteosclerotic lesion. CT scans with 1- to 2-mm cuts are of great value in identifying, localizing, and providing biopsy guidance in the diagnosis of osteoid osteomas (Fig. 2-44). MRI is also a common modality used to assist in the diagnosis (Fig. 2-45). The erosion of surrounding tissue and the presence of prostaglandin and nerve fibers in the nidus cause extreme pain, often at night, and the pain is readily relieved by NSAIDs. CT-guided laser ablation and surgical removal are common treatments for these benign lesions.

Giant Cell Tumor (Osteoclastoma)

Giant cell tumors (GCTs) are characterized by the presence of numerous, multinucleated osteoclastic giant cells. GCTs of the tendon sheath are the second most common benign soft tissue lesions of the hand and wrist. Unlike the previously mentioned neoplastic diseases, GCTs may be either benign or malignant. Approximately 50% of **osteoclastomas** are benign, 35% to 50% recur after surgical excision, and 15% are aggressively malignant from the beginning. This neoplasm affects women more often than

FIGURE 2-43 Anteroposterior hip radiograph of a 7-year-old girl, who complained of a 2-month history of pain. The radiograph demonstrates an osteoid osteoma as evidenced by the well-defined defect in the cortical area of the femoral neck.

FIGURE 2-45 Coronal magnetic resonance images demonstrating an osteoid osteoma in the right femoral neck.

FIGURE 2-44 Axial computed tomography (CT) scan demonstrating an osteoid osteoma **A,** in preparation for CT-guided needle biopsy **B.**

men and is found in individuals between the ages of 20 and 30 years. Anatomically, this disease tends to affect the ends or epiphyses of long bones, especially the lower femur, the upper tibia, and the lower radius. It begins in the medullary canal and expands outward, producing a clublike deformity of the end of the long bone. In addition, soft tissue extensions may be present, but the GCT does not involve the joint space.

Clinical signs and symptoms of a GCT are nonspecific and include pain, tenderness, an occasional palpable mass, and an occasional pathologic fracture. Because this is an osteoclastic disease process, bone and cartilage formation generally do not occur in these lesions; therefore, the radiographer must decrease exposure factors to avoid over-penetration of the affected bone. Radiographically, a GCT is a mass of osteolytic or cystic areas surrounded by a thin shell of bone, giving it the classic "soap bubble" appearance (Fig. 2-46). CT and MRI are also excellent modalities to image this neoplastic disease. GCTs are usually located in the epiphysis, producing erosion and thinning of the cortical bone without new bone growth. Treatment of an osteoclastoma consists of cryosurgery, surgical excision of

FIGURE 2-46 Lateral knee radiograph of a 30-year-old man who complained of a painful knee for approximately 2 months. The radiograph demonstrates a benign osteoclastoma of the knee.

the lesion, and bone grafting. The surgical site in the patient should be closely monitored radiographically at regular intervals.

Osteosarcoma (Osteogenic Sarcoma)

Except for myeloma, the most common primary malignancy of the skeleton is **osteosarcoma**, which arises from osteoblasts. The cause of osteosarcoma is linked genetically to deletion of genetic material on chromosome 13 and the oncogene *src*. Genetic instability is essential for the development of sarcomas. Patients with osteosarcoma frequently lose function of the proteins p53 and RB1, which are tumor suppressors and protect the genome from acquiring mutations that may lead to malignancy. Of osteosarcomas, 50% involve the proteins p53, RB, and MDM2, which may be utilized as genetic markers. Genetic syndromes associated with osteosarcoma include Li-Fraumeni, Rothmund-Thomson, and Werner syndromes. Li-Fraumeni syndrome is associated with mutation of the tumor suppressor gene *p53*; Rothmund-Thomson syndrome involves mutation of the *RECQL4* gene; and Werner syndrome, also referred to as *adult progeria*, may involve environmental factors such as exposure to radiation. This neoplasm is most frequently found in the metaphyses of long bones, with approximately 50% affecting the knee. Osteosarcoma may occur at any age, but 75% occur in patients younger than 20 years old. It is occasionally seen in older individuals with Paget disease or after high-level radiation exposure to bone, and the tumors are known as *postradiation sarcomas*. Clinically, the patient may have pain and swelling.

Osteosarcoma is a highly aggressive bone-forming neoplasm most often located in bone marrow (Fig. 2-47). As the tumor grows from the metaphysis, it lifts the periosteum from the cortical bone and lays down spicules of new bone radiating out from the origin, which gives the radiographic appearance of a sunray or sunburst. This appearance results from the radiopaque and radiolucent changes within the newly created space between the cortex of the metaphysis and the displaced periosteum and is termed a *periosteal reaction*. In some cases, a soft tissue mass that is not enclosed in bone may form as the neoplasm breaks through the cortex lifting the periosteum. MRI is an excellent modality for demonstrating this soft tissue extension (Fig. 2-48). Radiographic findings (Fig. 2-49) vary greatly in appearance because some osteosarcoma tumors produce very little osteoid tissue and contain no calcifications, whereas others are

FIGURE 2-47 Magnetic resonance image of the left femur is helpful in determining the medullary extension of the osteosarcoma.

densely opaque. 18F-Fluorodeoxyglucose positron emission tomography (FDG-PET) is the most frequently used imaging modality for assessing osteosarcoma, but its role in sarcoma analysis is not well delineated because of limited reimbursement. The most significant advantage is the simultaneous evaluation of bone and soft tissues with quantitative metabolic data.

Accurate diagnosis must be made through biopsy of the questionable lesion. Blood serum analysis often shows elevated serum alkaline phosphatase as a result of the osteoblastic activity.

Osteosarcoma is a highly malignant disease with a poor prognosis because lung metastasis almost always occurs via the bloodstream. This metastatic lung disease may appear as multiple, rounded, calcified shadows within the lung fields on a conventional chest radiograph. If the chest radiograph is clear, high-resolution CT of the chest often demonstrates micrometastases, which are commonly present in the lungs before the primary osteosarcoma is discovered. Secondary

FIGURE 2-48 A, Anteroposterior radiograph of the right knee demonstrates a tumor in the distal lateral femoral condyle. Interruption of the cortex and reactive sclerotic bone changes raise suspicion of metastatic disease or primary malignancy. **B,** Follow-up magnetic resonance image of the knee reveals an osteosarcoma that has replaced the distal femoral condyle.

FIGURE 2-49 Posteroanterior projection of the knee of a 14-year-old boy with painful swelling above the left knee. The radiograph demonstrates cortical destruction along the posteromedial margin of the distal femur consistent with an osteosarcoma of the left femur.

growths or spread to other bones is very rare with osteosarcoma. In the past, treatment of osteosarcoma included amputation of the limb followed by chemotherapy. Today, most physicians place the patient on preoperative chemotherapy after the initial diagnosis is confirmed by

bone biopsy. After initial chemotherapy, the patient undergoes limb salvage via a tumor resection with implantation of a cadaver allograft, vascularized grafts, or prostheses. This is followed by postsurgical chemotherapy involving high doses of methotrexate. This change in the management of osteosarcoma has increased 5-year survival rates from 20% to over 80%.

Ewing Sarcoma

Another primary malignant bone tumor is a **Ewing sarcoma.** This neoplasm occurs at a younger age than any other primary malignant bone neoplasm, usually between the ages of 5 and 15 years, and rarely after age 30 years. It is also more common in boys than in girls and shows a predilection for whites, with blacks rarely affected.

Unlike osteosarcoma, Ewing sarcoma arises from the medullary canal and involves bone more diffusely, giving rise to uniform thickening of bone. These lesions tend to be very extensive, often involving the entire shaft of a long bone. Also, unlike osteogenic sarcoma, Ewing sarcoma does not begin at the end of a long bone. It does, however, tend to affect the extremities and the pelvis. Although Ewing sarcoma is a fairly rare disease, it is extremely malignant. Clinical symptoms are nonspecific and include pain and tenderness of the affected area. Radiography, CT, and MRI are essential in establishing the diagnosis and identifying the extent of the disease. The lesions undergo a combination of bone formation in the early stages and destruction in the later stages, with new bone being formed on the surface (Fig. 2-50). This process often gives a classic onionskin or laminated appearance radiographically. Diagnosis is made by biopsy with the identification of an 11:22 chromosomal translocation within the tumor cells. Affirmation of this lesion is completed by immunohistochemistry or polymerase chain reaction (PCR) analysis, which demonstrates the presence of the *EWS-FLI1* fusion gene. The *EWS* gene is located on chromosome 22 and the *FLI-1* gene is located on chromosome 11. Cytologic analysis demonstrates

FIGURE 2-50 Lower leg radiographs of a 12-year-old boy complaining of left leg pain demonstrate a Ewing sarcoma of the tibia as indicated by the lytic defect in the proximal diaphysis of the fibula.

characteristic blue, round cell histology. Multidrug preoperative and postoperative chemotherapy, in combination with radiation therapy or surgical resection, has proven effective in improving the prognosis from a 60% 5-year survival rate to an 80% 5-year survival rate. Treatments based on newer research include the use of monoclonal antibodies, myeloablation therapy, or a combination of chemotherapy and hemopoietic stem cell transplantation.

Chondrosarcoma

A chondrosarcoma is a malignant tumor of cartilaginous origin and is composed of atypical cartilage. It is only half as common as osteosarcoma; approximately 10% of all malignant tumors of the skeletal system are chondrosarcomas. Common locations for chondrosarcoma are the pelvis, shoulder, and ribs. Men are three times more likely than women to develop chondrosarcoma, and it is more common in older

adults. As mentioned earlier in this chapter, benign exostoses and multiple endochondromas may be transformed into chondrosarcomas. However, this type of change accounts for only about 10% of the cases, with approximately 90% of chondrosarcomas arising afresh without prior cartilaginous lesions. Chondrosarcomas may be bulky, and they tend to destroy the bone as they extend through the cortex into surrounding soft tissue. These lesions have the ability to implant or seed into surrounding soft tissue, so careful excision is necessary. Radiographically, a chondrosarcoma shows irregular or circular radiolucencies in combination with granular areas of calcification. These tumors cause destruction and penetration of the cortex and extension into surrounding soft tissue. Often, the actual tumor may be larger than its radiographic appearance. Neither radiation therapy nor chemotherapy is particularly effective in the treatment of chondrosarcomas. Major surgery such as amputation or chest resection is often the treatment of choice, leading to a 5-year survival rate of approximately 40%.

Metastases from Other Sites

Virtually any type of cancer may metastasize to bone; metastatic disease from carcinomas is the most common malignant tumor of the skeleton, with secondary bone tumors of any origin far outnumbering primary bone tumors. Patients with skeletal metastases are usually older than 40 years. Principal signs and symptoms are pain and pathologic fracture.

The bones of the skeletal system that contain red bone marrow are the major bones affected by the metastatic disease because of their abundant vascularization. These include flat bones (such as the ribs, sternum, pelvis, and skull), the vertebrae, and the upper ends of the femora (Fig. 2-51) and humeri. The spine is the most common site for metastasis to occur, accounting for approximately 40% of all metastatic lesions. Radionuclide bone scans are more accurate than conventional radiography in the detection of metastasis because 3% to 5% bone destruction

FIGURE 2-51 Anteroposterior hip radiograph demonstrating metastatic disease from a primary breast cancer.

produces a "hot spot." Metastatic bone lesions appear as multiple, irregularly distributed areas of increased uptake that do not correspond to a single anatomic structure (Fig. 2-52). Bone scans are extremely helpful in assessing metastatic breast cancer because approximately 20% of women with breast cancer have a solitary area of increased activity, often without pain, in the site of the metastatic tumor. Radiographically, signs of bone metastasis include alteration of bone density and architecture. These may be osteolytic, osteoblastic, or mixed. Osteolytic metastases account for 75% of all metastatic lesions, and to be visible radiographically, the lesions must be greater than 1 cm in diameter with a loss of about 30% to 50% of bone density. CT is often employed, especially in the spine, to clear up discrepancies in which a bone scan may indicate metastatic disease that cannot be confirmed by plain radiographic analysis. MRI may also be used to differentiate between tumor tissue and normal bone marrow. Recently, whole body FDG-PET, whole body MRI, MRI-PET, and CT-PET have been advocated for imaging metastatic disease.

Certain characteristics help distinguish between a primary malignant neoplasm and a secondary one. Periosteal response is much more common with primary malignant tumors. Soft

FIGURE 2-52 Bone scan of the patient in Figure 2-45 demonstrating multiple areas of metastatic disease.

tissue masses are common in primary tumors and rare in metastases. Lesions longer than 10 cm often represent a primary malignant tumor; most metastatic tumors range between 2 and 4 cm in length. Tumors that expand bone are primary in nature, with rare exceptions. Most primary tumors are solitary, whereas metastatic lesions are usually multiple. Definitive diagnosis is obtained through biopsy.

The most common primary sites for metastatic bone cancer are the breast, lung, prostate, kidney, thyroid, and bowel, with the tumor spreading via proximity (direct extension), the bloodstream, or the lymphatic system. Treatment of metastatic disease is based on the primary disease, but radiation therapy in combination with either chemotherapy or hormone therapy is commonly used to manage such patients. Bone scans and PET scans are used to monitor the progress of therapy; a reduction in uptake on serial scans is a positive sign.

PATHOLOGY SUMMARY
The Skeletal System

Pathology	Imaging Modalities of Choice	Additive or Subtractive Pathology
Osteogenesis imperfecta	Radiography	Subtractive
Achondroplasia	Radiography	None
Osteopetrosis	Radiography	Additive
Anencephaly	Ultrasonography	None
Osteomyelitis	MRI, nuclear medicine, radiographs	Subtractive
Tuberculosis	Radiography	Subtractive
Infectious arthritis	Radiography	Subtractive (early)
Psoriatic arthritis	Radiography	Additive (healing) Subtractive
Reiter syndrome	Nuclear medicine, radiography	None Additive
Rheumatoid arthritis	Radiography	Additive Both
Ankylosing spondylitis	Radiography	Additive
Osteoarthritis	Radiography	Subtractive
Joint structures	MRI	None
Gouty arthritis	Radiography	Subtractive
Osteochondroma	Radiography, MRI	Additive
Osteoma	Radiography, MRI	Additive
Endochondroma	Radiography, MRI	Subtractive
Unicameral bone cyst	Radiography, MRI	Subtractive
Aneurysmal bone cyst	CT, MRI	Subtractive
Osteoid osteoma	CT	Subtractive
Osteoblastoma	Radiography, MRI	Subtractive
Giant cell tumor	Radiography, MRI	Subtractive
Osteosarcoma	Radiography, MRI	Additive
Ewing sarcoma	Radiography, MRI	Both
Chondrosarcoma	Radiography, MRI	Subtractive
Bone metastases from other sites	MRI, CT, FDG-PET	Subtractive

CT, Computed tomography; *MRI,* magnetic resonance imaging; *FDG-PET,* 18F-fluorodeoxyglucose positron emission tomography.

REVIEW QUESTIONS

1. Specialized cells responsible of the formation of bone are termed:
   a. Chondroblasts
   b. Osteoblasts
   c. Osteoclasts
   d. Both b and c

2. A freely movable joint is classified as:
   a. Amphiarthrodial
   b. Diarthrodial
   c. Synarthrodial
   d. Triarthrodial

3. Bone marrow is located anatomically within the:
   a. Cortex
   b. Medullary canal
   c. Periosteum
   d. Trabeculae

4. The end portion of a long bone is referred to as the:
   a. Epiphysis
   b. Diaphysis
   c. Diploë
   d. Metaphysis

5. One of the most common primary malignant tumors of the skeleton that arises from osteoblasts is:
   a. Giant cell tumor
   b. Osteoid osteoma
   c. Osteosarcoma
   d. Osteochondroma

6. The most common inherited disorder that results in dwarfism is:
   a. Achondroplasia
   b. Albers-Schönberg disease
   c. Osteogenesis
   d. Spina bifida imperfecta

7. A variant of rheumatoid arthritis associated with bacterial infections by organisms such as *Chlamydia trachomatis* or *Campylobacter* is:
   a. Juvenile arthritis
   b. Psoriatic arthritis
   c. Osteoarthritis
   d. Reiter syndrome

8. The formation of extra digits is termed:
   a. Adactyly
   b. Polydactyly
   c. Syndactyly
   d. Talipes

9. An abnormal lateral curvature of the spine is referred to as:
   a. Ankylosing spondylitis
   b. Scoliosis
   c. Spondylolisthesis
   d. Spondylolysis

10. Osteomyelitis is a disease of the skeletal system that is:
    a. Arthritic
    b. Congenital
    c. Inflammatory
    d. Neoplastic

11. Osteoarthritis affects the weight-bearing joints within the body and may be treated with:
    a. Exercise
    b. Medication
    c. Surgery
    d. All of the above

12. The type of arthritis believed to be an auto-immune disease is:
    a. Bursitis
    b. Gout
    c. Osteoarthritis
    d. Rheumatoid arthritis

13. Which of the following neoplastic diseases affects children more frequently than adults?
    a. Chondrosarcoma
    b. Ewing sarcoma
    c. Osteochondroma
    d. Osteoclastoma

14. The most common benign bone tumor is:
    a. Endochondroma
    b. Osteoid osteoma
    c. Osteoma
    d. Osteochondroma

15. All of the following are malignant neoplasms of the skeletal system except:
    a. Chondrosarcoma
    b. Ewing sarcoma
    c. Osteosarcoma
    d. Osteoma

16. A 60-year-old patient who was discharged from the hospital after knee replacement continued to complain of generalized pain in the area of the knee for several days. If you were this patient's physician, what imaging test might you order, and why?

17. A 35-year-old woman visits her family physician with complaints of swelling that comes and goes in her hands. What might be the initial suspicion, and what diagnostic procedure(s) might be ordered?

18. How may CT and MRI be used to complement skeletal radiography in the diagnosis and treatment of osteosarcoma?

19. A male construction worker sees his physician because of lower back pain. What are two possible causes that are unrelated to the bony vertebral column?

20. In diagnosing bone tumors, what are some of the characteristics taken into consideration?

Respiratory System

LEARNING OBJECTIVES

On completion of Chapter 3, the reader should be able to do the following:

- Describe the anatomic components of the respiratory system.
- Distinguish between the results obtained and uses for the various projections of the chest.
- Describe the various types of tubes, vascular access lines, and catheters used in relation to the respiratory system.

- Characterize a given condition as congenital, inflammatory, or neoplastic.
- Identify the pathogenesis of the chest pathologies cited and the typical treatments for them.
- Describe, in general, the radiographic appearance of each of the given pathologies.

OUTLINE

Anatomy and Physiology
Imaging Considerations
  Radiography
  Exposure Factor
    Conditions
  Position and Projection
  Chest Radiography
  Soft Tissues of the Chest
  Bony Structures of the
    Chest
  Mediastinum
  Computed Tomography
  Nuclear Medicine
    Procedures

Chest Tubes, Vascular Access
  Lines, and Catheters
Respiratory Failure
Congenital and Hereditary
  Diseases
  Cystic Fibrosis
  Hyaline Membrane
    Disease
Inflammatory Diseases
  Pneumonias
  Bronchiectasis
  Pulmonary Tuberculosis
  Chronic Obstructive
    Pulmonary Disease

Pneumoconioses
Fungal Diseases
Lung Abscess
Pleurisy
Pleural Effusion
Sinusitis
Neoplastic Diseases
  Bronchial Carcinoid
    Tumors
  Bronchogenic Carcinoma
  Metastases from Other
    Sites

KEY TERMS

Aspiration pneumonia
Asthma
Bronchial carcinoid
Bronchiectasis
Bronchogenic carcinoma

Chronic bronchitis
Chronic obstructive pulmonary disease
Coin lesion
Cystic fibrosis
Diffusion

Emphysema
Exudates
Hemothorax
Hypercapnia
Hypoxemia
Legionnaires' disease
Mediastinal emphysema
Miliary tuberculosis
Mycoplasma pneumonia
Pleural effusion
Pleurisy
Pneumococcal pneumonia

Pneumoconioses
Pneumonia
Progressive disseminated histoplasmosis
Pulmonary tuberculosis
Respiratory distress syndrome
Respiratory failure
Sinusitis
Subcutaneous emphysema
Transudates
Tuberculosis
Ventilation
Viral pneumonia

ANATOMY AND PHYSIOLOGY

The respiratory system is responsible for two major functions. **Ventilation** involves the movement of air in and out of the lungs, and **diffusion** relates to the gas exchange between the lungs and the circulatory system. This system is usually subdivided into the upper respiratory tract—the nose, mouth, pharynx, and larynx—and the lower respiratory tract—the trachea, bronchi, alveoli, and lungs (Fig. 3-1). The thoracic cavity consists of the right and left pleural cavities and the mediastinum. The parietal pleura lines the thoracic cavity, and the visceral pleura adheres directly to lung tissue.

Anatomically, the mediastinum is divided into the anterior, middle, and posterior portions. The anterior mediastinum contains the thyroid and thymus glands. The middle mediastinum contains the heart and great vessels, esophagus, and trachea. The posterior mediastinum contains the descending aorta and the spine.

The anatomic bony structures of the thorax assist in both inspiration and expiration. These bony structures include the ribs, sternum, and thoracic vertebrae.

The paranasal sinuses are lined with respiratory epithelium and communicate with the nasal cavities, hence their inclusion in this chapter. The maxillary and ethmoid sinuses are the only paranasal sinuses present at birth. The frontal sinuses generally develop shortly after birth and are fully developed by the age of 10 years. The sphenoid sinus begins to develop around the age of 2 or 3 years and is fully developed by late adolescence.

IMAGING CONSIDERATIONS

Radiography

The examination most frequently performed in any radiology department is chest radiography. Although this examination may seem routine, chest radiography provides important information about soft tissues, bones, the pleura, the mediastinum, and lung tissue.

Exposure Factor Conditions

Correct exposure factor selection is critical because an incorrect exposure factor may hide or appear to create pathologic findings. This is particularly true for serial mobile radiographs because the interpreting physician relies heavily on consistent exposure conditions to analyze the change in pathology after treatment. Institutions may record exposure techniques for mobile chest images so that different technologists can use similar exposure factors to

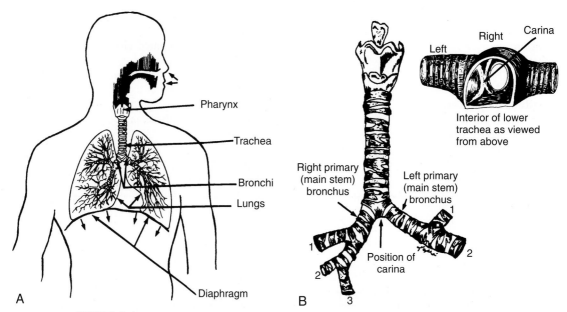

Pharynx

Trachea

Bronchi

Lungs

Diaphragm

A

Right primary
(main stem)
bronchus

Left primary
(main stem)
bronchus

Position of
carina

B

Left

Right

Carina

Interior of lower
trachea as viewed
from above

FIGURE 3-1 A, The respiratory system. **B,** The trachea and its bifurcation at the carina.

maintain consistency among the radiographs. Photostimulable phosphor–computed tomography (CT) imaging plates and direct readout (DR) image receptors are commonly used for mobile chest radiography to eliminate exposure repeats caused by the inadequacy or inconsistency of technical factors. Although accurate technical selection is important when using digital radiography systems to ensure that an appropriate exposure indicator is obtained, both systems offer wider latitude of error over conventional film or screen systems because of a wider dynamic range.

Some sources describe pathologies, including those in the chest, as *additive*, that is, they are harder than normal to penetrate or *subtractive* (destructive), that is, they are easier than normal to penetrate. In the respiratory system, any condition that adds fluid or tissue to the normally aerated chest (e.g., pneumonia) requires an increase in technical factors to afford proper penetration and exposure. Similarly, any condition that increases the aeration of the chest (e.g., emphysema) reduces the amount of radiation required for proper exposure to be achieved. Most experts agree that when chest radiography

is performed using a digital imaging system, the radiographer must use his or her knowledge of pathologic conditions and specific image receptor characteristics to assess whether a change in milliampere second (mAs) or kilovoltage peak (kVp) is required to adjust the radiographic exposure. The kilovoltage range should be chosen based on the energy level necessary to penetrate the part of interest, keeping in mind the presence of additive or subtractive pathologies.

The use of automatic exposure control (AEC) in chest radiography facilitates consistent radiographic exposures but requires careful analysis of the clinical history and conscious thought about the type of disease present and its location to ensure truly optimal diagnostic-quality radiographs. Activation of the sensor, for example, over an area of significant aeration or consolidation (tissue or fluid accumulation) may result in excessive or insufficient exposure, respectively. Although the image may look fine on initial visual examination, care must be taken to always utilize an exposure indicator to assess proper technique selection. Experience with AEC, combined with careful thought in selecting the proper sensor, eliminates these mistakes.

FIGURE 3-2 A, Normal erect posteroanterior chest. **B,** Normal erect lateral chest.

Position and Projection

Patient position and projection are also critical exposure conditions that may distort the final image. *Position* refers to the arrangement of the patient's body (e.g., erect, supine, recumbent), and *projection* refers to the path of the x-ray beam (e.g., anteroposterior [AP], i.e., entering through the body's anterior surface and exiting the posterior surface). The standard projections for chest radiography are the erect posteroanterior (PA) and left lateral (Fig. 3-2). Each of these serves to place the heart closer to the film because the heart lies in the anterior part of the chest and mostly to the left side. When combined with a standard 72-inch source-to-image distance (SID), magnification of the heart is minimized.

FIGURE 3-3 Recumbent anteroposterior chest demonstrating obscuring of the lower lung fields.

Chest Radiography

On a normal erect PA chest image, the costophrenic and cardiophrenic angles are demonstrated, with the right hemidiaphragm appearing 1 to 2 cm higher than the left because of the position of the liver. When a patient is radiographed in the recumbent position, the lower lung fields may be obscured because of abdominal pressure raising the level of the diaphragm (Fig. 3-3).

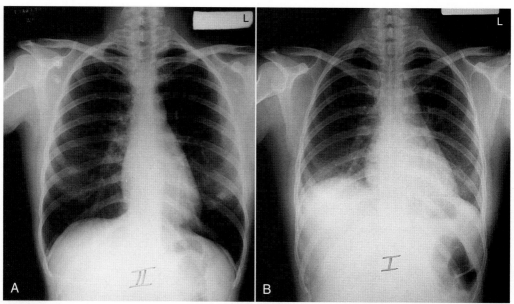

FIGURE 3-4 A, Normal appearance of chest on inspiration. **B,** Expiration film on the same patient demonstrates elevation of the diaphragm and a heart that is more transverse and appears larger.

Other projections of the thorax are used less frequently than the erect PA and left lateral projections. The AP projection is the method of choice for mobile radiography when the patient is too ill to tolerate a visit to the department and assume an erect position. As much as possible, it is important that mobile chest radiographs be taken with the patient sitting in bed in the erect position to demonstrate any air–fluid levels present. Maintenance of the beam perpendicular to the plane of the image receptor is essential to avoid any foreshortening of the heart. Furthermore, use of the 72-inch SID is very important for mobile radiography to minimize magnification of the heart, which is located farther from the image receptor in the AP projection. To improve image quality, many institutions commonly employ a short dimension grid when using a digital imaging system.

The AP and PA projections of the patient lying in the lateral decubitus position are useful under specific conditions such as diagnosing free air in the pleural space or pleural fluid. For example, for a right lateral decubitus chest radiograph, the

patient lies on his or her right side. In this position, any fluid present tends to layer out along the edge of the lung field on the dependent side, which enhances its visibility, whereas the free air rises toward the left side.

For evaluation of the standard PA chest radiograph, the size and radiolucency of both lungs should be compared. Criteria for adequate inspiration and penetration of chest radiographs vary from institution to institution; however, a rule of thumb is that adequate inspiration should provide visualization of 10 posterior ribs within the lung field. In addition, all thoracic vertebrae and intervertebral disk spaces should be faintly visible through the mediastinum on an adequately penetrated chest radiograph. The average movement of the lungs and diaphragm between inspiration and expiration is approximately 3 cm (Fig. 3-4).

Oblique projections of the thorax are useful in separating superimposed structures such as the sternum, esophagus, and thoracic spine. A lordotic chest radiograph is useful in demonstrating the apical regions of the lung, which are

FIGURE 3-5 Lordotic chest radiograph taken on expiration to demonstrate a possible pneumothorax.

FIGURE 3-6 Breast shadows are readily recognizable on the normal posteroanterior chest radiograph.

normally obscured by bony structures on the standard PA projection (Fig. 3-5). Certain diseases such as tuberculosis (TB) have a predilection for the apices.

Soft Tissues of the Chest

Various soft tissue densities are present on chest radiographs. They may vary with patient age, sex, and pathologic conditions. The pectoral muscles are normally demonstrated overlying and extending beyond the lung fields. Radiographs of both men and women demonstrate breast shadows in the midchest region (Fig. 3-6). These shadows are normally homogeneous in appearance, and female breasts may obscure the costophrenic angles. Elevation of the breasts may be necessary to better demonstrate the bases of the lungs. Surgical removal of one or both breasts is also evident on chest radiographs; breast prostheses, which appear as well-defined, circular, radiopaque densities, are also evident. Nipple shadows may be visible at the level of the fourth or fifth anterior rib spaces and may occasionally mimic nodules or masses in the chest. These soft tissue structures may be differentiated with nipple markers or oblique projections of the chest.

Bony Structures of the Chest

The ribs, sternum, and thoracic spine enclose the thoracic cavity. These structures assist the technologist in the assessment of the technical adequacy of chest radiographs. Congenital anomalies of the ribs may be demonstrated (Fig. 3-7), as well as calcified costal cartilages. This calcification generally occurs in patients in their late 20s and beyond. Rib fractures may be seen (Fig. 3-8), sometimes with an accompanying pneumothorax. A depressed sternum (pectus excavatum) may also be demonstrated, possibly displacing the heart (Fig. 3-9). The thoracic spine may be assessed for scoliosis, which may affect the chest cavity, and kyphosis or compression fractures of the vertebrae.

Mediastinum

The mediastinum contains all thoracic organs except the lungs. The heart occupies a large portion of the mediastinum, and the shape of the heart varies with age, degree of respiration, and

FIGURE 3-7 Congenital intrathoracic rib seen as curving, tubular density in the posterior thorax. Usually, these ribs are attached at one or both ends of a posterior rib and lie extrapleurally inside the thoracic cage.

FIGURE 3-9 Lateral projection of the chest demonstrating pectus excavatum, including compression of heart toward spine.

FIGURE 3-8 Right-sided rib fractures (*arrows*) in combination with a right clavicular fracture.

patient position. Other organs contained within the mediastinum include the thyroid and thymus glands and nervous and lymphatic tissues (Fig. 3-10).

Radiographically, the mediastinum is divided into three sections: (1) The anterior mediastinal masses generally arise from the thyroid gland, thymus gland, or lymphatic tissue; (2) the middle mediastinal masses are commonly lymphatic tissue; and (3) the posterior mediastinal masses usually arise from nervous or bony tissue.

In infants, the mediastinum appears wide because the thymus is normally large in a healthy infant. On frontal projections, it may extend beyond the heart borders and caudally to the diaphragm, and on a lateral projection, it may fill the anterior portion of the mediastinum, which is normally radiolucent later in life. This radiographic appearance is readily visible on both PA and lateral views and is referred to as the "sail sign" because of its characteristic appearance (Fig. 3-11). Diagnosis is difficult because the width of the upper mediastinum varies greatly with the phase of respiration. A crying child may present an opportune moment for the technologist to make an exposure, but the

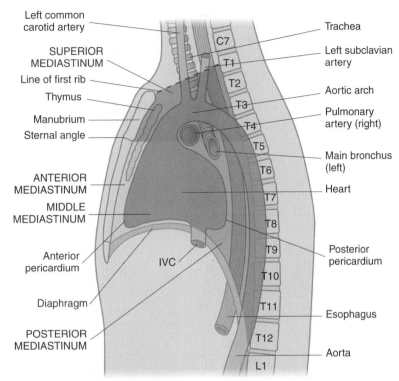

Left common
carotid artery

Trachea

SUPERIOR
MEDIASTINUM

Left subclavian
artery

Line of first rib

Aortic arch

Thymus

Pulmonary
artery (right)

Manubrium

Sternal angle

ANTERIOR
MEDIASTINUM

Main bronchus
(left)

MIDDLE
MEDIASTINUM

Heart

Anterior
pericardium

Posterior
pericardium

IVC

Diaphragm

Esophagus

POSTERIOR
MEDIASTINUM

Aorta

C7, T1, T2, T3, T4, T5, T6, T7, T8, T9, T10, T11, T12, L1

FIGURE 3-10 Sagittal view of mediastinum.

FIGURE 3-11 Normal enlargement of the thymus in a 3-month-old infant demonstrates the "sail sign," evidenced by the uniform density increase in the right upper lung area.

resultant Valsalva maneuver adds to the distortion of the thymus. The Valsalva maneuver increases both the intrathoracic pressure and the intraabdominal pressure by asking the patient to inhale deeply and hold the breath to force the diaphragm and chest muscles against a closed glottis. True mediastinal masses are rare in infants and generally represent congenital malformations or neoplasms. In the mediastinum of older adults, the aorta dilates, and the aortic knob becomes much more visible.

Mediastinal emphysema (pneumomediastinum) occurs when there has been a disruption in the esophagus or airway and air is trapped in the mediastinum (Fig. 3-12). It may result from chest trauma, endoscopy, or violent vomiting. When unaccompanied by a pneumothorax, spontaneous mediastinal emphysema is usually self-limiting, subsiding in a few days without complication. Air in the mediastinum from rupture of the esophagus (usually from vomiting) or a major bronchus (usually from trauma) is more serious and requires prompt diagnosis and surgical intervention. An esophagogram may be performed with a water-soluble contrast agent to verify that a leak has not occurred.

FIGURE 3-12 A, Portable pediatric anteroposterior chest radiograph demonstrating a pneumomediastinum; **B & C,** Oblique coronal chest computed tomography scan demonstrating a pneumomediastinum around the heart.

When the pneumomediastinum is extensive, air may pass from the mediastinum into the subcutaneous tissues of the chest or neck, resulting in **subcutaneous emphysema** (Fig. 3-13). Diagnosis of this may be made by feeling air bubbles in the skin of the chest or neck.

Glandular enlargements of the thyroid gland are demonstrated by a displacement or narrowing of the trachea. The thyroid gland is usually located superior to the lung apices, but an ectopic thyroid gland may also displace the trachea. Clinical manifestations of an ectopic thyroid gland are often absent, and the mass may be discovered accidentally when chest radiography is performed for some other purpose.

In some instances, a routine chest radiograph may be requested on admission to the hospital, but for stable patients, this must be based on specific clinical indications such as need for cardiac monitoring or the presence of extrathoracic disease. Although many institutions routinely obtain mobile chest radiographs for all patients in the intensive care unit, recent research indicates that the diagnostic and therapeutic value of routine chest radiography is low in this population. On the basis of current evidence, the American College of Radiology (ACR) suggests that routine mobile chest radiography is only indicated in patients with acute cardiopulmonary conditions and patients in respiratory failure

FIGURE 3-13 Significant subcutaneous emphysema seen throughout the thorax, especially extending along the right border of the chest.

FIGURE 3-14 High-resolution computed tomography scan of a normal chest.

who are on a mechanical ventilator. In cases involving the placement of an endotracheal tube, central venous line, arterial line, and chest tubes, radiographs should only routinely be obtained upon placement of the device. Follow-up chest radiography should not be routine for these patients and should be performed based on appropriate clinical indications.

Computed Tomography

Volumetric CT offers the advantage of imaging the entire chest with one breath hold, which allows better evaluation of the chest, especially the diaphragm area. Advances in CT software allowing high-resolution, thin-slice thicknesses ranging from 1 to 1.5 mm (Fig. 3-14) and faster scan times, in combination with dynamic scanning (Fig. 3-15), have greatly enhanced the role of CT in chest imaging. CT is the method of choice for evaluation of pulmonary adenopathy. Standard radiography is only about 50% sensitive to chest disease, typically displaying advanced pathologic conditions. The excellent specificity of CT, however, may be a problem because most people have granulomatous disease, which is often benign. A rule of thumb for evaluating the character of a visualized nodule relates to its size: Those less than 1 cm in size are usually benign,

and those larger than 1 cm may be malignant. Also, the presence of calcium within a nodule is a reasonable indication of benignancy, particularly in the middle of the lesion or diffusely within the nodule, but eccentric calcification may indicate malignancy.

CT is also sensitive in detecting emboli within the thoracic vessels (Fig. 3-16). In fact, the current standard of care when a pulmonary embolus is suspected is a computed tomographic angiogram (CTA) of the chest with contrast.

Chest CT is also indicated in the clinical staging of small cell lung carcinomas and in the detection of metastatic disease of the chest. Percutaneous transthoracic needle aspiration is commonly performed under CT guidance. Needle aspirations are performed to obtain cytologic specimens from lesions within the lungs (Fig. 3-17), pleural space, and mediastinum. Following the biopsy, chest radiographs may be obtained to check for a possible pneumothorax or hemorrhage.

Nuclear Medicine Procedures

Perfusion and ventilation scans, as performed in nuclear medicine, are useful in evaluating chest

FIGURE 3-15 Contrast enhanced computed tomography (CT) of the chest using CT software to track the bolus of intravenous contrast media.

FIGURE 3-16 Computed tomography scan of the lung demonstrating a massive embolism within the main pulmonary artery branches and smaller bronchial vessels.

FIGURE 3-17 Computed tomography–assisted core biopsy of a large right lung mass.

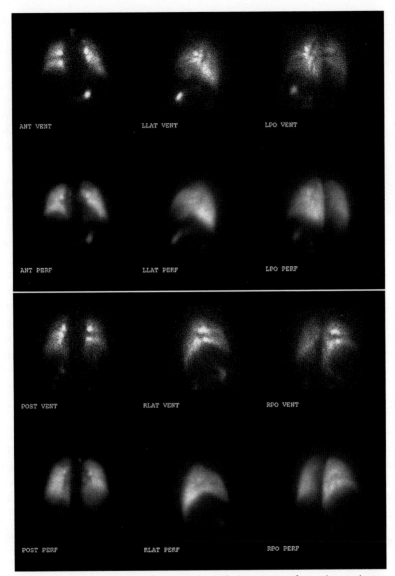

ANT VENT   LLAT VENT   LPO VENT

ANT PERF   LLAT PERF   LPO PERF

POST VENT   RLAT VENT   RPO VENT

POST PERF   RLAT PERF   RPO PERF

FIGURE 3-18 Example of a nuclear medicine perfusion and ventilation scan performed to evaluate a possible pulmonary embolism.

disease, particularly in the case of obstructive disease and in cases of suspected pulmonary emboli when a CTA is contraindicated. Injection of a radionuclide into the venous system for a perfusion causes it to become trapped in the pulmonary circulation, allowing for γ-camera visualization of its distribution. In a ventilation scan, the patient inhales a radioactive gas (such as xenon) and holds the breath while an image is taken of the gas distribution throughout the lungs (Fig. 3-18).

Positron emission tomography (PET) captures information regarding metabolic activity. The primary imaging agent used in PET of the lungs is fluorodeoxyglucose (FDG), making it useful in distinguishing benign and malignant lesions

FIGURE 3-19 Axial positron emission tomography and computed tomography of the abdomen used for staging bronchogenic carcinoma (same as Fig. 3-53, *A*).

within the chest because it has the capability of imaging an increase in glucose uptake from neoplastic cells. FDG whole body PET is useful in the evaluation of solitary pulmonary nodules and in the staging of bronchogenic carcinoma (Fig. 3-19).

CHEST TUBES, VASCULAR ACCESS LINES, AND CATHETERS

A variety of tubes, lines, and catheters can be placed in relation to particular parts of the respiratory system. It is important for the technologist to be familiar with each of these and exercise great caution in attempting patient movement with any of these in place. It is best to have assistance from another technologist or nursing personnel to ensure that the lines and tubes are free of any obstructions before patient movement occurs. Furthermore, the technologist who is unsure whether the patient is allowed to sit erect should always ask the patient's nurse. The x-ray tube, image receptor, and exposure technique should be established before the patient is moved. Patients in critical care units often can be erect for only a short period because of the instability of their blood pressure. Finally, it is necessary to cover cassettes with a plastic bag to limit infection transfer and keep the cold cassette surface from touching the patient's back.

An endotracheal (ET) tube is a large plastic tube inserted through the patient's nose or mouth into the trachea. It helps to manage the patient's airway, allows frequent suctioning, and allows mechanical ventilation. Its proper position is below the vocal cords and above the carina (Fig. 3-20). Movement of a patient with an ET tube should be done with great caution because inadvertent displacement or extubation may leave the patient without a patent airway.

A chest tube is a large plastic tube inserted through the chest wall between the ribs. It allows drainage of air (e.g., pneumothorax) or fluid (e.g., pleural effusion or hemothorax) from the thoracic cavity (Fig. 3-21) and allows the lungs to inflate to help the patient breathe normally. Those placed lower on the chest wall are usually for fluid drainage; those placed higher are usually for air removal. After open heart surgery, a chest tube may be placed in the mediastinum for proper fluid drainage. Its location is midline, just below the sternum. The collection device attached to the chest tube must be kept below the level of the chest to allow for proper drainage. The amount of time a chest tube remains in the thorax is dependent on the amount of deflation of the lung.

Central venous pressure (CVP) lines are usually inserted via the subclavian vein, but they may also be placed through the jugular vein, antecubital vein, or femoral vein. Proper insertion places the tip of the CVP catheter in the distal superior vena cava (SVC) just above the right atrium (Fig. 3-22). This catheter provides an alternative injection site to compensate for loss of peripheral infusion sites or to allow for infusion of massive volumes of fluids. In addition, it allows for measurement of CVP, which indicates the patient's fluid status and provides information about the function of the heart's right side. However, pulmonary artery catheters have largely supplanted the use of CVP lines for these purposes because they provide even greater accuracy in measurements. Chest radiographs are generally requested following the insertion of a CVP line to check for proper placement and the presence of a pneumothorax or hemothorax.

FIGURE 3-20 A, Incorrect endotracheal (ET) tube placement creates shift of heart and mediastinum to the left with loss of air volume in the left lung. The ET tube tip lies in the proximal right main stem bronchus inferior to the carina. **B,** Correct placement of the ET tube demonstrating balanced lung ventilation.

FIGURE 3-21 Portable chest radiograph demonstrating proper chest tube placement in the right lung near the apex.

Improperly placed catheters may result in cardiac arrhythmias.

A pulmonary artery catheter (Swan-Ganz catheter) is usually inserted via the subclavian vein, but other injection sites include the antecubital vein, jugular vein, and femoral vein. It is a multilumen catheter that serves to evaluate cardiac function. The pulmonary artery catheter measures pulmonary wedge pressure, reflecting left atrial pressure. It does not enter the heart's left side but is positioned in the pulmonary artery (Fig. 3-23). Inflation of the balloon at the tip of the catheter allows the tube to float into a smaller pulmonary artery capillary. Diagnosis and management of heart failure resulting from myocardial infarction and cardiogenic shock represent the most common use of the catheter.

Access catheters such as a Hickman catheter or a Port-a-Cath are usually inserted via the subclavian vein. Hickman catheters are open to the outside of the body with the tip of the catheter placed in the SVC. Port access devices are placed under the skin, just below the clavicle (Fig. 3-24). Because these devices are not open to the outside, a port access device is less likely to become infected and requires little maintenance. Access catheters allow multiple tapping for injection of various agents, typically chemotherapeutics. Patients in whom these catheters are used typically have poor peripheral venous access because of the toxic effects of chemotherapeutic drugs. Location in the subclavian vein provides ready

FIGURE 3-22 A, Central venous catheter entering the left subclavian vein is positioned with the tip properly placed in the distal superior vena cava. **B,** Inverted image of same patient.

FIGURE 3-23 A, Swan-Ganz catheter placement from the right interjugular vein (IJ) with the tip in the proximal right pulmonary artery. **B,** Inverted image of same patient.

access to the venous circulation and its blood flow return to the heart. An intraaortic balloon pump (IABP) catheter is a specialized device typically inserted in surgery or percutaneously at the bedside in critical care units. A 40-mL balloon at the distal end of the catheter allows inflation and deflation by a pump that is synchronized to the patient's cardiac cycle to provide mechanical support of the left ventricle. These devices reduce

the workload of the heart and help improve systemic blood flow, including increased blood supply to the cardiac muscle. The balloon is placed in the descending aorta below the subclavian artery and above the renal arteries (Fig. 3-25). Particular caution should be used in moving affected patients because movement may cause the balloon to float downward, possibly blocking the lower circulation.

FIGURE 3-24 Portable anteroposterior chest radiograph demonstrating the placement of a double port.

FIGURE 3-25 Portable anteroposterior chest radiograph demonstrating an intraaortic pump placement.

FIGURE 3-26 A, Portable chest radiograph taken after pacemaker insertion demonstrating proper placement of lead wires. **B,** Inverted image of same patient.

Ventricular pacing electrodes may be placed for temporary or permanent purposes. Temporary pacing electrodes are inserted via the antecubital vein into the right ventricle. They provide electrical pacing of the heart in patients experiencing a very slow heart rate (i.e., bradycardia) as a result of misfiring of the heart's electrical system. Also, patients who have had open heart surgery may have these electrodes placed directly on the heart's surface and brought externally beneath the sternum at midline as a temporary precaution against heart arrhythmia problems. Permanent electrodes are used for permanent

heart pacing needs. The pacemaker generator is inserted under the skin below the right clavicle, with the electrodes placed into the right ventricle (Fig. 3-26).

RESPIRATORY FAILURE

Respiratory failure is a term used to describe lack of respiratory function or the lack of oxygen and carbon dioxide exchange. This may occur at two levels: (1) within the lungs (intrapulmonary gas exchange) or (2) as a result of impaired breathing (inability to move air into and out of the lungs).

This may occur following acute trauma to the chest or as a result of an acute or chronic lung disease. When ventilation is normal carbon dioxide (CO_2) is removed from the lungs to maintain homeostasis with the cell metabolism thus ensuring that the CO_2 level in arterial blood (PCO_2) is approximately 40 mm Hg. When PCO_2 levels are above 40 mm Hg, this signals that the CO_2 is not being removed properly, which denotes hypoventilation that can cause hypoxemia and hypercapnia. **Hypoxemia** denotes low oxygen levels within arterial blood and results from a failure of the gas exchange function. Common causes include toxic gas or smoke inhalation, chronic obstructive pulmonary disease (COPD), atelectasis, severe pneumonia, high altitudes, hypoventilation, or impaired diffusion (a physical separation of gas and blood) resulting from pulmonary edema or an acute lung injury. In cases of congenital heart defects, hypoxemia may also be caused by shunting of blood from the right side to the left side of the heart without passing through the lungs. The term **hypercapnia** refers to failure of ventilation resulting in the inability to move air into and out of the lungs, with consequent increased blood CO_2 content. Hypercapnic or hypotoxic respiratory failure may be caused by upper airway obstruction, insufficient respiratory drive, respiratory muscle fatigue or paralysis, or a dysfunction of the central nervous system (CNS) resulting in a defective ventilatory pump. Individuals in respiratory failure usually exhibit tachypnea, tachycardia, irregular or gasping breathing patterns, and paradoxic abdominal motion. If the hypoxemia is acute, it may cause cardiac arrhythmias and alteration of consciousness ranging from confusion to coma.

Arterial blood gas (ABG) measurement is the primary method for diagnosing respiratory failure and for determining the severity of the failure. An arterial oxygen level (PO_2) less than 60 mm Hg, an arterial PCO_2 greater than 45 mm Hg, or both are indicative of respiratory failure. Chest radiographs are often obtained to help identify the cause of respiratory failure. The treatment of respiratory failure includes establishing a patent airway, administration of bronchodilating drugs, and controlled oxygen therapy with the use of specialized, nonventilator masks termed *continuous positive airway pressure* (CPAP) and *bilevel positive airway pressure* (BiPAP) devices. Individuals may also be intubated and placed on a mechanical positive pressure ventilator (PPV). Care must also be taken to maintain cardiac output and to assist the failing circulation secondary to cardiac dysfunction.

CONGENITAL AND HEREDITARY DISEASES

Cystic Fibrosis

Cystic fibrosis is a generalized disorder resulting from a genetic defect transmitted as an autosomal recessive gene that affects the function of exocrine glands. The recessive gene responsible for the development of cystic fibrosis has been localized to 250,000 base pairs of genomic deoxyribonucleic acid (DNA) on chromosome 7q. Mutations to this cystic fibrosis transmembrane regulator (*CFTR*) gene make the epithelial membrane impermeable to the chlorine ion, which leads to an increase in the absorption of sodium and water from the bronchi to blood, thus lowering the water content within the mucociliary portion of the respiratory epithelium. This dehydration of the mucous layer leads to an accumulation of viscous secretions that obstruct the airway. Cystic fibrosis involves many organs in addition to the respiratory system, and nearly all exocrine glands are affected in varying distribution and degree of severity. These glands and other organs affected include the salivary glands, small bowel, pancreas, biliary tract, female cervix, and male genital system. In the respiratory system, evidence suggests that the lungs are histologically normal at birth. Pulmonary damage is initiated by gradually increasing secretions from the hypertrophy of bronchial glands, leading to obstruction of the bronchial system. The resultant plugging promotes staphylococcal infection, followed by more tissue damage, as well as atelectasis (collapse of lung tissue) and emphysema. Once the cycle is in motion, it is difficult to stop.

The signs and symptoms of cystic fibrosis usually include a chronic cough and wheezing associated with recurrent or chronic pulmonary infections. The cough is often accompanied by sputum, gagging, vomiting, and disturbed sleep. Barrel-chest deformity, clubbing of fingers, and cyanosis occur as the disease progresses. In adolescents and adults, pulmonary complications associated with cystic fibrosis include pneumothorax, hemoptysis, and right-sided heart failure secondary to pulmonary hypertension.

Despite increasing life spans to the age of 30 years or older, CF remains the most common lethal genetic disease in white children. Its diagnosis rests largely on a medical history of a sibling with cystic fibrosis, laboratory findings indicating elevated sodium and chloride levels in sweat, and genetic testing for *CFTR* gene mutation. Chest radiography aids in the diagnosis of cystic fibrosis. Radiographs taken over a period of years demonstrate gradually worsening structural abnormalities. Early changes of bronchial thickening and hyperinflation (Fig. 3-27) progress to extensive bronchiectasis, cyst formation, lobar atelectasis, scarring, pulmonary artery and right ventricular enlargement, and overinflation of the lung and chest wall. Conventional sinus radiography and CT studies of the paranasal sinuses demonstrate persistent opacification of the paranasal sinuses.

The prognosis associated with cystic fibrosis is determined by the degree of pulmonary involvement and varies greatly. However, respiratory failure resulting from deterioration of the lungs is inevitable and eventually leads to death in the 40s. Treatment methods include antimicrobial drugs to combat infection, bronchodilators administered through inhalers, respiratory physical therapy, and in some cases, a lung transplant may be performed in patients with end-stage lung disease. At this time, gene therapy is not available for cystic fibrosis.

Hyaline Membrane Disease

Also known as **respiratory distress syndrome** (RDS), hyaline membrane disease affects infants

FIGURE 3-27 Increased lung volume resulting from generalized obstructive disease and air trapping, which is characteristic of cystic fibrosis, as seen in this 9-year-old boy. Also seen are areas of irregular aeration with cystic and nodular densities.

and is a disorder of premature infants or those born at less than a 37-week gestation. Incomplete maturation of the type II alveolar cells within the surfactant-producing system causes unstable alveoli, the structures in which gas exchanges occur in the lungs. Infants are particularly in need of a low surface tension in the alveoli, and surfactant (an agent that lowers surface tension) provides this. Its deficiency results in alveolar collapse with widespread atelectasis. RDS occurs more frequently in premature, white, male infants. It also occurs in premature infants of mothers with diabetes because insulin may inhibit the production of surfactant. When an increased risk is assumed prior to birth, corticosteroid drugs may be administered to the mother before delivery.

The signs of RDS include rapid and labored breathing within the first 24 hours after delivery with the atelectasis and respiratory failure progressively worsening. Because of the rigid lung

FIGURE 3-28 Respiratory distress syndrome in a preterm infant. Note the "ground glass" appearance of the lungs, especially in the right perihilar area.

structure, resistance develops in the pulmonary circulatory system. This may result in the development of patent ductus arteriosus, which allows blood to be shunted between the ventricles of the heart. In severe cases, respiratory and metabolic acidoses develop because blood passing through the lungs is not adequately oxygenated and its CO_2 is inadequately eliminated.

Chest radiography demonstrates severe atelectasis with an air-bronchogram sign, characterized by bronchi surrounded by nonaerated alveoli (Fig. 3-28). This is a life-threatening condition, but if the infant's ventilation is adequately supported, surfactant production should begin within a few days. Treatment consists of maintenance of a proper thermal environment and satisfactory levels of tissue oxygenation, which is monitored frequently via ABG measurements. In some instances, pulmonary surfactant may be introduced intratracheally to reduce the severity of the disease. Once the surfactant is present, RDS will resolve in 4 or 5 days.

INFLAMMATORY DISEASES

Pneumonias

Pneumonia is the most frequent type of lung infection, resulting in an inflammation of the lung (pneumonitis) and compromised pulmonary

function. Pneumonia ranks eighth among the leading causes of death in the United States and is the most common lethal nosocomial infection. The main causes of pneumoniae are bacteria, viruses, and mycoplasmas. In adults, bacteria such as *Streptococcus pneumoniae* (*Pneumococcus*), *Staphylococcus aureus*, *Haemophilus*, *H. influenzae*, and *Legionella pneumophila* are the most common causes of typical pneumonia. *Chlamydia pneumoniae* and *Mycoplasma pneumoniae* are common causes of atypical pneumonias in adolescents and young adults. Atypical pneumonias present less obvious radiographic signs compared with typical bacterial pneumonias. Viral pathogens such as influenza virus, parainfluenza virus, adenovirus, and respiratory syncytial virus may cause pneumonias. In addition, fungal pneumonias may result from *Pneumocystis carinii*, especially in individuals with compromised immune systems.

The inflammation may affect the entire lobe of a lung (lobar pneumonia), a segment of a lung (segmental pneumonia), the bronchi and associated alveoli (bronchopneumonia), or interstitial lung tissue (interstitial pneumonia). Chest radiography is important in determining the location of the inflammation, with the pneumonias appearing as soft, patchy, ill-defined alveolar infiltrates or pulmonary densities. Alveolar infiltration results when the alveolar air spaces are filled with fluid or cells. Symptoms associated with pneumonia include a cough, fever, and sputum production, usually developing over days. Individuals with pneumonia often exhibit tachypnea, and on physical evaluation, crackles may be heard in conjunction with bronchial breath sounds.

Pneumococcal (lobar) **pneumonia** is the most common bacterial pneumonia because this type of bacteria is often present in healthy throats. This infection is generally preceded by an upper respiratory infection. When the body defenses are weakened, the bacteria multiply, work their way into the lungs, and inflame the alveoli. This disease is usually accompanied by chills, cough, and fever. Pneumococcal pneumonia generally affects the alveoli of an entire lobe of a lung,

FIGURE 3-29 Posteroanterior, **A,** and lateral, **B,** chest radiographs demonstrating pneumococcal pneumonia infiltrates in the upper lobe of the right lung. Note that the lateral projection clearly demonstrates the segment of the lobe affected, and the posteroanterior projection shows a faint outline of the air-filled bronchi.

without affecting the bronchi themselves (Fig. 3-29). Chest radiography demonstrates collection of fluid in one or more lobes, with the lateral view serving to identify the degree of segmental involvement. Pleural fluid may often be seen in lateral decubitus projections of the chest. Antibiotics—based on Gram stain laboratory results, patient age, and epidemiology—and bed rest are the treatment for pneumococcal pneumonia, which usually resolves in approximately 1 week. Immunization with the polysaccharide pneumococcal vaccine is recommended in children under 2 years of age and in older adults, especially residents of nursing homes and extended care facilities.

Staphylococcal pneumonia occurs sporadically except during epidemics of influenza, when secondary infection with staphylococci is common. It is severe and may be fatal, especially in infants. A pneumatocele (a thin-walled, air-containing cyst) is the characteristic radiographic lesion and is more typically seen in children. These may enlarge and form abscesses in the later stages of the disease. Another characteristic sign is the spread of patchy areas localized in and around the bronchi (Fig. 3-30). Drug therapy with particular chemotherapeutic agents is the treatment of choice.

FIGURE 3-30 Staphylococcal pneumonia in a 20-year-old man, indicated by multiple large pneumatoceles in the right lung and consolidation of the left lower lobe of the lung. An empyema in the lower left lung was later drained surgically.

FIGURE 3-31 Legionnaires' disease in a 55-year-old woman, showing rounded opacities in the upper half of the right lung and lower two thirds of the left lung.

FIGURE 3-32 Aspiration pneumonia caused by aspiration of gastric contents.

Legionnaires' disease is the name given to a severe bacterial pneumonia that became known after it caused the deaths of four people attending an American Legion convention in Philadelphia in 1976. The causative bacterium (*L. pneumophila*) was unknown at the time of the 1976 outbreak, and its explosive effects attracted significant attention. *L. pneumophila* thrives in warm, moist places and may be transmitted through heating and cooling systems. Clinically, patients complain of malaise, muscular aches, chest pain with a nonproductive cough, and occasional vomiting and diarrhea. Outbreaks of this disease occur in large buildings such as hotels and hospitals, most frequently in late summer to early fall. *L. pneumophila* tends to affect middle-aged men more frequently than it does other groups of individuals. Risk factors include smoking, alcohol abuse, and immunosuppression from corticosteroids. Its radiographic appearance is similar to those of other bacterial pneumonias, with patchy infiltrates throughout the lungs (Fig. 3-31). Diagnosis is made by one of four methods. The two more common methods include culturing the *L. pneumophila* organism from sputum or bronchoscopy brushings and

performing urinary antigen assays. Direct fluorescent antibody stain of exudate or serology using the indirect fluorescent antibody assay may also detect the presence of this disease, but both of these diagnostic methods require a high level of technical expertise. Treatment consists primarily of antibiotic administration (erythromycin or azithromycin) and oxygen therapy.

Mycoplasma **pneumonia** is caused by mycoplasmas, the smallest group of living organisms. They have characteristics of both bacteria and viruses. Because they do not have a typical bacterial cell wall, some confusion existed in the scientific community with regard to their classification. Currently, they are classified as "bacteria-like." *Mycoplasma* pneumonia is most common among older children and young adults. Radiographically, this disease appears as a fine reticular pattern in a segmental distribution, followed by patchy areas of air space consolidation. In severe cases, the radiographic appearance may mimic TB. The morbidity rate associated with mycoplasma pneumonia is very low, even when the disease is not treated.

Aspiration (chemical) **pneumonia** is caused by acid vomitus aspirated into the lower respiratory tract, resulting in a chemical pneumonitis. It may follow anesthesia, alcoholic intoxication, or stroke that causes loss of the cough reflex. Chest radiography reveals edema produced by irritation of air passages (Fig. 3-32), appearing as densities radiating from one or both hila into the dependent segments. The treatment of aspiration pneumonia is strictly supportive and includes correction of hypoxia, control of secretions, and replacement of fluids. Further infection is treated by antimicrobial drugs based on laboratory results.

Viral (interstitial) **pneumonia** is caused by various viruses, most commonly influenza virus A and B. It is more common than bacterial pneumonia but less severe. This disease is spread by an infected person shedding the virus, which is transmitted to a nonimmune individual. Most cases of viral pneumonia are mild, and radiographic findings are often minimal. The diagnosis of this disease is based on clinical findings and serologic tests. Symptoms include a dry cough and fever. Complications include secondary bacterial infections, termed *superinfections,* which result from a lowered resistance brought on by the inflammatory response to the virus. Otherwise, treatment of viral pneumonia usually focuses on relief of symptoms because viral infections do not respond to antibiotic agents.

Bronchiectasis

Bronchiectasis is a permanent, abnormal dilatation of one or more large bronchi as a result of destruction of the elastic and muscular components of the bronchial wall. The basic pathogenesis is either congenital or an acquired weakness, typically following inflammation of the bronchial walls, because of a viral or bacterial infection. In the early stage of the disease, the most common symptom is a chronic cough; however, some individuals may initially remain asymptomatic. As the bronchiectasis progresses, the cough becomes more productive because the weakened wall allows the bronchus to become dilated, forming a saclike structure that harbors the pathogenic organism. As the infection grows, the bronchial wall is destroyed, resulting in an abscess. Nonreversible bronchiectasis results in saccular and varicose dilations and constrictions which are permanent alterations to the bronchial tree (Fig. 3-33). These individuals may also complain of

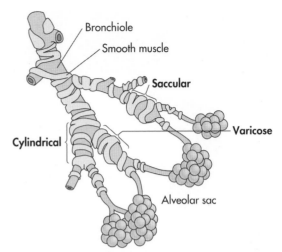

FIGURE 3-33 Types of bronchiectasis.

FIGURE 3-34 Bronchiectatic changes are seen peripherally on this computed tomography scan of the lungs from the 9-year-old patient with cystic fibrosis.

pleuritic pain, demonstrate recurrent fevers, wheezing, and shortness of breath, or both on physical examination.

Conventional chest radiography generally demonstrates increased bronchovascular markings and parallel lines outlining the dilated bronchi ("tram lines") because of peribronchial fibrosis and inflammation and intrabronchial secretions (Fig. 3-34). Occasionally, areas of honeycombing or cystic areas may be present. Bronchography is rarely performed in cases of

FIGURE 3-35 High-resolution computed tomography scan demonstrating bilateral lung bronchiectasis with associated left lung pneumatoceles.

FIGURE 3-36 Tuberculosis of left upper lobe in a 49-year-old man admitted with esophagitis and dull pain in the left subclavicular region.

bronchiectasis; it has been replaced by high-resolution CT (HRCT) of the chest, through which 1- to 2-mm slice images are obtained. HRCT, with or without contrast enhancement, is able to demonstrate bronchiectasis better than clinical findings and conventional radiography alone. It clearly shows dilated airways (those with a luminal diameter more than 1.5 times that of the adjacent vessel in cross-section), extension of the bronchi as a result of the destruction of lung parenchyma, thickening of bronchial walls, and obstruction of airways either by a mucous plug or by air trapping (Fig. 3-35).

Pulmonary Tuberculosis

Pulmonary tuberculosis is an infection caused by inhalation of *Mycobacterium tuberculosis*. Although *M. tuberculosis* generally affects the lungs, it may also affect other systems of the body such as the genitourinary system, the skeletal system, and the CNS. *M. tuberculosis* organisms are captured by macrophages within the alveoli but are not killed. This creates a cell-mediated immune response, which results in granulomatous lesions that infiltrate the tracheobronchial lymph nodes. These lesions eventually result in necrosis, fibrous scarring, and calcifications, which are visible on chest radiographs. It is more prevalent in persons born outside the United States, individuals in correctional facilities and homeless shelters, and intravenous (IV) drug users. An estimated 1.7 billion people worldwide (including 10 million Americans) are carriers of *M. tuberculosis*.

Early pulmonary TB is asymptomatic in 90% to 95% of cases and may be identified only with a skin test. Signs appear when the lesion or nodular scars are large enough to be seen on a chest radiograph. Lesions are most commonly seen in the apical region of the chest (Fig. 3-36); therefore, the apical lordotic projection of the chest is useful in the evaluation of TB.

The primary means for diagnosing TB requires identifying the organism from a sputum culture or by using a microbacterial nucleic acid amplification technique for laboratory confirmation. A positive response to intradermal injection of purified protein derivative (the Mantoux test) is the primary means of diagnosing latent TB. Because reading the results of this test is not conclusive, a two-step testing procedure may be used if the first step is negative. The most common symptom is a morning cough producing minimal mucus. As the disease progresses, the cough becomes more productive, the patient may complain of dyspnea, and a spontaneous pneumothorax or pleural effusion may develop.

If the patient is in good health, and the bacterial load is fairly small, healing with scarring of the lung tissue is the most common result of infection. The presence of tuberculous scars may be demonstrated radiographically in the apex of one or both lungs. These scars result from the body's immune system surrounding the bacilli with fibrous tissue, which invades and destroys the infectious agent. Fibrocaseous TB is usually the course of the disease if the patient demonstrates active signs of TB. Necrosis is a prominent feature of the disease because its infiltration affects the lung parenchyma. This infiltration may expand and produce the formation of a cavity (cavitation) (Fig. 3-37). If these cavities spread to communicate with the bronchus, the bacteria are spread throughout the lung. In older adults, dormant TB may reactivate and remain undiagnosed for weeks or months. Infection spreads to the lobar or segmental bronchus, causing a persistent pneumonia resistant to antibiotic therapy. As a result, these individuals are especially susceptible to **miliary tuberculosis,** which occurs when large numbers of bacteria are picked up and carried via the bloodstream throughout the body. *Miliary* refers to its characteristic resemblance to millet seeds, which are small, white grains (Fig. 3-38). Initially, the disseminated miliary pattern may not be radiographically identifiable, but when disseminated TB is suspected, chest radiography should be repeated in a few days to better visualize the millet-sized tubercles.

In immunocompromised patients, the infection is much more aggressive. It overwhelms the immune system and progresses through the lungs at a rapid rate to cause acute tuberculous

FIGURE 3-37 Cavitation in the right lung resulting from expansion of tubercular lesion.

FIGURE 3-38 Miliary tuberculosis (TB) resulting from hematogenous spread of TB, demonstrating small, distinct nodules throughout the lung fields.

pneumonia. The body does not develop fibrous tissue to surround the bacteria, so the infection spreads quickly. Without medical treatment, acute tuberculous pneumonia may result in death within a few months. If the particular bacterial strain is resistant to drug therapy, the result is a 50% mortality rate within a median time of 60 days.

Patients with pulmonary TB are contagious and should be placed in isolation. The bacteria are spread through sputum and airborne droplets expelled on coughing. Modern treatment of TB consists primarily of various chemotherapeutic agents that are effective and usually curative if the full course is taken. TB must be treated with at least two antituberculous drugs, including both bactericidal and bacteriostatic drugs that act through different mechanisms. In extreme cases where the disease shows drug resistance, surgical resection of a persistent TB may be performed to eliminate the bacteria.

Chronic Obstructive Pulmonary Disease

Chronic obstructive pulmonary disease (COPD) refers to a group of disorders that cause chronic airway obstruction. The most common forms are chronic bronchitis and emphysema, which frequently coexist and may be associated with varying degrees of asthma and bronchiectasis—two other causes of airway obstruction.

Because it may be difficult to determine whether the pulmonary obstruction is caused by chronic obstructive bronchitis, emphysema, or a combination of the two diseases, the designation COPD is commonly used. This disease is irreversible and results in limited airflow and, in the case of emphysema, decreased elastic recoil of the alveoli. Statistics show that the mortality rate of COPD has dramatically increased over the past 20 years, and it is ranked as the fourth most common cause of death in the United States. In addition, the number of individuals diagnosed with COPD in the United States continues to increase each year. The predominant risk factor associated with COPD is cigarette smoking. Air pollution, airborne chemical fumes, and inhalation of hazardous dust such as silica may also increase the risk of COPD but are minimal compared with the effects of cigarette smoke.

Chronic obstructive bronchitis most often arises from long-term, heavy cigarette smoking or prolonged exposure to high levels of industrial air pollution. Cigarette smoke and industrial air pollutants irritate the mucous lining of the bronchial tree and increase the susceptibility to both bacterial and viral infections. Chronic exposure to these respiratory irritants leads to hyperplasia of the mucous glands, hypertrophy of the smooth muscle, and thickening of the bronchial wall.

Persistent cough and expectoration (expulsion of mucus or phlegm from the throat) are the primary symptoms of chronic bronchitis. The effects of the disease develop slowly and progressively over months and years, gradually resulting in bronchial obstruction from excess secretion of mucus. Eventually, the lungs remain in a chronically inflated state because more air is inhaled than is exhaled. Additional signs and symptoms of chronic bronchitis include wheezing, shortness of breath, and arterial hypoxemia leading to right-sided heart hypertrophy and failure (cor pulmonale). No dependable radiographic criteria exist for a definitive diagnosis of chronic bronchitis.

Chest radiography may demonstrate hyperinflation of the lungs. Elimination of the causative agent (e.g., cigarettes) is an important first step in treatment. Pulmonary rehabilitation, including breathing exercises and physical conditioning, helps manage the disease. Antibiotics may reduce the presence of infection; adrenergic and anticholinergic bronchodilators are used to reduce bronchospasm; and oxygen therapy may be prescribed for patients with severe hypoxemia.

Emphysema is a condition in which the lung's alveoli become distended, usually from loss of elasticity or interference with expiration. It is characterized by an increase in the air spaces distal to the terminal bronchioles, with destruction of the alveolar walls.

The primary symptom of emphysema is dyspnea, which at first occurs only during exertion but eventually even at rest. In the early stages of emphysema, chest radiography may show normal results. However, as the disease progresses, hyperinflation results (Fig. 3-39), and

FIGURE 3-39 Posteroanterior chest radiograph demonstrating hyperinflation and blunting of costophrenic angles caused by emphysema.

FIGURE 3-40 Pulmonary emphysema with a giant emphysematous bleb occupying the upper half of the right lung.

the AP diameter of the chest increases because of increased air in the lungs. Emphysema appears radiographically as a depressed or flattened diaphragm, abnormally radiolucent lungs, and an increased retrosternal air space (barrel-shaped chest). Conventional chest radiography helps differentiate emphysema from other lung disorders such as TB or lung cancer, which have similar symptoms. Conventional chest radiography may demonstrate large bullae (>1 cm in diameter), prominent hilar markings, or blisters filled with air (Fig. 3-40), but smaller lesions are best demonstrated by CT examinations of the chest. HRCT using thin section cuts (1 to 2 mm) clearly demonstrate areas of hypovascularity and bullae associated with emphysema (Fig. 3-41).

Treatment for emphysema is much like that for chronic obstructive bronchitis. The goals are to alleviate the symptoms, treat any reversible elements (e.g., infection), and prevent further progression of the disease, if possible.

FIGURE 3-41 High-resolution computed tomography scan of the chest demonstrating parenchymal changes associated with emphysema.

Because these two forms of COPD represent chronic deterioration of the pulmonary system, the continued problems eventually lead to heart failure. The heart begins to wear out over time in its effort to increase blood flow to compensate for the decreased airflow caused by COPD. This may result in death from associated complications such as respiratory failure, pneumonia, cardiac arrhythmias, or pulmonary embolism. However, some individuals may live for many years with COPD and will eventually develop pulmonary edema and cor pulmonale. Both these conditions are discussed in Chapter 4.

Asthma is a chronic inflammation of the bronchial system resulting in airway obstruction and bronchial hyperresponsiveness. It may affect individuals at any age, most commonly before the age of 40 years. The incidence of asthma has increased over the past 20 years, and it is estimated that over 22 million individuals in the United States have this pathologic condition. Genetics play a major role in the development of asthma. Additional risk factors include exposure to allergens, air pollution, cigarette smoke, and recurrent viral respiratory infections. The signs and symptoms of asthma include intermittent attacks of coughing, wheezing, dyspnea, and chest tightness caused by airflow obstruction. Radiography plays a limited role in the diagnosis of asthma. Diagnosis is made through the assessment of ABGs and expiratory flow rates. Management of asthma most frequently includes the use of inhaled bronchodilators and oral corticosteroids and the administration of oxygen.

Pneumoconioses

Pneumoconioses result in pulmonary fibrosis from inhalation of foreign inorganic dust, most commonly from a particular work environment. The effects of an inhaled foreign material depend on its physical and chemical properties, the dose of the agent, and the site of deposition within the bronchial tree. The size of the dust particle inhaled is of particular importance. Most occupationally generated dusts and those occurring naturally are too large to cause pneumoconioses. Dusts greater than 10 micrometers (μm) are filtered out in the nasal passages or the mucous lining of the tracheobronchial tree; those smaller than 1 μm generally remain suspended in the air and are exhaled. Those most likely to be trapped are 1 to 5 μm. In addition to the size criterion, exposure to a substance capable of causing disease for a sufficient duration (dose) and the susceptibility of the host are factors required to cause pneumoconiosis. Fibrogenic inorganic dusts responsible for pneumoconiosis generally include silica, coal, asbestos, and beryllium.

Radiography assists in the detection and follow-up of this disease group. Lesions produced by the different pneumoconioses vary but may include nodules, cavitation, and pleural thickening. The three primary types of pneumoconioses are (1) silicosis, (2) anthracosis, and (3) asbestosis. Treatment is focused on preventing infection, relieving any respiratory symptoms, and maintaining adequate oxygenation.

Silicosis, the oldest known pneumoconiosis, results from inhaling silica (quartz) dust and is common among miners, grinders, and sandblasters. It is the most widespread and most serious type of pneumoconiosis. This disease occurs following 10 to 30 years of exposure to silica dust. Phagocytes located within the bronchioles carry silica dust into the septa of the alveoli. In response to the foreign dust particles, the alveoli form large amounts of fibrous connective tissue, thus destroying normal lung tissue. This disease is clearly visible on conventional chest radiographs as multiple small, rounded, opaque nodules throughout the lungs, resulting from the creation of the fibrous tissue. With the exception of lung transplantation, no treatment exists for silicosis. Therefore, prevention through the use of protective masks and adequate ventilation is the key to controlling this occupational disease.

Anthracosis (black lung disease) results from inhalation of coal dust (Fig. 3-42) over an extended period of about 20 years. As coal dust is deposited in the lungs, "coal macules" develop around the bronchioles and cause their dilation. This dilation does not affect the alveoli or the

FIGURE 3-42 Chest radiograph demonstrating large perihilar nodules. Thoracotomy revealed heavy anthracotic pigmentation, with two largest nodules containing black fluid, consistent with anthracosis.

airflow; thus, impairment of the function of the lungs and the lung architecture is limited. Other than suppressing coal dust in the work environment to prevent anthracosis, no real treatment for anthracosis exists, and usually efforts to treat this condition are futile.

Asbestosis results from the inhalation of asbestos dust, which causes chronic injury to the lungs. Asbestos dust is found in building materials and insulation. Radiographically, diffuse, small irregular or linear opacities may be demonstrated in the lower lungs, and diaphragmatic pleural calcifications suggest asbestosis. Pleural changes in asbestosis are considered far more striking than parenchymal changes. Pleural thickening may also be present. This disease may be prevented by effectively suppressing asbestos dust in the air of the work environment. Because of a heightened awareness of asbestosis, advances in industry, and the use of occupational face mask ventilators, the incidence of asbestosis has decreased, and further advances are likely to eliminate it in the United States. A cumulative,

extended exposure to asbestos dust has been shown to increase the risk of mesothelioma, a rare malignant neoplasm of the pleura. This neoplasm develops at least 15 years after a high exposure to asbestos.

Fungal Diseases

Fungi are plants without chlorophyll and are widely found in nature. Many fungi found in nature are not usually pathogenic unless they enter a compromised host. Therefore, most severe fungal infections are termed *opportunistic.* They are more likely to disseminate, causing severe illness in patients undergoing therapy with corticosteroids or immunosuppressants or in individuals with human immunodeficiency virus (HIV) infection, diabetes mellitus, bronchiectasis, emphysema, TB, lymphoma, leukemia, or serious burns.

Histoplasmosis is a systemic fungal infection caused by a dimorphic fungus, *Histoplasma capsulatum,* which thrives in the soil, especially soil that is fueled by bird or bat excreta. The infectious agent, which is particularly endemic to the Ohio, Missouri, and Mississippi River valleys, enters the body through the respiratory system. Most cases are classified as acute primary histoplasmosis and are so mild that they may go undiagnosed. Symptoms of acute primary histoplasmosis are nonspecific and include fever, cough, and general malaise. However, if the immune system is not effective at controlling and overcoming the fungal infection, it may spread from the lungs to other parts of the body. This condition is termed **progressive disseminated histoplasmosis.** This is considered an opportunistic infection in acquired immunodeficiency syndrome (AIDS), often leading to severe acute pneumonia. Disseminated histoplasmosis that leads to cavitary formations (chronic cavitary histoplasmosis) is more serious. The cavities resemble those in TB, often affecting the apical portion of the lungs. Dyspnea, cough, and fatigue may persist for months or even years. Diagnosis of histoplasmosis is made by histologic laboratory analysis. Chest radiography eventually may

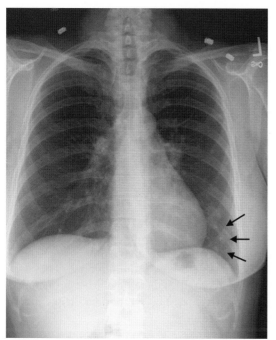

FIGURE 3-43 Posteroanterior chest radiograph demonstrating old histoplasmosis with calcified nodes in left lower lobe.

disruptions. For this reason, agricultural and construction workers are particularly at risk. As with histoplasmosis, most primary coccidioidomycosis infections are mild, usually self-limiting, and may go unrecognized. The most common radiographic finding of primary coccidioidomycosis, if present, is a small area of pulmonary consolidation. Lesions may comprise nodules of varying sizes that appear similar to malignant nodules and thus require biopsy or surgical excision. The typical treatment is bed rest because most occurrences are mild. However, in a few cases, progressive coccidioidomycosis may develop weeks or months after the primary infection, especially in immunosuppressed individuals. If disseminated coccidioidomycosis is not treated, it may lead to meningitis. The treatment for meningeal coccidioidomycosis must be continued for many months or years. Progressive coccidioidomycosis could be a deadly disease, as over 70% of individuals infected with HIV who develop this disease die from disseminated coccidioidomycosis within 1 month of initial diagnosis.

Lung Abscess

A lung abscess is a localized area of dead (necrotic) lung tissue surrounded by inflammatory debris. These abscesses may result from periodontal disease, pneumonia, neoplasms, or other organisms that invade the lungs. Lung abscess is more common in the right lung because of the vertical orientation of the right main bronchus. When the abscess reaches a bronchus, it drains into the bronchus forming a cavity (cavitation), which is visible on a chest radiograph. Clinical manifestations of a lung abscess include fever, cough, expectoration of pus, and foul sputum. Radiographically, an abscess generally appears as a lobar or segmental consolidation that becomes globular in shape as pus accumulates, or it may appear as a round, thick-walled capsule containing air and fluid. CT may be used to provide better anatomic information or to detect cavity formations. Empyemas consist of an accumulation of pus in the pleural cavity, usually caused by some primary lung infection. They may be

reveal small calcifications as a late manifestation of the disease, although these do not usually appear for 4 or 5 years (Fig. 3-43).

Less than 1% of those who acquire histoplasmosis require treatment because most forms of the disease (acute primary histoplasmosis) are self-limiting and may remain undiagnosed. If undiagnosed, however, advanced cases such as chronic cavitary histoplasmosis may result in death. Antifungal therapy is used to treat progressive disseminated histoplasmosis on diagnosis, and patients with AIDS often receive intermittent doses of IV antifungal medications necessary for chronic suppression of the infectious agent.

Coccidioidomycosis is also a systemic fungal infection. It is caused by a dimorphic fungus, *Coccidioides immitis*, which thrives in semiarid soil, particularly the southwestern United States and northern Mexico. Infective spores in the soil become airborne by winds, digging, or other caused by the invasion of a lung abscess that results in a bronchopleural fistula.

Treatment of an abscess and empyema centers on treatment of the primary condition causing it, including antibiotic therapy, chest physical therapy, postural drainage, and possible drainage of fluids via bronchoscopy. If the abscess is resistant to antibiotics, surgical resection of the abscess may be necessary, and in cases of multiple drug-resistant abscesses, the entire lobe may be surgically removed.

Pleurisy

Inflammation of the pleura is loosely termed *pleurisy*, a word often used to indicate inconsequential thoracic pain. True **pleurisy** is often indicative of a serious condition such as pneumonia, pulmonary embolism, TB, or malignant disease. Pain, varying in intensity, is usually distributed to one side or the other and along the intercostal nerve roots. Because the parietal layer of the pleura contains sensory receptors (the visceral layer does not), pain indicates that the parietal layer is involved in the inflammatory process.

Chest radiography does not generally demonstrate pleurisy, but it is helpful in confirming the presence of pleural fluid associated with the disease. Diagnosis and treatment of any underlying condition are important in relieving the symptoms of pleurisy.

Pleural Effusion

Pleural effusion results when excess fluid collects in the pleural cavity. It is a frequent manifestation of serious thoracic disease, usually pulmonary or cardiac in origin. It should be regarded not as a disease entity but rather as a sign of an important underlying condition. Pleural effusion may be caused by inflammation, as in pleurisy, a pulmonary embolism, or a neoplasm. These pleural effusions are termed **exudates**. Pleural effusions may also result from microvascular changes such as those associated with heart failure or ascites and are termed **transudates**. A pleural effusion containing blood is called a

FIGURE 3-44 Posteroanterior erect chest radiograph demonstrating bilateral pleural effusions with right lower lobe atelectasis.

hemothorax and most frequently follows trauma to the thorax or thoracic surgery.

Conventional chest radiography is commonly used in the diagnosis of pleural effusion. The radiographic signs of pleural effusion include a blunting of the costophrenic angles (Fig. 3-44), which is often best demonstrated on an erect lateral chest radiograph. The blunting occurs as part of the healing process, and the fibrous changes in the lung tissue may remain even after the pleural effusion has resolved. Lateral decubitus chest radiographs are also valuable (Fig. 3-45) because they can better demonstrate smaller amounts (<100 mL) of fluid in the pleural space compared with either erect PA radiographs or lateral chest radiographs. In severe cases, an entire lung may be opacified, and the mediastinum may be shifted to the contralateral side of the chest. Because a pleural effusion is indicative of an underlying medical problem, CT may be used to evaluate the lung parenchyma in search of a neoplasm, abscess, or pneumonia hidden by the effusion. Diagnostic sonography is also an excellent modality for locating or localizing pleural effusion (Fig. 3-46) and assisting the clinician in performing thoracocentesis.

Thoracocentesis or interventional techniques may be used to remove excess fluids for symptom

FIGURE 3-45 Left lateral decubitus chest shows free pleural fluid layering out against the chest wall.

FIGURE 3-46 Sonograms demonstrating pleural effusion, which help the clinician in preparation for performing a thoracocentesis.

FIGURE 3-47 Chest computed tomography scan for placement of a pigtail catheter into the pleural space to drain a large, loculated pleural effusion.

alleviation and laboratory analysis and to confirm the presence and type of fluid present in the pleural cavity (Fig. 3-47, *A* and *B*). In the case of a hemothorax, blood rarely clots within the pleural cavity, so a water-sealed chest tube is placed within the pleural cavity to drain blood, provided the bleeding has stopped.

Sinusitis

The communication with the nasal cavities that subjects the paranasal sinuses to infection and inflammation is called **sinusitis**. Common causes of acute sinusitis include streptococcal, pneumococcal, *H. influenzae,* and staphylococcal bacteria. Sinusitis often follows acute viral infection of the respiratory tract, and the ethmoid sinuses tend to be the most commonly affected sinuses because of their proximity to the nose. Exposure to extremes in humidity or temperature, poor oral hygiene, the presence of a deviated septum, or all of these factors may exacerbate the condition. The symptoms of sinusitis include nasal discharge, headache, tenderness over the affected area, a toothache, and general malaise.

Radiography is important in the diagnosis of sinusitis. CT is the modality of choice because it clearly demonstrates the swollen mucous membrane and retained exudate caused by the infection. Although upright sinus radiographs do demonstrate the increased density and possible air–fluid levels (Fig. 3-48) from both mucosal swelling and fluid accumulation, CT provides better definition of the extent and degree of the sinusitis (Fig. 3-49). Chronic sinusitis may cause nasal polyps.

Treatment of sinusitis typically involves saline nasal sprays, antibiotic therapy, and analgesics for pain relief. A deviated septum that contributes to sinusitis can be corrected surgically, if necessary.

NEOPLASTIC DISEASES

Bronchial Carcinoid Tumors

Bronchial carcinoid tumors (adenomas) are usually considered benign but are included in the World Health Organization's classification of "lung cancer" because they tend to invade local tissues, sometimes metastasize to regional lymph nodes, and are treated much like other malignant neoplasms. They are rare in occurrence, accounting for less than 1% of all lung tumors. Bronchial carcinoid tumors occur equally in both sexes,

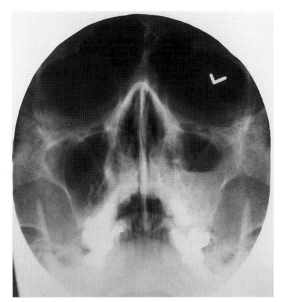

FIGURE 3-48 Air–fluid level present in the left maxillary sinus reflects sinusitis secondary to an oral–antral fistula in this 26-year-old woman.

generally affecting adults in their mid-40s, and often have a prolonged course of disease. Although they are adenomas, they rarely produce the endocrine symptoms associated with most carcinoid tumors. Bronchial carcinoid tumors are slow growing and often asymptomatic. The radiographic appearance of this neoplasm shows opacity; bronchial narrowing, obstruction, or both; and possible collapse of the affected segment of the lung. Bronchial obstruction is the most common presentation, and recurrent pneumonia within the same area of the lung, in combination with pleural pain, is a common occurrence in affected individuals. If the disease is discovered prior to metastasis, surgical resection may be curative.

Bronchogenic Carcinoma

Bronchogenic carcinoma, the most common fatal primary malignancy in the United States, accounts for over 90% of all lung tumors and has a very low 5-year survival rate (20%). It accounts for 31% of cancer-related deaths in males and 26% in females and usually occurs in individuals

FIGURE 3-49 A, Axial and **B,** coronal computed tomography scans of paranasal sinuses, demonstrating bilateral mucosal thickening of the maxillary sinuses and opacification of the nasal cavity.

FIGURE 3-50 Posteroanterior chest radiograph demonstrating advanced small cell lung carcinoma.

between the ages of 45 and 70 years, especially among cigarette smokers. Lung cancers are divided into two major categories: (1) non–small cell lung cancer (NSCLC) and (2) small cell lung cancer (SCLC). The four main histologic types of bronchogenic cancer are (1) squamous cell carcinoma, (2) adenocarcinoma, (3) undifferentiated large cell carcinoma (NSCLC); and (4) undifferentiated small cell carcinoma (SCLC) (Fig. 3-50). These tumors arise from epithelial tissue in the major bronchi near the hilar area and metastasize via the lymph nodes, the bloodstream, or both. Adenocarcinomas are the most common type of bronchogenic cancers, accounting for almost 40% of the cases diagnosed in the United States. A decline in the incidence of squamous cell carcinoma has been noted over the past 20 years, with this tumor currently accounting for about 30% of all bronchogenic cancers. Undifferentiated large cell carcinomas and small cell carcinomas occur equally in approximately 10% to 15% of individuals diagnosed with bronchogenic cancer; however, small cell carcinoma has a much higher mortality rate, accounting for about one quarter of deaths from lung cancer in the United States.

In addition to a thorough patient history, chest radiography is essential for the diagnosis of bronchogenic carcinoma. The most common radiographic presentation of squamous cell carcinomas is airway obstruction caused by a unilateral hilar mass (Fig. 3-51); however, the lesion must be larger than 6 mm to be visible on a conventional radiograph. As the tumor grows, it may occlude the bronchus, producing atelectasis and pneumonitis. These secondary effects provide more opacity radiographically than does the actual tumor. Adenocarcinomas usually are relatively small and are found in the peripheral regions of the lung parenchyma. The radiographic presentation of this neoplasm consists of a solitary radiopaque lung nodule, sometimes called a **coin lesion**. Histologic confirmation is necessary to make a definitive diagnosis.

CT is essential in demonstrating nodules smaller than 6 mm, which are not visualized with conventional chest radiography. CT has the ability to show calcifications to help differentiate malignant and benign tumors of the lung and is useful in staging the disease by demonstrating the presence or absence of spread to the lymph nodes in the thoracic and upper abdominal areas. Malignant lesions are rarely calcified (Fig. 3-52), whereas benign lesions generally have a calcified center. Staging bronchogenic carcinoma is critical to the selection of treatment of the disease. CT or PET can assist in determining metastases to the liver, brain, and adrenal glands (Fig. 3-53, A and B), so it is now a common practice to include a portion of the upper abdomen on oncologic CT examinations of the chest and from the base of the skull through the midfemur on PET scans. Advances in technology have made it possible to perform virtual bronchoscopy to assess the location and extent of the carcinoma. Thoracic magnetic resonance imaging (MRI) is of limited value, but it is helpful in assessing tissue planes and the chest wall before surgery and in cases where apical tumors have invaded the vertebral column. Nuclear medicine bone scans may be used to screen for bone metastases, which are often confirmed with either conventional skeletal radiography or MRI.

FIGURE 3-51 A, Bronchogenic carcinoma on posteroanterior projection indicated by large right hilar mass. **B,** Chest computed tomography scan demonstrating a large bronchogenic mass in the anteromedial aspect of the right lung with a cavitary lesion just above the level of the right main stem bronchus.

FIGURE 3-52 Chest computed tomography scan of a bronchogenic lesion (*arrow*) in the upper lobe of the right lung.

The patient may undergo percutaneous lung biopsy, bronchoscopy, or brush biopsy. In brush biopsy, a device with tiny brushes is introduced through a bronchoscope or bronchial catheter to procure cells and tissues under fluoroscopic guidance.

The prognosis is very poor for bronchogenic carcinoma, with a 5-year survival rate of only 12% to 14%. Fairly good results are associated with a lobectomy in individuals with peripheral nodular lesions; however, second primary lesions occur in 6% to 10% of survivors. Small cell tumors tend to be the most deadly because the cancer almost always has metastasized before diagnosis. Cigarette smoking is, by far, the most important etiologic factor, accounting for over 90% of cases in men and over 80% of cases in women. Exposure to potentially carcinogenic substances from air pollution and occupational exposure are also etiologic factors.

FIGURE 3-53 A, Axial and **B,** coronal positron emission tomography and computed tomography demonstrating metastasis of bronchogenic carcinoma to the left adrenal gland.

FIGURE 3-54 Axial magnetic resonance imaging of the brain, demonstrating metastatic spread from a primary bronchogenic neoplasm.

led to developments in targeted growth factor receptor therapy, gene therapy, antiangiogenic therapy, and immunotherapeutic treatments. As mentioned earlier, CT, MRI, and PET scans are all vital in staging the carcinoma and determining the optimal treatment. In addition, CT of the chest and upper abdomen should be performed for all patients before surgical resection.

Metastases from Other Sites

Pulmonary metastases are much more common than primary lung neoplasms. Many malignancies progress to pulmonary metastases, which are detectable on chest radiographs. The most common primary sites for these tumors are the breast, the gastrointestinal tract, the female reproductive system, the prostate, skin (melanoma), and the kidneys.

Malignancy spreads to the lungs from a primary site via five different routes: (1) through

This disease process may be treated with surgery, chemotherapy, external radiation therapy, brachytherapy, or any combination of these modalities, depending on the type, location, and stage of disease. Chemotherapy, radiation therapy, or a combination of both may be administered before surgical resection, and radiation therapy may also be used for palliative treatment to control the pain associated with skeletal metastasis, spinal cord compression, or brain metastasis (Fig. 3-54). Recent research has the bloodstream in hematogenous metastases, (2) through the lymph system in lymphogenous metastases, (3) by direct extension in local invasion, (4) through the tracheobronchial system in bronchogenic metastases, and, rarely, (5) by direct implantation from biopsies or other surgical procedures. Radiographically, these metastatic lesions appear as single or multiple rounded opacities throughout the lungs (Fig. 3-55, *A* and *B*). CT is more sensitive than conventional chest radiography in the detection of small metastatic lesions.

FIGURE 3-55 A, Pulmonary metastases from uterine cancer demonstrate multiple lesions with characteristic "cotton ball" appearance. **B,** Lateral projection of pulmonary metastases resulting from uterine cancer.

PATHOLOGY SUMMARY
The Respiratory System

Pathology	Imaging Modalities of Choice	Additive or Subtractive Pathology
Cystic fibrosis	Chest radiography	Additive
Hyaline membrane disease	Chest radiography	Additive
Pneumonias	Chest radiography	Additive
Bronchiectasis	Chest radiography, high-resolution chest CT	Additive
Tuberculosis	Chest radiography, chest CT	Additive
COPD	Chest radiography, high-resolution chest CT	Subtractive
Pneumoconioses	Chest radiography	Additive
Fungal disease	Chest radiography	Additive
Lung abscess	Chest radiography, chest CT	Additive
Pleurisy	None	None
Pleural effusion	Chest radiography, chest CT, sonography	Additive

PATHOLOGY SUMMARY
The Respiratory System—cont'd

Pathology	Imaging Modalities of Choice	Additive or Subtractive Pathology
Sinusitis	Sinus CT	Additive
Bronchial adenoma	Chest CT	Additive
Bronchogenic carcinoma staging	Chest CT, FDG-PET	Additive
Metastatic lung disease	Chest CT, FDG-PET, brain MRI	Additive

COPD, Chronic obstructive pulmonary disease; *CT,* computed tomography; *FDG-PET,* fluorodeoxyglucose–positron emission tomography; *MRI,* magnetic resonance imaging.

REVIEW QUESTIONS

1. By use of what radiographic position can bony structures such as clavicles be removed from the apices of the lungs?
   a. AP
   b. Lateral decubitus
   c. Lordotic
   d. 45-degree oblique
2. The "sail sign" in an infant is commonly associated with enlargement of the:
   a. Heart
   b. Pulmonary arteries
   c. Thymus
   d. Thyroid
3. Posterior mediastinal masses most commonly originate from_____tissue.
   a. Lymphatic
   b. Nervous
   c. Thymus
   d. Thyroid
4. An infant born after only 6 months of gestation could have:
   a. Cystic fibrosis
   b. Hyaline membrane disease
   c. Mediastinal emphysema
   d. Pectus excavatum
5. Lack of respiratory function or lack of proper oxygen and carbon dioxide exchange best describes:
   a. Cardiac arrest
   b. Cardiac arrhythmia
   c. Respiratory failure
   d. Tachypnea

6. Which of the following is the most common type of bacterial pneumonia?
   a. Aspiration pneumonia
   b. Legionnaires' disease
   c. Pneumococcal pneumonia
   d. Streptococcal pneumonia
7. Loss of elasticity of the bronchial walls as a result of bacterial infection may result in:
   a. Bronchiectasis
   b. Bronchogenic carcinoma
   c. Pneumococcal pneumonia
   d. Tuberculosis
8. Pulmonary fibrosis resulting from occupationally inhaled dusts is characteristic of:
   a. Atelectasis
   b. Chronic bronchitis
   c. Pleural effusion
   d. Pneumoconiosis
9. An accumulation of pus in the pleural cavity is known as a(n):
   a. Coin lesion
   b. Empyema
   c. Pleural effusion
   d. Pleurisy
10. The most common etiologic factor in the development of bronchogenic carcinoma is:
    a. Automobile emissions
    b. Cigarette smoking
    c. Dust
    d. Iatrogenic treatment

11. Explain how technical exposure factors must be changed to compensate for the additive and subtractive pathologies of the chest. Give one example of each type of pathology.

12. Specify the reasons for obtaining chest radiographs taken in the erect position at a 72-inch source-to-image distance.

13. What specialized radiographic projection of the chest is used to demonstrate tuberculosis? Why is this projection of benefit?

14. Chronic obstructive pulmonary disease (COPD) includes both emphysema and chronic bronchitis. Compare and contrast these two pathologic conditions, and explain how both can be considered COPD.

15. Metastasis to the lungs from other primary tumors occurs via five routes. What are they?

4

Cardiovascular System

Doppler echocardiography
Ductus arteriosus
Embolization
Endocardium
Epicardium
Foramen ovale
Fusiform aneurysm
Gated cardiac blood pool scans
Heart
Infarct
Intima
Ischemia
Lumen
Media
M-mode echocardiography
Murmur
Myocardial perfusion scan
Myocardium
Patent ductus arteriosus
Percutaneous transluminal angioplasty
Permanent catheterization

Phlebitis
Pulmonary embolus
Rheumatic fever
Right and left atria
Right and left ventricles
Saccular aneurysm
Sinoatrial node
Stent
Systole
Tetralogy of Fallot
Thrombolysis
Thrombophlebitis
Thrombus
Transesophageal echocardiography
Transjugular intrahepatic portosystemic shunt
Transposition of great vessels
Valvular stenosis
Veins
Venous thrombosis
Ventricular septal defects

ANATOMY AND PHYSIOLOGY

The cardiovascular system consists of the heart, arteries, capillaries, and veins and may be further divided into two subsystems of circulation: (1) The *pulmonary circulation* transports blood between the heart and lungs for exchange of blood gases, and (2) the *systemic circulation* transports blood between the heart and the rest of the body.

Heart

The **heart** acts as a pump to propel the blood throughout the body via the circulatory vessels. It lies in the anterior chest within the mediastinum and is generally readily visible on a chest radiograph. The interior of the heart is divided into two upper chambers, termed the **right and left atria**, and two lower chambers, termed the **right and left ventricles** (Fig. 4-1). Note that the heart lies in an oblique plane within the

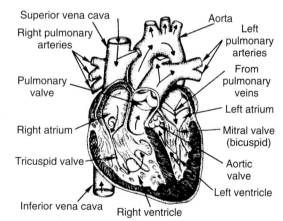

FIGURE 4-1 Blood flow through the heart.

mediastinum; therefore, a conventional postero-anterior (PA) chest radiograph does not clearly demonstrate all chambers of the heart.

A frontal projection of the chest shows a cardiac silhouette, with two thirds of the heart lying to the left of midline; the right side is

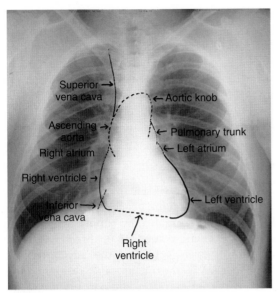

FIGURE 4-2 Posteroanterior chest radiograph with heart chambers and great vessels outlined.

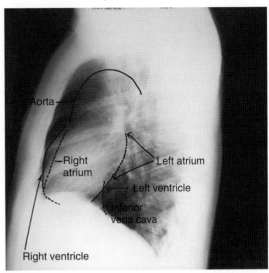

FIGURE 4-3 Lateral chest radiograph with heart chambers and great vessels outlined.

composed mainly of the right atrium, and the left side is composed mainly of the left ventricle. The right ventricle lays midline within the cardiac shadow and is located anterior to the right atrium and left ventricle. The left atrium is located midline and is the most posterior aspect of the heart (Fig. 4-2). Therefore, it is necessary to obtain a lateral projection of the chest to best demonstrate the right ventricle and the left atrium. On a lateral projection of the chest, the right ventricle constitutes the anterior portion of the cardiac silhouette, and the left atrium and the left ventricle constitute the posterior portion of the cardiac shadow (Fig. 4-3).

The heart contains three tissue layers. The innermost layer, termed the **endocardium**, is smooth. The valves located within and between the various chambers are also composed of endocardium. Although the valve tissue is relatively thin, in a normal heart, it is able to prevent the backflow and passage of blood when the valve is closed. The middle layer is muscular and is termed the **myocardium**. This is the thickest layer of heart tissue, and the cardiac muscle receives blood supply from the right and left coronary

arteries, which arise directly from the aorta, just superior to the aortic valve. When the myocardium contracts (systole), blood is pumped out of the heart. The outermost layer is a protective covering termed the **epicardium**. The entire heart is enclosed within a pericardial sac, which contains a small amount of fluid to lubricate the heart as it contracts and relaxes, thus reducing friction between the heart and other mediastinal structures.

In the normal heart, the right atrium receives deoxygenated blood from the body via the superior and inferior venae cavae. The deoxygenated blood passes through the right atrioventricular or tricuspid valve into the right ventricle. The right ventricle contracts during systole, thus propelling blood to the lungs through the pulmonary valve and pulmonary trunk, which bifurcates into the right and left main pulmonary arteries, respectively. Approximately 60% of deoxygenated blood enters the right lung, and approximately 40% enters the left lung.

The exchange of gases occurs at the capillary–alveolar level within the lungs, and the now-oxygenated blood is returned to the left atrium via the four pulmonary veins. Oxygenated blood flows from the left atrium to the left ventricle via the left mitral valve. The left ventricle is responsible for pumping oxygenated blood throughout the systemic circulatory system; therefore, the left ventricle has a thicker layer of myocardium and contracts with greater force than does the right ventricle. Oxygenated blood flows through the aortic valve into the aorta when the left ventricle contracts.

Cardiac Cycle

The contraction of the myocardium is termed **systole**, and the subsequent relaxation is termed **diastole**. The pacemaker of the heart is the **sinoatrial** (SA) **node,** which is located in the upper portion of the right atrium near the superior vena cava. An electrical current is transmitted through the myocardium, resulting in a heartbeat.

Electrocardiography graphically demonstrates this electrical activity. The elements of an electrocardiogram (ECG) include the P wave, PR interval, QRS complex, T wave, and QT duration (Fig. 4-4). The P wave is the graphic display of the spread of the electrical impulse from the atria. The PR interval shows the amount of time required for the electrical impulse to travel from

the SA node to the ventricular muscle fibers. The spread of the electrical impulse through the ventricles is displayed by the QRS complex, and the period in which the ventricles recover from the spent electrical impulse is graphically displayed by the T wave. The QT duration represents the total time from ventricular depolarization (QRS) to ventricular repolarization (T).

Circulatory Vessels

Arteries are blood vessels that carry blood away from the heart and are generally named for their location or the organ they supply (e.g., splenic artery). They are composed of three layers. The outermost layer is termed the **adventitia**, the middle layer is the **media**, and the innermost layer is the **intima**. The internal, tubular structure of the vessel is termed the **lumen**. **Veins** are blood vessels that carry blood to the heart. They are composed of the same three layers; however, venous walls are thinner than arterial walls, and veins contain valves at set intervals to help with blood return to the heart. **Capillaries** are microscopic vessels that connect arteries and veins (Fig. 4-5). They are responsible for the exchange of substances necessary for nutrient and waste transport.

FIGURE 4-4 Electrocardiogram demonstrating P wave, QRS wave, and T wave.

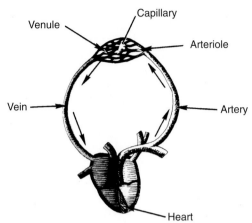

FIGURE 4-5 General systemic circulation.

IMAGING CONSIDERATIONS

Radiography

Several imaging modalities play an important role in the evaluation of the cardiovascular system and the management of cardiovascular disease. Chest radiography provides information about heart shape and size. Chest radiography is also excellent for demonstrating the great vessels and vascular changes within the lung fields. Radiographers do need to be aware that many factors may affect the cardiac image.

Factors that the radiographer can control include patient posture, degree of inspiration, correct positioning, geometric factors, and exposure technique selection. Whenever possible, chest radiographs should be taken with the patient in the erect position. If a patient is semi-recumbent or recumbent, the heart appears to be enlarged because abdominal organs push the diaphragm and the heart up into the thoracic cavity. It is important to identify cases in which the patient is not able to assume the erect position to aid the physician in diagnosis and interpretation.

Chest radiographs obtained without a good inspiration also distort heart shape and size (Figs. 4-6 and 4-7). Keep in mind that at least 10 posterior ribs should be visible within the lung fields on a chest radiograph taken with a good

FIGURE 4-6 Posteroanterior chest radiograph with adequate level of inspiration.

inspiration. The sternoclavicular joints should be an equal distance from the spine, and the scapulae should be rolled forward out of the lung fields on a well-positioned PA chest radiograph. To position a patient for a lateral chest radiograph, the arms and shoulders should be placed above the patient's head to ensure that they are above the apices.

Geometric factors affecting heart shape and size include source-to-image receptor distance (SID) and object-to-image receptor distance (OID). Conventional chest radiographs are generally obtained using a 72-inch SID to decrease magnification of the heart to an approximate factor of 10%. Again, it is important to document variations in SID to aid in the proper diagnosis of heart disorders. Because the heart is fairly anterior in the mediastinum, it is preferable to obtain PA chest images, whenever possible.

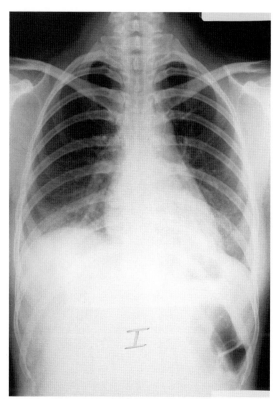

FIGURE 4-7 Posteroanterior chest radiograph with expiration on the same patient as in Fig. 4-6; note the enlargement of the cardiac shadow on this radiograph.

FIGURE 4-8 Posteroanterior chest radiograph demonstrating cardiomegaly secondary to congestive heart failure.

This places the heart closest to the image receptor, allowing for the smallest OID. Positioning the patient for a PA projection also helps decrease magnification of the cardiac silhouette. A third geometric factor that is frequently overlooked is the anode-heel effect. Radiographers can use this phenomenon to their advantage by placing the anode over the apical region and the cathode toward the base of the lungs, when possible, thus distributing the radiographic density more evenly throughout the chest radiograph.

Adequate penetration of the mediastinal structure is also critical in chest radiography and requires the use of a relatively high kilovoltage. A minimum of 100 kilovolts peak (kVp) should be used. Vascular markings within the chest help the physician assess ventricular function. The pulmonary vessels also provide information about pulmonary artery pressure. Dilatation of these vessels often indicates problems with the right ventricle. Exposure times of one tenth of a second or less should be used, whenever possible, to decrease involuntary cardiac motion. It has been documented that heart motion may increase the size of the cardiac shadow. The heart may look larger if the radiograph is exposed during diastole.

In most institutions, chest radiography is the most commonly performed procedure, and radiographers all too often underestimate the importance of these basic radiographic principles. Well-positioned diagnostic chest radiographs are crucial in the diagnosis and treatment of cardiovascular disorders. In a normal adult, the transverse diameter of the cardiac shadow should be less than half the transverse diameter of the thorax on a PA erect chest radiograph. An enlarged heart is termed **cardiomegaly** (Fig. 4-8), which is indicative of many cardiovascular disorders and is a nonspecific finding.

Factors affecting cardiac shape and size that are not under the technologist's control include patient body habitus, bony thorax abnormalities, and pathologic conditions such as pneumothorax or pulmonary emphysema. Bone abnormalities of special concern include scoliosis and

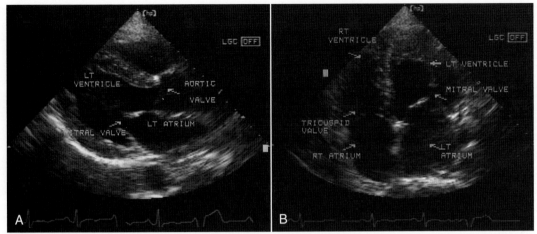

FIGURE 4-9 A, Echocardiographic visualization of heart anatomy of a 47-year-old man as seen in a parasternal sagittal view. **B,** Coronal view of the same heart demonstrated by echocardiography.

pectus excavatum. Individuals with pectus excavatum present a funnel-shaped depression of the sternum. The abnormal placement of the xiphoid causes displacement of the heart to the left and distortion of the cardiac shadow. Vascular lines and tubes are discussed in Chapter 3 of this text.

Echocardiography

Echocardiography encompasses a group of non-invasive sonographic (ultrasound) procedures that can provide detailed information about heart anatomy, function, and vessel patency (Fig. 4-9). Sonographic imaging may be performed using M-mode, two-dimensional (2-D) imaging, spectral Doppler, color Doppler, or stress echocardiography.

M-mode echocardiography uses a stationary ultrasound beam to provide an examination of the atria, ventricles, heart valves, and aortic root, allowing evaluation of left ventricular function. The "M" refers to motion, as this technique allows for the recording of the rate of motion and the amplitude of moving objects. This technique has the advantage of being able to demonstrate subtle motion of the cardiac structures. M-mode cardiac sonography is also used to measure the thickness of the ventricular walls; however, it has largely been replaced by 2-D

echocardiography. Use of 2-D imaging allows for spatially correct, real-time imaging of the heart. It provides multiple tomographic projections of the heart and great vessels in a cinelike (dynamic imaging) presentation. In addition, it is an excellent modality for visualizing the ascending and abdominal aorta in cases of suspected aneurysm. Both M-mode and 2-D images are obtained by placing the transducer over the thorax at the sternal borders, at the cardiac apex, between the ribs, or at the suprasternal notch. Smaller transducers have been developed to allow for **transesophageal echocardiography** (TEE), in which the patient swallows a mobile, flexible probe containing the transducer. With TEE, the heart's structure can be readily visualized without interference from such structures as skin, the rib cage, and chest muscles. It is especially helpful in imaging the aortic arch and aortic root. Smaller transducers are placed on intravascular catheters to assess vessel anatomy and blood flow.

Stress echocardiography combines an exercise test with an echocardiogram to check the heart's contraction ability and its pumping efficiency. If exercise is not possible, a drug, dobutamine, may be used to increase cardiac output to assess how well the heart pumps during infusion.

Doppler sonography is an adjunct, noninvasive procedure used to study the peripheral

FIGURE 4-10 Doppler effect with normal arterial flow in the internal carotid artery depicted above a graph of the arterial flow.

FIGURE 4-11 Doppler sonogram of an abnormal internal carotid artery spectrum caused by heterogeneous calcified plaque. Note the difference in appearance of the graphic representation compared with Fig. 4-10.

vasculature. It has been a mainstay of vascular imaging since the 1970s and is used to determine the direction and velocity, as well as the presence or absence, of blood flow in both arteries and veins. The Doppler Effect is the principle that the sound coming toward you has a higher pitch than the sound going away from you. The return of pulsed ultrasound allows calculation of the shift in the direction of blood flow and creates a spectral display from which velocity is calculated (Fig. 4-10). The spectral signal is displayed on a strip chart or videotape. With Doppler sonography the flow of blood is not affected until any obstruction present is at least 60% complete. The percentage of stenosis present dictates the treatment of vascular disease, and usually this consists of surgery (e.g., endarterectomy). Such vascular imaging is said to be *duplex* in that it helps reveal physiologic characteristics, and the imaging component defines anatomy (e.g., plaque morphology). The most common conditions imaged by 2-D Doppler sonography are carotid stenosis (significantly reducing carotid angiography) (Figs. 4-11 and 4-12), lower extremity arterial stenosis, and deep venous thrombosis (Figs. 4-13 and 4-14), largely supplanting traditional venography. Blood flow may be encoded with color to differentiate blood flowing toward the transducer (red) from blood flowing away from the transducer (blue); this is termed *color Doppler echocardiography.*

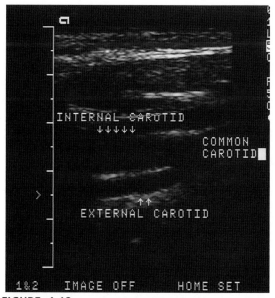

FIGURE 4-12 Doppler sonogram of a normal carotid bifurcation from the common carotid into the internal and external carotid arteries.

Nuclear Cardiology

Nuclear medicine procedures used in the assessment of cardiovascular disease include myocardial perfusion scans, gated cardiac blood pool scans, and positron emission tomography (PET). They are useful in assessing coronary artery

FIGURE 4-13 Doppler sonographic portrayal of normal flow on the left of the image through the greater saphenous vein (*GSV*), common femoral vein (*CFV*), and common femoral artery (*CFA*). Compression on the right side of the image depicts normal closure of the common femoral vein and greater saphenous vein, as expected.

FIGURE 4-15 Appearance of a normal heart on a nuclear medicine perfusion scan, with the isotope distribution equal throughout the myocardium at rest.

FIGURE 4-14 Transverse view of the greater saphenous vein and common femoral vein indicating failure to close on compression because of the large venous thrombus contained within.

disease (CAD), congenital heart disease, and cardiomyopathy.

A **myocardial perfusion scan** is the most widely used procedure in nuclear cardiology. It may be performed on patients with chest pain of an unknown origin, to evaluate coronary artery stenosis, and as a follow-up to bypass surgery, angioplasty, or thrombolysis. It is especially useful in detecting regions of myocardial ischemia and scarring (Figs. 4-15 and 4-16). In this study, a radionuclide, usually radioactive technetium sestamibi or thallium, is injected through a vein. It concentrates in the areas of the heart that have the best blood flow. Those areas lacking blood flow demonstrate filling defects, visualized between images taken at rest and under stress. Stress may be induced by exercise on a treadmill or by the use of pharmaceuticals such as regadenoson. Myocardial perfusion scanning is performed using single photon emission computed tomography (SPECT), allowing the camera to rotate around the patient to obtain tomographic images of the heart parallel to the short and long axes of the left ventricle. SPECT myocardial perfusion scans can detect significant CAD in 90%

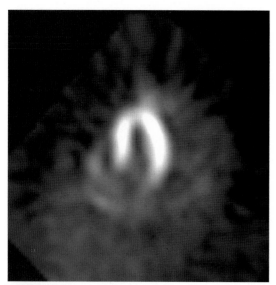

FIGURE 4-16 The appearance of a normal heart on a nuclear medicine perfusion scan on the same patient as in Fig. 4-15 during exercise. Notice the increased activity in the myocardium

of patients presenting with CAD. PET may also be used for imaging myocardial perfusion employing a variety of positron perfusion and metabolic agents. A PET unit is more sensitive than conventional nuclear medicine cameras, and spatial resolution is superior to that of conventional cameras. It is highly accurate for detecting CAD that interferes with blood flow to the heart muscle and can identify injured but viable heart muscle. PET can also provide quantitative data about the distribution of the radionuclide within the body.

Gated cardiac blood pool scans, sometimes called *radionuclide ventriculograms* or *multiple gate acquisition scans (MUGA)*, are used to evaluate ventricular function and ventricular wall motion. These images are obtained with the patient at rest and during exercise. They are synchronized with the patient's heartbeat using electrocardiography to image the heart during specific phases of the cardiac cycle with the use of the radionuclide technetium-99. Images are obtained over a 5- to 10-minute period. The images are displayed in a cinelike format, allowing the wall motion of the beating heart to be evaluated. Ventricular function is assessed by calculating the ejection fraction, ejection and filling rates, and left ventricular volume.

Computed Tomography

Computed tomography (CT) is a noninvasive modality used to assess cardiac and vascular disease. Multidetector (or multislice) scanners provide the highest image quality, and electron beam CT (EBCT) may also be used to image the heart. Cardiac scoring is performed without the use of a contrast agent. It was introduced in 1990, and a scoring algorithm was developed for evaluating the amount of calcium (hard plaques) present in the coronary arteries.

EBCT was introduced in the mid-1980s and is a technique used primarily to examine the heart, particularly as related to coronary artery calcifications. It uses a scanning focused x-ray beam to provide complete cardiac imaging in 50 milliseconds (ms)—fast enough to "freeze" heart motion without the need for ECG gating. An electron gun produces an electron stream that is magnetically focused onto four tungsten targets. Each target emits two fan beams of x-rays, which are directed through the patient and registered on detectors arranged in a semicircle above the patient. The net result is that extremely thin slices are readily demonstrated, either as a cine loop or as single images. This allows for coronary calcium scoring, which may represent a predictor of atherosclerosis and current heart disease. A low calcium score implies a low risk for obstructing coronary disease. EBCT should not be relied on for a final diagnosis of CAD, as it is limited in its ability to detect noncalcified (soft) plaques. EBCT is not of value in patients with a history of a previous heart attack, angioplasty, or bypass surgery.

Multidetector volumetric CT units with specialized cardiac software are most commonly used to perform calcium scoring and have better reproducibility compared with EBCT examinations. The software enables ECG gating and fast, multiple-section scans to obtain images without interference from the normal heart motion.

Images are generally captured during the R wave to acquire the image during the diastolic phase of the heart. The gating may occur prospectively or retrospectively. Images of 2.5 mm are obtained, generally at 2.5-mm intervals. Images can also be obtained at much smaller thicknesses such as 0.6 mm and then reconstructed at a larger thickness. As with EBCT, multidetector CT cardiac scoring uses software to analyze the histogram information obtained during the scans and computes image and region scores.

ECG-gated CT is also used to perform noninvasive angiography (CT angiography [CTA]) allowing evaluation of the right and left coronary arteries, the circumflex artery, and the anterior descending artery. Currently, by using CTA, it is possible to identify a stenotic cardiac vessel in almost 70% of cases because of CTA's ability to image soft atherosclerotic plaque. Postprocessing software can reproduce three-dimensional (3-D) images of the heart to assess the coronary arteries, heart chambers, coronary stents, and coronary anomalies and to assess bypass grafts. Contrast-enhanced CT images may also be reviewed in a cine loop to allow evaluation of heart motion and assessment of cardiac function and perfusion.

Contrast-enhanced CTA is approved by the U.S. Food and Drug Administration (FDA). It is noninvasive (requiring only a peripheral intravenous [IV] line for contrast administration) and is more cost-effective than conventional angiography. In combination with 3-D reconstruction, it is used to image vascular structures for organ donors, to diagnose pulmonary embolisms, to evaluate vascular stenosis and peripheral vascular disease, and to image abdominal aortic aneurysms (Fig. 4-17). CTA helps the surgeon determine the necessary stent type and size in the presurgical planning of abdominal aortic aneurysms and in the evaluation after surgery to assess the stent's effectiveness.

Magnetic Resonance Imaging

Magnetic resonance imaging (MRI) is also a common imaging modality used to evaluate many cardiac, mediastinal, and great vessel anomalies (Fig. 4-18). It may be used to evaluate myocardial wall thickness and chamber volumes and is especially helpful in diagnosing right ventricular dysplasia. MRI is highly effective in the evaluation of viable versus nonviable myocardium. Most protocols involve obtaining imaging sequences and putting them into motion using a cine loop to evaluate how well the valves of the heart are functioning. Like nuclear cardiology, contrast-enhanced MRI can demonstrate myocardial perfusion, and blood flow velocities within the heart can be measured. The advantage of MRI is the production of images with high spatial resolution and, thus, higher quality images. As with many other imaging modalities, information may be ECG gated to acquire the images during specific portions of the cardiac cycle. MRI is a valuable tool for imaging the anatomy, function, and disease of the heart and is fast becoming a "one-stop shop" for noninvasive cardiac imaging.

MRI is also used to evaluate aortic aneurysms, dissections, and aortic stenosis, especially in patients who are unable to have contrast-enhanced CT scans because of renal failure. Contrast-enhanced magnetic resonance angiography (MRA) is widely used to evaluate the vasculature from the aorta to the brain (Fig. 4-19). This technology takes only about 1 minute to acquire data and is considered noninvasive. The larger coronary arteries may also be assessed with MRA.

Angiography

Angiography is a procedure commonly performed to evaluate cardiovascular disease. It may be performed for diagnostic purposes or for therapeutic reasons. As discussed earlier, traditional diagnostic angiography is being challenged by less invasive procedures such as MRA and CTA. Cardiac catheterization is an invasive procedure specific to the heart and the great vessels. It is performed in patients with CAD, conduction disturbances, or congenital heart disease and provides information about heart and vessel anatomy.

FIGURE 4-17 Computed tomography angiogram demonstrating an abdominal aortic aneurysm in three planes: **A,** axial. **B,** coronal. **C,** sagittal.

FIGURE 4-18 Normal magnetic resonance image of the heart. **A,** axial. **B,** coronal. **C,** sagittal.

FIGURE   4-19 Contrast-enhanced   three-dimensional magnetic resonance angiography image of the aortic arch, carotid and vertebral arteries, and circle of Willis.

Intracardiac and arterial pressures are measured as the catheter passes through the various areas of the heart. This provides information about the function of the cardiac valves. Angiocardiography is performed by injecting the contrast material into the heart chambers and obtaining cine images of the heart and the great vessels in motion.

Therapeutic angiography continues to steadily increase through expanded use of interventional procedures. Percutaneous transluminal coronary angioplasty (PTCA) is a therapeutic procedure commonly performed to open stenotic coronary vessels and place a **stent** in a narrowed vessel to maintain its patency. **Thrombolysis** is a procedure in which a high-intensity anticoagulant such as streptokinase is dripped over a period of hours directly onto a clot to dissolve it (Fig. 4-20). With **embolization**, devices such as coils are used to clot off vessels (Fig. 4-21). Common examples of the use of embolization include clotting of vessels feeding brain tumors, arteriovenous malformations, or other abnormalities of the brain to prevent excessive bleeding during open cranial

FIGURE 4-20 A, An apparent embolus in the right popliteal artery prevents blood flow to the foot in this 91-year-old woman. **B,** In this thrombolysis procedure, urokinase is sprayed onto the embolus and allowed to drip over a 30-minute period. Patency is restored.

FIGURE 4-21 A, A large aneurysm is seen angiographically in the left common iliac artery of this 74-year-old man. **B,** Embolization of this large aneurysm was accomplished by progressive insertion of a variety of coils and guidewire fragments.

FIGURE 4-22 A, A specialized catheter is used to create an opening through a cirrhotic liver of a 69-year-old man for the beginning of a transjugular intrahepatic portosystemic stent procedure. **B,** After dilation of the pathway using standard angioplasty technique, a shunt is installed to connect the right hepatic vein to the right portal vein, restoring blood flow.

surgery. In a **transjugular intrahepatic portosystemic shunt** (TIPSS) procedure, a catheter is used to connect the jugular vein to the portal vein to reduce the flow of blood through a diseased liver (Fig. 4-22). Arterial stents are devices placed in arteries (Fig. 4-23), typically the iliac, aorta, renal, or coronary arteries, to open occluded vessels. Insertion of a stent is often preceded by

percutaneous transluminal angioplasty (PTA) with a balloon catheter to open up the vessel's occlusion before stent placement (Fig. 4-24). In **permanent catheterization,** a catheter is placed in the subclavian or jugular vein and tunneled under the skin to allow for improved dialysis access. Vena caval filters are basketlike devices placed in the inferior vena cava to catch clots before they

FIGURE 4-23 A, Bilateral lower extremity arteriogram reveals stenosis of both external iliac arteries. **B,** After balloon angioplasty, stent placement in each external iliac artery results in restored flow of blood.

FIGURE 4-24 A, Catheterization and angiography of the left brachiocephalic vein of this 56-year-old man reveal significant narrowing. **B,** Balloon angioplasty and a stent are used to open up the stenotic left brachiocephalic vein. Excellent blood flow was restored in subsequent images.

enter the heart (Fig. 4-25). Besides typical contrast media, some of these procedures use carbon dioxide as the contrast agent in patients who do not tolerate normal agents (Fig. 4-26). The role of interventional angiography will continue to grow and reduce costs and complications associated with certain surgical procedures it replaces.

CONGENITAL AND HEREDITARY DISEASES

Because fetal circulation and blood–gas exchange occur within the placenta, certain characteristics are present in the fetal circulatory system that should normally disappear at birth. These characteristics include an opening in the septum between the atria, termed the **foramen ovale,** which allows the blood to bypass the pulmonary circulatory system, and a small vessel termed the *ductus arteriosus,* which connects the pulmonary artery and the descending aorta. If these anatomic structures persist, a variety of congenital anomalies may develop in the newborn. The incidence of congenital cardiovascular anomalies is approximately 1 per 120 live births.

FIGURE 4-25 A, Greenfield filter placement in the inferior vena cava, as seen on an anteroposterior abdominal radiograph. **B,** Greenfield filter placement in the inferior vena cava, as seen on a lateral abdominal radiograph.

Etiology of congenital heart disease includes inherited genetic disorders, chromosomal aberrations (such as Down syndrome), and environmental factors (such as drugs, alcohol, infection, radiation, and maternal disease). In addition, individuals with congenital anomalies of the heart are at an increased risk for developing endocardial infections. Immediate diagnosis to determine the type and severity of the anomaly and treatment of the cardiac anomaly are vital to survival. The outcome of the disease depends on the pressure differences created between the right and left sides of the heart, abnormal ventricular load, and defects that obstruct blood flow.

Radiography and diagnostic medical sonography play a critical role in the diagnosis and treatment of congenital anomalies, along with the diagnosis of heart murmurs by physical examination, and abnormal heart rates and ventricular hypertrophy demonstrated by ECG. Although echocardiography is generally used to diagnose congenital heart disease, MRI and CT have

become valuable tools for the continued evaluation of congenital heart diseases as affected patients are living longer. Three-dimensional reconstructions allow for visualization of defects as well as any repair of the defect.

A **murmur** is an abnormal heart sound resulting from disturbed or turbulent flow, often through malformed valves. Common signs of heart failure include tachycardia, respiratory distress, cyanosis, and a weak or impalpable pulse.

Patent Ductus Arteriosus

The **ductus arteriosus** is a temporary vessel that is used during in utero life. It shunts blood from the pulmonary artery into the systemic circulation because the pulmonary circulation is not needed during this time. If it does not close at birth, **patent ductus arteriosus** results (Figs. 4-27 and 4-28). This condition is more common in premature infants, occurring in approximately 80% of infants born before 28 weeks of

FIGURE 4-26 Use of carbon dioxide as a contrast medium demonstrated in inferior vena cavogram (appearing white along the right of the spine) on a frail 75-year-old man.

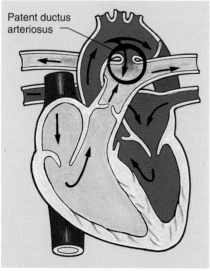

FIGURE 4-27 Patent ductus arteriosus.

gestation, especially in those with respiratory distress syndrome.

Because the left ventricle contracts with more force compared with the right ventricle, arterial blood within the aorta is shunted into the pulmonary trunk via the open ductus arteriosus instead of out into the systemic circulation. This increases the volume of blood propelled into the lungs, thus increasing pulmonary vascular congestion and the volume of blood returning to the left atrium. Infants with this condition generally have a heart murmur and display cyanotic features resulting from the shunting. Echocardiography is the imaging method of choice for evaluating the severity of this anomaly and usually demonstrates a left atrial diameter larger than the aortic root. Color Doppler technology demonstrates the reverse pulmonary artery flow during diastole and shows the full length of the ductus arteriosus. Chest radiography demonstrates cardiomegaly with prominence of the left side of the heart and ascending aorta and increased pulmonary vascular congestion. In premature infants, treatment includes fluid restriction and diuresis, the use of drugs, or surgical intervention. Surgery is used as a last resort in premature infants and generally is not performed until the child is 1 to 2 years of age. In full-term infants, surgical ligation is necessary in cases of heart failure. In full-term infants without distress, elective surgery is generally performed between the ages of 6 months and 3 years to decrease the risk of the infant developing infective endarteritis.

Coarctation of the Aorta

Although the ductus arteriosus may close normally at birth, a narrowing of the aorta may occur at the junction site. This anomaly is termed **coarctation of the aorta** (Fig. 4-29); it is the cause of 7% to 8% of all congenital cardiac anomalies and is more common in boys. It occurs anatomically inferiorly to the vessels responsible for circulation to the head, neck, and upper extremities, so circulation to these anatomic regions is not affected. However, blood flow to the abdomen

FIGURE 4-28 A, Aortogram demonstrating patent ductus arteriosus. Note filling of the pulmonary vessels as well as the aorta. **B,** Magnetic resonance imaging demonstrating patent ductus arteriosus.

FIGURE 4-29 A, Coarctation of the aorta. **B,** Computed tomography volume three-dimensional rendering of coarctation of the aorta.

and lower extremities is compromised, and the femoral pulse is very weak in most individuals with this anomaly. This anomaly may lead to heart failure. Radiographically, two bulges of the aorta are demonstrated in the aortic arch region, one superior to and one inferior to the stenosis. *Rib notching,* another radiographic indication of coarctation of the aorta, refers to well-defined bone erosions along the lower rib margins as a result of the enlargement of anastomotic vessels. Coarctation of the aorta may be successfully treated surgically by removing the narrowed region of the aorta and reattaching the normal aorta superiorly and inferiorly to the coarctation.

Septal Defects

A defect in either the ventricular septum or the atrial septum allows the blood to be shunted between the two chambers (Figs. 4-30 and 4-31), mixing pulmonary and systemic blood. Blood is generally shunted from the left chamber to the right chamber because of increased pressure on the left side of the heart. This shunting of the blood results in an enlargement of the right side of the heart and increased pulmonary vascularity as the lungs overload with blood.

If the foramen ovale does not close at birth, an opening remains between the right and left atria. **Atrial septal defects** are the most common congenital heart defect, responsible for about 10% of all cases of congenital heart disease. Such defects occur twice as frequently in girls as in boys and are generally detected clinically by an audible heart murmur at the upper left sternal border around the age of 1 year as well as by atrial dysrhythmias on ECG evaluation. Doppler and 2-D echocardiography may also be performed to confirm the diagnosis. Radiographically, the right atrium and ventricle are enlarged, resulting in cardiomegaly. Evidence of increased pulmonary blood flow within the lung fields is also present. In most cases, this does not require surgical intervention. However, if surgical intervention is necessary, a preoperative cardiac catheterization may be performed to evaluate the size of the defect, left ventricular function, and the vessel anatomy.

Ventricular septal defects involve defects between the two ventricles and are more serious because the pressure difference is greater between

Atrial septal defect

FIGURE 4-30 Atrial septal defect.

Ventricular septal defect

FIGURE 4-31 Ventricular septal defect.

FIGURE 4-32 Chest radiograph depicting ventricular septal defect. Note the enlargement of the right heart border.

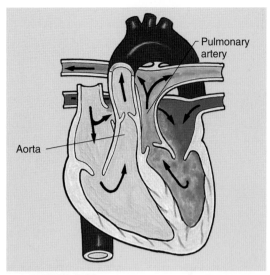

FIGURE 4-33 Transposition of great vessels.

the ventricles than between the atria. Clinically, patients with these defects also have an audible heart murmur; however, it is heard a little lower on the left sternal border and at a younger age than the murmur associated with an atrial defect. In significant cases of ventricular septal defect, the murmur may be audible in infants as young as 2 to 3 weeks old. In these cases, intervention is necessary, as signs of heart failure may develop between 6 and 8 weeks of age. In addition, these infants are at an increased risk for developing severe viral or bacterial pneumonia and infective endocarditis. Again, color flow **Doppler echocardiography** is the imaging method of choice. Radiographically, the left atrium and ventricle are enlarged, resulting in cardiomegaly (Fig. 4-32). Increased pulmonary flow is also evident in the lung fields. Surgical intervention depends on the size of the defect and the risk of developing bacterial endocarditis at the site of the defect.

Transposition of the Great Vessels

Transposition of the great vessels is an anomaly in which the aorta arises from the right ventricle instead of the left ventricle, and the pulmonary trunk arises from the left ventricle instead of the right ventricle (Figs. 4-33 and 4-34). This serious congenital defect does not allow the pulmonary and systemic subsystems to communicate and comprises over 5% of all cardiac anomalies. Deoxygenated blood returns to the right atrium, travels through the right ventricle, and is pumped through the aorta back into the systemic subsystem without becoming oxygenated. Oxygenated blood returns to the left atrium, travels through the left ventricle, and is pumped through the pulmonary trunk back to the lungs for gas exchange to occur. Conventional chest radiography demonstrates a narrow mediastinum because the vessels are superimposed and the main pulmonary trunk is not in the usual location. Pulmonary congestion is also visible in the lung fields. Obviously, this anomaly is incompatible with life. Because immediate recognition and treatment of this defect are imperative, echocardiography is performed to confirm the diagnosis. Emergency cardiac catheterization and balloon septostomy must be performed to enlarge the opening between the atria to increase mixing of venous and arterial blood and to decompress the left atrium. Surgical correction of this anomaly is indicated within the first 10 days of life.

FIGURE 4-34 Angiogram demonstrating transposition of great vessels. Note the "closed" system of the right side of the heart. Blood is returned via the venae cavae and redistributed via the aorta, thus bypassing the lungs.

Tetralogy of Fallot

Tetralogy of Fallot is a combination of four defects: (1) pulmonary stenosis, (2) ventricular septal defect, (3) overriding aorta, and (4) hypertrophy of the right ventricle (Fig. 4-35). Narrowing of the pulmonary valve prevents passage of a sufficient volume of blood from the right ventricle to the lungs and results in the most common cause of cyanosis in infants with cardiovascular anomalies. Normally, the aorta should arise from the left ventricle, but in patients with tetralogy of Fallot, the aorta arises from a ventricular septal defect. In other words, it overrides the right ventricle, which, in turn, results in hypertrophy of the right ventricle. Enlargement of the right ventricle is demonstrated radiographically as a boot-shaped cardiac shadow caused by displacement of the heart apex (Fig. 4-36). Corrective surgery is usually performed after the age of 1 year.

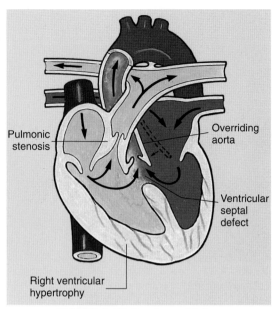

FIGURE 4-35 Tetralogy of Fallot.

FIGURE 4-36 Chest radiograph on an infant with tetralogy of Fallot. Note the "boot-shaped" cardiac shadow.

VALVULAR DISEASE

Abnormalities of the heart's valves often cause cardiac symptoms such as dyspnea, fatigue, syncope, or chest pain and signs such as murmurs. In addition, lesions of the valves often result in abnormal pulses detectable through palpation. Clinicians are often able to diagnose most valve abnormalities by assimilating historical and physical findings. Noninvasive techniques add to the precision of diagnosis, and invasive studies are reserved for surgical candidates.

The most common cause of chronic valve disease of the heart is **rheumatic fever**. This condition most frequently affects the bicuspid (mitral) and aortic valves and is more common in women than in men. Because of advances in pharmaceuticals, technology, and medical care, the incidence of rheumatic heart disease is on the decline. Rheumatic fever produces inflammatory changes within the connective tissues of the body, thus affecting the valves within the heart. It may result in stenosis, insufficiency, or incompetency. Individuals with rheumatic heart disease have a distinct heart murmur audible on physical examination.

Valvular stenosis (Fig. 4-37) is caused by a scarring of valve cusps that eventually adhere to one another. The results of valvular stenosis become apparent in adult life because it generally takes years for the scarring to affect valve function. Mitral valve stenosis inhibits blood flow from the left atrium into the left ventricle. It slows the blood flow through the lungs and the right side of the heart, resulting in an enlargement of the right side of the heart and the left atrium. Insufficiency and incompetency occur when the valves do not close properly and allow blood to reflux during systole. This complication often follows endocarditis or is seen in the case of mitral valve prolapse. Mitral valve prolapse, a genetic disease caused by an autosomal dominant inheritance, occurs in about 6% of the population and is generally diagnosed by clinical examination. Echocardiography, which is usually performed to confirm the diagnosis, has an accuracy rate of approximately 95%. Patients with mitral valve prolapse are at an increased risk for developing endocarditis, so prophylactic treatment is necessary.

Damaged valves are often replaced surgically, especially in patients experiencing symptoms of heart failure. Patients with a reduced ejection fraction diagnosed by either nuclear medicine studies or echocardiography are also candidates for surgery. These patients must receive prophylactic medication to prevent endocarditis both preoperatively and postoperatively. Cardiac catheterization is performed before surgery to assess valve function and to detect CAD. After surgery, patients are generally placed on a regimen of medications to help maintain proper cardiac function.

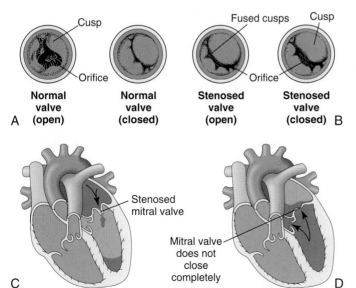

FIGURE 4-37 Valvular stenosis and regurgitation. **A,** Normal position of the valve leaflets, or cusps, when the valve is open and closed. **B,** Open position of a stenosed valve (*left*) and open position of a closed regurgitant valve (*right*). **C,** Hemodynamic effect of mitral stenosis. The stenosed valve is unable to open sufficiently during left atrial systole, inhibiting left ventricular filling. **D,** Hemodynamic effect of mitral regurgitation. The mitral valve does not close completely during left ventricular systole, permitting blood to reenter the left atrium.

Radiographically, manifestations of mitral stenosis may be subtle. More progressed cases may show the heart silhouette as enlarged, with a straightening of the left cardiac border and a prominent main pulmonary artery. The diseased valves may contain small calcifications visible during echocardiographic or CT evaluation. Mitral valve insufficiency appears radiographically as an enlargement of the left atrium and ventricle with right upper lobe pulmonary congestion. Color Doppler echocardiography provides quantification or grading of the severity of regurgitation; however, TEE provides the most information in terms of mitral valve function. In cases of aortic valvular disease, both conventional chest radiography and echocardiography may demonstrate calcification of the cusps of the valve and hypertrophy of the septum. Left ventricular enlargement is generally present only when the left ventricular myocardium is damaged. In cases of tricuspid damage, the right side of the heart is affected, and chest radiography will reveal enlargement of the superior vena cava, right atrium, and right ventricle. The right ventricular enlargement is best demonstrated on the lateral projection of the chest. Doppler and 2-D echocardiography confirm the diagnosis by demonstrating increased dimensions in the right side of the heart. After valve replacement, the prosthetic devices are clearly visible on conventional chest radiographs (Fig. 4-38).

CONGESTIVE HEART FAILURE

Congestive heart failure (CHF) occurs when the heart is unable to propel blood at a sufficient rate and volume. This results in congestion of the circulatory subsystems and does not allow a sufficient supply of blood to reach the tissues of the body. CHF is most commonly caused by hypertension but may result from other disease processes that overburden the heart, such as valvular disease. CHF may affect either side of the heart, but both sides are commonly affected together. It may develop gradually or have a quick onset in combination with pulmonary edema. Regardless of the side affected initially, prolonged strain on

FIGURE 4-38 Lateral chest radiograph demonstrating two prosthetic valve replacements clearly visible within the heart.

the heart eventually affects the entire organ. Signs and symptoms may vary with the extent and location of the disease. The treatment of CHF is usually medical but depends on the cause and severity of the disease and may include surgical intervention, especially in cases of valvular disease.

Left-Sided Failure

When the left ventricle of the heart cannot pump an amount of blood equal to the venous return in the right ventricle, the pulmonary circulatory subsystem becomes overloaded. The fluid that accumulates in the capillaries of the lungs leaks into the interstitial tissue within the lungs. This results in rales and pulmonary edema, which may be a life-threatening condition. Radiographically, the heart is enlarged, and the hilar region of the lungs is congested with increased vascular markings (Fig. 4-39). On physical examination, individuals with left-sided heart failure are found to have an increased heart rate because the heart tries to compensate for the deficiency. Individuals commonly complain of difficulty breathing or shortness of breath on exertion and respiratory distress severe enough to awaken them during

FIGURE 4-39 Chest radiograph demonstrating cardio-megaly resulting from congestive heart failure.

the night. As the disease progresses, sleeping in a recumbent position becomes impossible. The most common cause of left-sided failure is hypertension, but other causes include aortic and mitral valvular disease and CAD.

Right-Sided Failure

Right ventricular failure is not as common as left-sided failure and occurs when the right ventricle cannot pump as much blood as it receives from the right atrium. This causes the venous blood flow to slow down, producing engorgement of the superior and inferior venae cavae and edema of the lower extremities. A common complaint from individuals with right-sided failure is swelling of the ankles. Radiographically, the right atrium and the right ventricle appear enlarged. Common causes of true right-sided failure are pulmonary valve stenosis, emphysema, and pulmonary hypertension secondary to pulmonary emboli.

COR PULMONALE

Cor pulmonale results from a lung disorder producing hypertension in the pulmonary artery and an enlargement of the right ventricle of the heart. It may be acute, in the case of a pulmonary

embolism, or chronic, as a result of chronic obstructive pulmonary disease (COPD). This disease results from alveolar hypoxia, and common symptoms include dyspnea and syncope on exertion. Patients may also experience chest pain. Conventional chest radiography reveals enlargement of the right ventricle and a proximal pulmonary artery. Echocardiography and nuclear medicine examinations are performed to demonstrate and evaluate right ventricular function. Right-sided heart catheterization may be performed to confirm the diagnosis. Patients with cor pulmonale are at an increased risk for venous thrombosis and may be placed on long-term anticoagulants.

DEGENERATIVE DISEASES

Atherosclerosis

Atherosclerosis is a degenerative condition that affects the major arteries of the body, often termed *hardening of the arteries*. It is the most prevalent disease in humans and occurs in epidemic proportions in the United States. It tends to affect men at an earlier age compared with women. Atherosclerosis may occur in any artery (Fig. 4-40), but it has a predilection for the aorta, coronary arteries, and cerebral arteries (Fig. 4-41). Risk factors associated with this disorder that cannot be controlled include increased age and a strong family history of atherosclerosis. Risk factors that can be altered include increased serum low-density lipoprotein (LDL), reduced levels of high-density lipoprotein (HDL), hypertension, cigarette smoking, obesity, and a sedentary lifestyle. In addition, some other disease processes such as diabetes mellitus predispose individuals to atherosclerotic disease.

Atheroma formations (fibrofatty plaques) are composed of intracellular and extracellular lipids, muscle, and connective tissue. They begin as fatty streaks and progress to fibrous plaque, which collects within the vessel and reduces its ability to expand during systole (Fig. 4-42). The cause of the development of these formations within the vessel is currently being debated, but

FIGURE 4-40 Arteriogram from a 47-year-old man demonstrates atherosclerosis occluding the femoral artery.

FIGURE 4-41 Digital subtraction arteriogram demonstrating atherosclerotic disease of the carotid artery. Note that the carotid artery is almost completely occluded.

FIGURE 4-42 Development of arteriosclerosis.

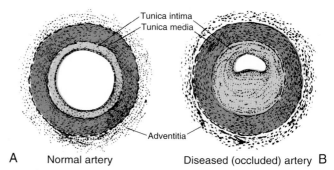

A   Normal artery   Diseased (occluded) artery B

two hypotheses, the chronic endothelial injury theory and the lipid theory, are most prominent. The chronic endothelial injury theory suggests that the disease process first affects the intima, or inner layer, of the artery as a result of injury, resulting in an accumulation of platelets, monocytes, and T-cell lymphocytes at the site of injury.

These cells cause a migration of the smooth muscle tissue from the media, forming a fibrous plaque. The lipid theory suggests that an increase in LDL within blood plasma causes lipid accumulation in smooth muscle cells. The LDL becomes oxidized, and this modification affects the monocytes, creating fat-laden macrophages

FIGURE 4-43 Computed tomography of chest demonstrating extensive coronary artery calcification. The patient's major complaint was shortness of breath.

and foam cells. As these cells enlarge and project into the vessel lumen, platelets aggregate to the site. Oxidized LDL has been found to be toxic to endothelial cells and may be responsible for their dysfunction. The reality may be a combination of the two theories because the oxidized LDL may injure the endothelium, attracting the monocytes and macrophages as described in the endothelial injury hypothesis. As the disease slowly progresses, the vessel becomes stenotic, and the atheroma may calcify (Fig. 4-43), hemorrhage, ulcerate, or include a superimposed thrombosis. These arterial changes often occur silently, and symptoms may not manifest until atheroma formation occludes more than two thirds of the vessel. In some cases, this slow narrowing allows enough time for the formation of collateral vessels to maintain blood supply distal to the stenotic site. If normal blood supply is decreased or stopped completely, **ischemia** occurs. Unfortunately, the most common signs and symptoms associated with atherosclerotic disease result from ischemia of a vital organ such as the heart or the brain or a weakening of a vital artery resulting in an aneurysm. Atherosclerotic disease is the most common cause of coronary heart disease (CHD) and cerebrovascular accidents (CVAs).

Cardiovascular angiography is often used in the diagnosis and treatment of atherosclerosis

FIGURE 4-44 Multislice computed tomography angiogram image demonstrating soft plaque (*arrow*) in the left anterior descending artery.

through the use of PTA. CTA is becoming more popular for imaging atherosclerosis and provides results rapidly (Fig. 4-44). Doppler sonography also plays a major role in the diagnosis of atherosclerosis (Fig. 4-45). MRI (Fig. 4-46) and echocardiography are both noninvasive modalities that may also visualize blood flow without the use of contrast agents.

Some researchers believe that a simple blood test, cross-reactive protein (CRP), may be helpful in determining who is at risk for developing atherosclerosis. CRP is a marker of inflammation and it is now believed that inflammation plays a major role in the formation of atherosclerosis. This particular blood test (specifically the high sensitivity test, hs-CRP) is sometimes ordered in conjunction with a lipid profile (cholesterol,

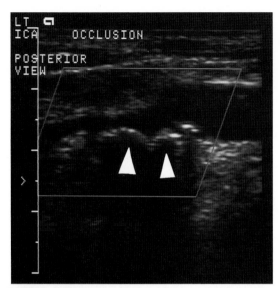

FIGURE 4-45 Atherosclerosis as seen in Doppler sonography of the internal carotid artery in a 75-year-old man. Arrows point to the "hilly" plaque deposit on the lower surface of the artery; the lack of echo signal beneath them indicates calcium contained within the plaque.

FIGURE 4-46 Two-dimensional time flight magnetic resonance imaging of normal venous blood flow of the brain within the sagittal and transverse sinuses.

triglycerides, LDL, HDL). An increased level of CRP may point to an increased future risk of heart attack, stroke, and peripheral arterial disease (PAD). It is important to note that an increased CRP may also indicate inflammation associated with another disease process such as infection or an autoimmune disease.

Coronary Artery Disease

CAD results from the deposition of atheromas in the arteries supplying blood to the heart muscle. As plaques accumulate in the coronary arteries, blood supply to the heart muscle is decreased, resulting in ischemia, a local and temporary impairment of circulation caused by obstruction of circulation, and myocardial damage as an **infarct**, which is an area of ischemic necrosis (Fig. 4-47). Major complications of CAD include angina pectoris (chest pain), myocardial infarction (MI), and subsequent myocardial necrosis, if the patient survives the heart attack. CAD is responsible for over 30% of all deaths annually in the United States and is the single most

FIGURE 4-47 Posteroanterior chest radiograph on patient with known coronary artery disease. The radiograph demonstrates cardiomegaly with left ventricular configuration and mild dilatation of the thoracic aorta.

frequent cause of death in both men and women. Most cases, on autopsy, demonstrate significant widespread atherosclerotic disease of the coronary arteries.

As noted earlier, the exact cause of plaque formation is unknown. However, risk factors for CAD are well known and include tobacco use, diets high in fats and calories and low in phytochemicals and fiber, and poor physical fitness. Recent research has demonstrated the possibility that a common variant of the platelet fibrinogen receptor may also be a strong predictor of CAD.

Medical treatments of CAD may include antianginal drugs to improve circulation and decrease the amount of oxygen consumed by the myocardium. Other cases may be treated surgically with coronary artery bypass grafting (CABG), which involves bypassing the obstruction with a segment of the saphenous vein. A portion of the saphenous vein is removed from the patient's leg, and one end is attached to the aorta above the level of the coronary arteries. The lower end of the graft is attached to the coronary artery, beyond the site of the occlusion.

Nuclear medicine studies such as myocardial perfusion scans and gated examinations are important noninvasive methods of determining the presence and extent of CAD; these studies also assist in the clinical management of patients after an MI. In addition, echocardiography may be used to provide needed clinical information in the diagnosis, treatment, and management of CAD. It is also helpful in demonstrating abnormalities in the left ventricular wall motion when the diagnosis of MI is uncertain. Highly advanced MRI and CT are noninvasive, efficient methods of diagnosing CAD.

Myocardial Infarction

MI is most commonly caused by an acute thrombus of the coronary arteries and primarily affects the left ventricle of the heart. The ability of the heart to continue pumping blood depends on the extent of muscle damage. Clinical signs and symptoms of MI include a sudden onset of severe, crushing chest pain that may radiate down the

left arm or up into the neck. It may be accompanied by profuse sweating, shortness of breath, nausea, or vomiting. In milder cases, it may be dismissed as indigestion. It is important to note that while the signs and symptoms are similar in men and women, women often experience atypical chest discomfort. Immediate medical attention is critical to the survival of individuals experiencing an MI. Approximately 20% to 25% of these patients die before reaching the hospital, primarily from ventricular fibrillation. Early medical intervention significantly increases survival. Survival rates are approximately 85% in those having the first attack and receiving medical attention within the first 30 minutes after the attack. The prognosis of CAD is variable, depending largely on the location of the occlusion, the extent of damage to the heart muscle, and the amount of collateral circulation available.

Cardiac angiography plays a major role in the diagnosis of stenotic or occluded heart vessels (Figs. 4-48 and 4-49). PCTA with stent placement is routinely performed to open stenotic vessels and is quite effective. Thrombolytic therapy may also be used, and it is most effective if administered within hours of the onset of an MI. If therapy is started within 3 hours, the chances of survival are better. The most common thrombolytic agents include streptokinase, anistreplase, alteplase, and reteplase.

FIGURE 4-48 Coronary angiography demonstrating a normal left anterior descending artery as shown in this right anterior oblique projection.

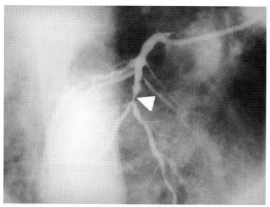

FIGURE 4-49 A major stenosis is seen in this coronary arteriogram in a left anterior oblique projection, just as the left coronary artery bifurcates into the left anterior descending artery to the right and a major diagonal branch to the left.

Acute coronary syndrome (ACS) may be diagnosed by performing cardiac biomarker tests. A biomarker is a characteristic that can be measured and evaluated as an indicator of a normal biologic process or a pathogenic process. Common cardiac biomarkers include troponin I or T, creatine kinase (CK), and CK–muscle-type or brain-type (CK-MB). Troponins are proteins found in skeletal and heart muscles. Troponin I and T are specific to cardiac muscle and are normally present in very small quantities. When heart muscle is damaged, troponins I and T are released into the circulation. Thus, an elevated level of troponin indicates that an individual has suffered a heart attack. CK is an enzyme found in the heart, brain, skeletal muscle, and other tissues. Enzymes are proteins that help cells perform their normal functions. CK-MB is found mostly in the heart and its levels are elevated when muscle or heart cells are injured. These tests are completed with a simple blood draw from a vein.

ANEURYSMS

A localized "ballooning" or outpouching of a vessel wall is called an **aneurysm**. It results when the vessel wall has been weakened by atherosclerotic disease, trauma, infection, or congenital defects. Aneurysms are usually classified as saccular, fusiform, or dissecting (Fig. 4-50). A **saccular aneurysm** is a localized bulge involving one side of the arterial wall (Fig. 4-51). Usually, it occurs in a cerebral artery. If this bulging includes the entire circumference of the vessel wall, it is termed a **fusiform aneurysm**. This type is often found in the distal abdominal aorta. A **dissecting aneurysm** results when the intima tears and allows blood to flow within the vessel wall, thus forming an intramural hematoma (Fig. 4-52). Symptoms of a dissecting aneurysm often mimic those of a heart attack.

Although an aneurysm may occur anywhere in the aorta, the majority (75%) occur in the abdominal aorta, with 90% of those occurring below the level of the renal arteries. Abdominal aortic aneurysms (AAAs) may cause pain, or the patient may remain symptom-free. Conventional abdominal images are of little value; however, a cross-table lateral abdomen radiograph may show enlargement of the aorta with calcification of the vessel wall. Diagnostic medical sonography, MRI, and CT are fairly noninvasive and are of value in determining the size and extent of the aneurysm (Figs. 4-53 and 4-54). Aortography is an invasive procedure that also helps delineate the aneurysm, especially in cases in which the aneurysm extends above the renal arteries. Surgical repair is necessary for AAAs larger than 6 cm in diameter. The aneurysm is removed, and the section of the vessel is replaced with a synthetic graft (Fig. 4-55), possibly extending to the iliac arteries.

Thoracic aortic aneurysms most commonly result from congenital anomalies or blunt chest trauma. These are visible on conventional chest radiographs (Fig. 4-56); however, CT, MRI, and transesophageal ultrasonography are most helpful in assessing the size and extent of the aneurysm. As in the case of AAAs, thoracic aortic aneurysms are surgically repaired if they are 6 cm or larger in diameter. Aneurysms may also occur in the extremities, most commonly in the popliteal artery. These often are bilateral and occur in conjunction with an abdominal aortic

FIGURE 4-50 Types of aneurysms.

FIGURE 4-51 Abdominal aortogram from a 53-year-old man demonstrating a saccular abdominal aneurysm and bilateral areas of stenosis at the bifurcation of the aorta into the common iliac arteries.

aneurysm. Popliteal aneurysms are generally confirmed by ultrasonic evaluation or CT. Arteriography may also be performed.

VENOUS THROMBOSIS

The formation of blood clots within a vein is called **venous thrombosis**. These clots commonly form in the veins of the lower extremities (Fig. 4-57) and result from a slowing of the blood return to the heart. The contraction of leg muscles assists with venous blood return; therefore, postoperative or bedfast patients are especially prone to this disorder. **Phlebitis**, an inflammation of the vein, is often associated with venous thrombosis. The medical term used to specify the combination of these disorders is **thrombophlebitis**. The thrombus formation generally begins in the valves of the deep calf veins, where thromboplastin traps red blood cells to create the blood clot. Patients may be placed on anticoagulant drugs or receive thrombolytic therapy.

Sonography is performed to determine the location and the extent of this disease, primarily

FIGURE 4-52 A, A dissecting aneurysm in a 79-year-old man seen in a coronal magnetic resonance imaging (MRI) scan, with clear depiction of the extraluminal flow. **B,** A dissecting aneurysm in a 79-year-old man, seen as extraluminal flow in this transverse MRI scan, which represents a view looking down into the aorta.

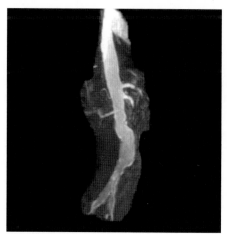

FIGURE 4-53 Three-dimensional reconstruction of a magnetic resonance angiogram demonstrating an abdominal aortic aneurysm below the level of the renal arteries.

FIGURE 4-54 Contrast-enhanced axial computed tomography image showing an infrarenal abdominal aortic aneurysm approximately 4 cm in diameter.

in the lower extremities, and venography may be of use in confirming the diagnosis. One major complication associated with deep vein thrombosis (DVT) is the development of a pulmonary embolism. Filters may be placed in the patient's inferior vena cava to prevent these clots from reaching the kidneys and the chest. These filters may be inserted under fluoroscopic control and

are clearly visible on plain radiographs of the abdomen (Fig. 4-58).

PULMONARY EMBOLI

A **pulmonary embolus** (PE), or thromboembolism, occurs when a blood clot forms or becomes lodged in a pulmonary artery. Most commonly,

FIGURE 4-55 Computed tomographic examination of a patient after graft placement for abdominal aortic aneurysm.

FIGURE 4-56 A, Posteroanterior chest radiograph demonstrating a widened mediastinum as a result of a thoracic aortic aneurysm. **B,** Lateral projection of the chest on the same patient as in **A.**

this arises from a **thrombus** that originates in a lower extremity, migrates to the lungs, and becomes lodged there, resulting in an obstruction of blood supply to the lungs. Pulmonary emboli are also caused by fat emboli resulting from skeletal fractures or from amnionic fluid emboli. The resulting decrease in blood supply to the lungs may lead to acute respiratory distress and heart failure or cardiogenic shock, depending on the extent of the obstruction and the individual's cardiovascular status before the embolism. Pathophysiologically, the pulmonary embolus

FIGURE 4-57 Venogram of the left lower extremity demonstrating deep vein thrombosis.

FIGURE 4-58 Abdominal radiograph from an older woman demonstrating the proper placement of a vena caval filter.

changes the pulmonary hemodynamics and the gas exchange capabilities of the lungs. Prolonged periods of inactivity or bed rest increase the risk for pulmonary embolism. Symptoms generally occur abruptly and include a sudden onset of coughing, acute shortness of breath, and chest pain.

Pulmonary angiography and nuclear perfusion and ventilation lung scans (VQ scan) are commonly used in the diagnosis of a PE; however, multidetector CT has been demonstrated to be the most time-saving and cost-effective imaging modality for diagnosis of pulmonary emboli (Fig. 4-59). The prognosis is dependent on the size and location of the PE as well as the patient's prior

FIGURE 4-59 Computed tomographic angiogram demonstrating a large pulmonary embolism in the right pulmonary artery.

cardiovascular status. Thrombolytic agents such as streptokinase, urokinase, or tissue plasminogen activator (tPA) and placement of inferior vena caval filters may be used in the treatment of a PE. In some cases, a pulmonary embolectomy may be required. Anticoagulant therapy with agents such as heparin or warfarin is always indicated after the initial episode because it decreases the probability and intensity of recurrent pulmonary emboli. Approximately 50% of patients who survive the initial PE experience a recurrent episode.

Thrombolytic therapy (with streptokinase or urokinase) is used in life-threatening situations and is administered in the cardiovascular or interventional area of the radiology department. In less severe cases, patients may be treated with anticoagulation medications.

PATHOLOGY SUMMARY
Cardiovascular System

Pathology	Imaging Modalities of Choice	Additive or Subtractive Pathology
Patent ductus arteriosus	Echocardiography	
Coarctation of the aorta	Echocardiography, chest radiography	Additive because of enlarged mediastinum
Septal defects	Echocardiography, MRI heart, chest radiography, CT heart, cardiac catheterization	Additive because of enlarged mediastinum
Transposition of great vessels	Echocardiography and cardiac catheterization	
Tetralogy of Fallot	Echocardiography, chest radiography	Additive because of enlarged mediastinum
Valvular disease	Echocardiography, cardiac catheterization, chest radiography	Additive because of enlarged mediastinum
Congestive heart failure	Chest radiography	Additive because of fluid in great vessels and lungs
Cor pulmonale	Echocardiography, nuclear medicine cardiac studies, chest radiography	Additive because of enlarged right ventricle and pulmonary artery
Atherosclerosis	Sonography and angiography	
Coronary artery disease	Echocardiography, nuclear medicine cardiac studies, CT	
Myocardial infarction	Cardiac catheterization, nuclear medicine, SPECT, MRI rest and stress, echocardiography rest and stress, CTA coronary arteries	
Aneurysm	Sonography, MRI, CT	
Aortic dissection	Chest radiography, CTA chest and abdomen, transesophageal sonography, MRA chest and abdomen, sonography	Additive because of widened mediastinum
Venous thrombosis		
Pulmonary embolism	CTA chest, chest radiograph, nuclear medicine, V/Q lung scan, angiography	

CT, Computed tomography; *CTA,* computed tomographic angiography; *MRI,* magnetic resonance imaging; *SPECT-MRI,* single photon emission computed tomography-MRI.

REVIEW QUESTIONS

1. The heart chamber located most anteriorly and forming the anterior border of the cardiac shadow on a lateral chest radiograph is the:
   a. Left atrium
   b. Left ventricle
   c. Right atrium
   d. Right ventricle

2. The bicuspid valve is also known as the:
   a. Left atrioventricular valve
   b. Right atrioventricular valve
   c. Aortic valve
   d. Pulmonary valve

3. Contraction of the myocardium is termed:
   a. Diastole
   b. Systole
   c. Peristole
   d. Myostole

4. How many posterior ribs should be visible on a good inspiration PA chest radiograph?
   a. 12
   b. 10
   c. 8
   d. 6

5. In a fetus, the ductus arteriosus connects the:
   a. Aorta and the superior vena cava
   b. Aorta and pulmonary trunk
   c. Right and left atria
   d. Right and left ventricles

6. Which of the following defects are included in tetralogy of Fallot?
   a. Pulmonary stenosis
   b. Ventricular septal defect
   c. Hypertrophy of right ventricle
   d. a and c
   e. a, b, and c

7. A condition in which the left ventricle cannot pump an amount of blood equal to the venous return of the right ventricle is:
   a. Coronary artery disease
   b. Left-sided congestive heart failure
   c. Right-sided congestive heart failure
   d. Patent ductus arteriosus

8. Risk factors associated with atherosclerosis include:
   A. Low blood sugar levels
   B. Hypertension
   C. Cigarette smoking
   a. A and B
   b. A and C
   c. B and C
   d. A, B, and C

9. A decrease in tissue blood supply is termed:
   a. Atheroma
   b. Infarction
   c. Ischemia
   d. Necrosis

10. The single most frequent cause of deaths in the United States is:
    a. Congestive heart failure
    b. Coronary artery disease
    c. Transposition of the great vessels
    d. Valvular disease

11. Clinical signs of a myocardial infarction include:
    A. Shortness of breath
    B. Crushing chest pain
    C. Neck pain
    a. A and B
    b. A and C
    c. B and C
    d. A, B, and C

12. Which type of vessel is used as the graft material for coronary artery bypass grafts?
    a. Arteries
    b. Capillaries
    c. Veins

13. Aortic aneurysms most commonly occur in the:
    a. Abdominal aorta above the level of the renal arteries
    b. Abdominal aorta below the level of the renal arteries
    c. Thoracic aorta

14. Imaging procedures that may be used to demonstrate an abdominal aneurysm include:
    A. Angiography
    B. CT
    C. Sonography
    a. A and B
    b. A and C
    c. B and C
    d. A, B, and C
15. Venous thrombosis most often affects the:
    a. Deep veins of the upper extremities
    b. Deep veins of the lower extremities
    c. Superficial veins of the upper extremities
    d. Superficial veins of the lower extremities
16. What common imaging procedures provide functional information regarding the heart?
17. Which type of aneurysm results when the intima tears and allows blood to flow within the vessel wall?
18. An older adult has shortness of breath on exertion and overall respiratory distress. The chest radiograph reveals an enlarged heart and a congested hilar region, with some pulmonary edema. What is the likely cause?
19. Identify at least two common sites where atherosclerosis occurs.
20. What is the cause of ischemia in coronary artery disease?

Abdomen and Gastrointestinal System

KEY TERMS

Achalasia	Granulomatous colitis
Adenocarcinomas	Hernia
Adynamic ileus	Hiatal hernia
Anal agenesis	Hirschsprung disease
Appendicitis	Hypertrophic pyloric stenosis
Atresia	Ileostomy
Carbohydrate intolerance	Imperforate anus
Colostomy	Intussusception
Crohn disease	Leiomyomas
Diverticulitis	Malrotation
Diverticulum	Mechanical bowel obstruction
Dysphagia	Paralytic ileus
Endoscopy	Peptic ulcer
Esophageal varices	Reflux esophagitis
Gallstone ileus	Regional enteritis
Gastroenteritis	Situs inversus
Gastroesophageal reflux disease	Ulcerative colitis
Gluten-sensitive enteropathy	Volvulus

ANATOMY AND PHYSIOLOGY

Abdomen

The abdomen is composed of the abdominal and pelvic cavities and is often divided into nine anatomic regions: (1) right hypochondriac, (2) epigastric, (3) left hypochondriac, (4) right lumbar, (5) umbilical, (6) left lumbar, (7) right iliac, (8) hypogastric, and (9) left iliac (Fig. 5-1). It may also be described in terms of quadrants: right-upper (RUQ), right-lower (RLQ), left-upper (LUQ), and left-lower (LLQ) (Fig. 5-2). The abdominal cavity contains organs of the digestive system (stomach and intestines), the hepatobiliary system (liver, gallbladder, and pancreas), the urinary system (kidneys and ureters), and the circulatory system (spleen). The pelvic cavity contains the bladder, portions of the intestines, and the reproductive organs.

The abdominal cavity is lined by the peritoneum, a serous membrane (Fig. 5-3, *A*). The serous lining attached to the abdominal organs

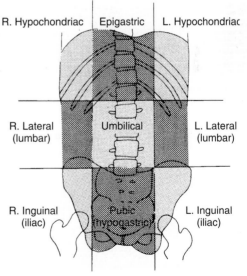

FIGURE 5-1 The nine regions of the abdomen.

is the visceral peritoneum. The peritoneum attached directly to the abdominal wall is the parietal peritoneum. The mesentery is a double fold of parietal peritoneum projecting from the posterior abdominal wall in the lumbar region (see Fig. 5-3, *B*). Most of the small bowel is attached to the outer edge of the mesentery.

The greater omentum is a double fold of peritoneum that attaches to the duodenum, stomach, and transverse colon. It hangs loosely over the intestines. The lesser omentum is a fold of peritoneum that attaches the liver to the lesser curvature of the stomach and the duodenum (Fig. 5-4).

Gastrointestinal System

A major portion of the gastrointestinal (GI) system is the alimentary tract, which serves to digest and absorb food. Extending from the

FIGURE 5-2 The four quadrants of the abdomen.

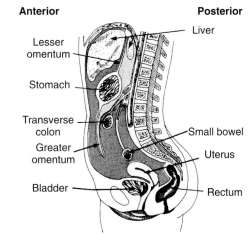

FIGURE 5-4 A cross-sectional drawing of the abdominal cavity demonstrates the omentum.

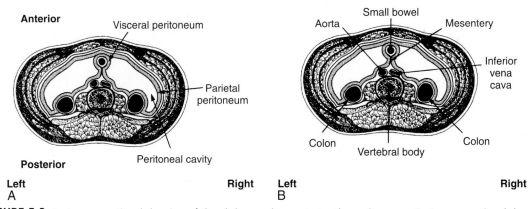

FIGURE 5-3 A, A cross-sectional drawing of the abdomen demonstrates the peritoneum. **B,** A cross-sectional drawing of the lower abdomen demonstrates the mesentery.

Indentation:
Aortic arch
Left bronchus
Heart
Esophagus
T10 level

Frontal View   **Lateral View**

FIGURE 5-5 The esophagus in the mediastinum.

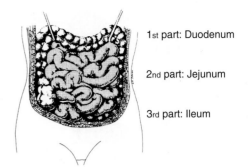

1st part: Duodenum

2nd part: Jejunum

3rd part: Ileum

FIGURE 5-7 The small bowel and its divisions.

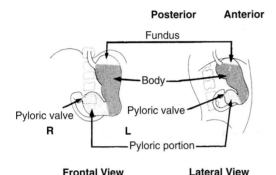

Posterior   **Anterior**

Fundus

Body

Pyloric valve   Pyloric valve

R   L

Pyloric portion

Frontal View   **Lateral View**

FIGURE 5-6 The stomach depicted in its average orientation when empty.

mouth to the anus, the alimentary tract consists of the mouth, pharynx, esophagus, stomach, small bowel and large bowel, and rectum.

The esophagus is the first part of the GI system. It is approximately 10 to 12 inches long and extends from the posterior pharynx to the stomach (Fig. 5-5). The upper esophagus is midline, but it courses to the left to pass behind the aortic arch, which indents the esophagus. Other indentations occur at the level of the left main stem bronchus and at the gastroesophageal junction. As it passes downward, the esophagus follows the curvature of the thoracic spine and thoracic descending aorta.

The stomach occupies the body's LUQ, with the cardiac orifice at the level of the tenth or eleventh thoracic vertebra and the pyloric canal just to the right of the first or second lumbar vertebra (Fig. 5-6). Peristalsis churns the gastric

content and propels it toward the pylorus. Gastric emptying of liquids is accounted for by the peristalsis initiated in the fundus of the stomach; gastric emptying of solids requires a to-and-fro action of the antrum and pylorus. In the presence of masses, inflammation, or diabetes, the peristaltic activity may be diminished. When the stomach is filled with barium, its curvatures are visible as generally smooth contours. The rugae appear as longitudinal ridges within the stomach.

The small bowel includes the duodenum, jejunum, and ileum. It arises from the stomach at the duodenal bulb and courses to the ileocecal valve (Fig. 5-7), over a length of nearly 21 feet. The duodenal C-loop moves posteriorly from the gastric antrum to its ending at the ligament of Treitz. The jejunum begins here and coils in the LUQ before terminating at the ileum in the RUQ. The ileum then courses through the RLQ and LLQ to terminate at the ileocecal junction. When filled with barium the segments of the small bowel are distinguishable by their appearance. The duodenal mucosa is indicated by its transverse rigid appearance. The jejunal mucosa appears delicate and feathery. Ileal folds look like those of the duodenum, although not as large.

The large bowel extends from the terminal ileum to the anus for a length of about 6 feet (Fig. 5-8). Its distinct regions are the cecum, orifices for the terminal ileum and the appendix, ascending colon and hepatic flexure, transverse colon and splenic flexure, descending colon, sigmoid, rectum, and anus. The cecum is usually retroperitoneal and anterior and lies against the

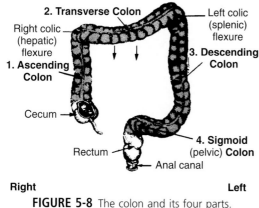

FIGURE 5-8 The colon and its four parts.

abdominal wall. The ascending colon is also retroperitoneal and becomes more posterior as it ascends to lie adjacent to the undersurface of the liver. The hepatic flexure, transverse colon, and splenic flexure are all intraperitoneal. They lie more anteriorly and are attached to the posterior abdominal wall by the mesocolon, a double layer of peritoneum. The descending colon is retroperitoneal, moving posteriorly as it descends. The peritoneal sigmoid colon lies in the pelvis and is quite mobile. Structures located anterior to it include the bladder and, in women, the uterus. Posterior structures include the iliac arteries and sacral nerves. The rectum is extraperitoneal, beginning at the third sacral segment and following the sacrococcygeal curve to the anus. The valves of Houston are prominent transverse folds in the distal rectum, where it dilates. The anus forms the distal 1 to 2 inches of the large bowel and contains no peritoneal covering.

IMAGING CONSIDERATIONS

Radiography

Abdomen. Abdominal radiography is often performed for survey purposes, without contrast agents. The usual starting point is a supine radiograph taken to include the kidneys, ureters, and bladder ("KUB"). The frequency of abnormal findings on a conventional abdominal radiograph is fairly low and nonspecific, but it is of

most value for patients complaining of severe abdominal tenderness and to rule out bowel obstructions and perforations. In addition, abdominal radiographs are invaluable in assessing the placement of various tubes and catheters, as discussed later in this chapter.

Anteroposterior (AP) projections of the abdomen are generally taken in the supine position. An AP radiograph allows examination of air distribution within the bowels and of the size of the viscera, serves to evaluate vascular and other types of calcifications and body or soft tissue trauma, and, finally, serves as a preliminary radiograph for other procedures.

On initial inspection of the abdominal radiograph, the technologist should verify that the technique chosen is correct or diagnostic, motion is nonexistent, and the anatomy under consideration has been properly visualized. As with other body areas, evaluation of the abdomen should be done systematically. This should include inspection of the renal outlines, ureters, psoas muscles, spleen, liver, gallbladder, and peritoneal fat stripes.

In a normal abdomen (Fig. 5-9), varying amounts of gas and fecal material are always present in an unprepared patient. The liver, kidney, spleen, and psoas muscle shadows are variably outlined because of the lucent layer of fat surrounding them. Properitoneal fat stripes are visible as radiolucencies extending laterally from the costal margins down to the iliac crests. The aorta and pancreas are not normally seen unless they are calcified, as might be expected in an older patient in the case of the aorta or in a patient with chronic calcific pancreatitis. The inferior margin of the liver should lie at or above the level of the right twelfth rib. The left kidney is usually slightly higher than the right kidney because of the presence of the liver superior to it. The top of the left kidney generally lies at the vertebral level of T11-T12, whereas the top of the right kidney is approximately 1 cm lower in position. In terms of renal size, the kidneys are generally the length of three vertebrae in children over 1 year of age. By adulthood, the kidneys reach the length of approximately two and a half vertebrae.

FIGURE 5-9 Radiographic appearance of a normal abdomen, demonstrating kidney shadows, liver shadow, psoas muscles, and transverse processes of the lumbar spine.

FIGURE 5-10 A left lateral decubitus abdomen demonstrating free air over the dome of the liver.

Few, if any, air–fluid levels are present in the normal patient who is radiographed in the erect position. Limited fluid levels in the small bowel and large bowel, however, may be considered normal. Fluid levels are abnormal when they are seen in dilated bowel loops or when they are numerous. The intestinal gas pattern may be confusing to the diagnostician. In infants and children, gas may be scattered throughout the bowel, but in adults gas is normally seen only in the stomach and colon. Small bowel gas in an adult, therefore, may indicate a pathologic process. In some patients, gas may be recognizable only on erect radiographs because of the presence of intraluminal fluid. Free air should not be visible in the peritoneal cavity and is indicative of a bowel perforation or other pathologic entities that introduce air into the peritoneum. Erect abdominal radiographs must include the diaphragm to assess for free air, and in instances in which the patient is unable to stand, a left lateral decubitus abdomen should be obtained (Fig. 5-10).

Gastrointestinal System. Some contents of the abdomen can be seen without contrast media, as explained earlier. However, most of the GI tract cannot be examined directly. The internal surfaces of both ends can be visualized through endoscopy, the use of lighted instruments with optics to visualize disease of the esophagus, stomach and duodenum, rectum and distal colon, and, occasionally, the terminal ileum. Endoscopy allows abnormal areas to be visualized, biopsied, and examined histologically. Computed tomographic (CT) colonoscopy is becoming more common in health care as the technology continues to improve and allows for more detailed studies. Virtual endoscopic studies are less invasive than conventional endoscopic procedures and provide greater patient comfort.

Radiographic investigation of the GI system is commonly a combination of fluoroscopy and radiography. Fluoroscopy provides dynamic information, whereas radiography provides a permanent static record of the examination. Fluoroscopic examination of the GI system requires positive and negative contrast agents for visualization of body parts. Barium sulfate is generally used as the positive contrast agent but is contraindicated in cases of GI tract perforation. If a perforated bowel is suspected, a water-soluble contrast agent should be used. Although infrequently used alone, a negative contrast agent (e.g., air or carbon dioxide) may be used to distend the stomach and bowel for better visualization of the mucosal lining. A combination of both positive and negative contrast agents is commonly used so that the thicker barium sulfate adheres to the mucosa while the carbon dioxide expands the stomach or bowel, thus allowing optimal visualization of small variances in the walls of the GI organs.

Esophagus. Most upper GI studies begin with the patient in the erect position to evaluate air and fluid levels in the alimentary tract. An esophageal or barium swallow study may be performed to demonstrate anomalies and abnormalities of the esophagus. Transport of the food or liquid bolus through swallowing is the sole function of the esophagus and is accomplished by gravity and peristalsis. If it is studied as part of a GI tract examination, thin barium sulfate may be used. Thick barium sulfate is used if the esophagus is the only object of study. Barium sulfate tablets may also be administered to patients who complain that food seems to be getting stuck after swallowing. The chief complaint from most patients undergoing a traditional esophagram is **dysphagia,** or difficulty swallowing. The causes for dysphagia are numerous and are discussed later in this chapter.

During fluoroscopy, the radiologist is able to visualize mechanical problems presented while the patient is swallowing the barium sulfate mixture. When assessing motor disorders such as achalasia or cricopharyngeal spasms the barium swallow may be recorded for dynamic viewing. For patients with motor disorders, care needs to be taken to avoid aspiration of the barium sulfate into the bronchus, which could lead to aspiration pneumonia.

Stomach. One common radiologic procedure of the GI tract is an "upper GI," in which barium sulfate flows from the esophagus and into the stomach and small bowel. Once the barium reaches the stomach, the radiologist evaluates the stomach contour, position, and rugae and the

FIGURE 5-11 Normal stomach as seen on this radiograph of an 18-year-old man.

peristaltic changes occurring as the stomach fills and empties.

If the radiologist wishes to diminish peristalsis, glucagon is given to relax the stomach musculature. In many instances, a gas-producing substance (carbon dioxide crystals) is used with barium sulfate to produce a double-contrast examination. The purpose is to expand the stomach and promote coating of the stomach mucosa. The duodenal bulb is studied as it fills with barium sulfate and empties into the small bowel. Compression may be used for better visualization of specific anatomic areas of the upper GI tract.

A series of images are obtained during or after fluoroscopy, with the projections differing from one institution to another. Typical patient positions include recumbent posteroanterior (PA) projection to demonstrate the entire stomach and duodenal bulb, right anterior oblique (RAO) to highlight the pyloric canal and duodenal bulb (Fig. 5-11), right lateral to show the duodenal bulb, duodenal loop, and retrogastric space, and left posterior oblique (LPO) to demonstrate the gastric fundus. Proper positioning relates significantly to the patient's body habitus. Generally, the more hypersthenic a patient is, the higher and more transverse the stomach tends to lie. For other body habitus (i.e., sthenic, hyposthenic, and asthenic), the stomach is more J-shaped, lying lower and closer to the spine.

Small Bowel. In some instances, the barium sulfate mixture may be followed as it progresses through the small intestines. Radiographs are exposed at set intervals to determine GI motility and to demonstrate abnormalities within the small bowel. Once the contrast agent reaches the ileocecal valve, the small bowel study is complete, typically within 2 to 3 hours (Fig. 5-12).

The small intestines may also be studied radiographically by means of enteroclysis, a small-bowel enema. This is accomplished by advancing an intestinal tube through the patient's mouth to the end of the duodenum at the ligament of Treitz. Contrast agents, both positive and negative (barium sulfate and methylcellulose, respectively), are directly injected into the small bowel.

Large Bowel. The lower GI tract is examined by administering a barium enema through the rectum. This examination demonstrates abnormalities of the large bowel and intraluminal neoplasms. The barium enema is performed in a single-contrast fashion with only barium or as a double-contrast study using barium sulfate in combination with a negative contrast agent (e.g., air). The negative contrast agent distends the lumen, allowing improved visualization of the mucosal lining (Fig. 5-13), especially small polyps and intraluminal tumors. In either case, the radiologist typically obtains a series of images during fluoroscopy, with the patient in various positions to highlight certain areas of the colon (e.g., flexures). The radiographer may also expose a series of radiographs of the contrast-enhanced large bowel per the radiologist's instructions (Fig. 5-14). After evacuation of the barium sulfate mixture, the radiographer will obtain a "postevacuation" radiograph to visualize colon contraction and to demonstrate the mucosa.

Abdominal radiography may often depict abnormalities in patients with known inflammatory bowel disease (IBD). Since negative findings will rarely preclude the need for further imaging studies, radiography typically is reserved for evaluating the presence of obstruction, perforation, or toxic colon distention associated with

B

FIGURE 5-12 A, Small-bowel radiograph demonstrating barium filled terminal ileum. **B,** Spot image demonstrating ileocecal junction.

advanced disease. Although small bowel barium studies were, at one point, the primary method for diagnosing suspected IBD cases, the introduction of capsule endoscopy is playing an increasingly larger role in making the initial diagnosis.

FIGURE 5-13 Normal air-contrast enema as demonstrated on this anteroposterior projection.

FIGURE 5-14 Normal air contrast barium enema as demonstrated on this left lateral decubitus posteroanterior projection.

If a patient has had a surgical enterostomy procedure, the contrast medium may be administered through the opening in the abdominal wall to the specific area of the GI system. A **colostomy** is a procedure in which a stoma is surgically created on the abdominal wall to allow drainage of bowel contents into a closed pouch hung outside the body. Those in the sigmoid and descending colon are most frequently placed because of rectal or sigmoid cancer. Those placed in the transverse or ascending colon are often for indications that allow the colostomy to be placed for temporary purposes for diversion of flow of colonic contents (e.g., sigmoid diverticulitis, rectovaginal fistula, colon obstruction).

An **ileostomy** is a similar opening but is placed from the ileum, with the most common indication being ulcerative colitis. As with colostomies, patient problems with ileostomies include proper skin protection and odor control. Proper fit of the appliance for drainage is essential to prevent problems caused by excoriating digestive enzymes. Other enterostomies (i.e., jejunostomies and duodenostomies) are more rarely used, and only under very specific circumstances because of the loss of electrolytes that occurs before their absorption through the small bowel. Affected patients often require total parenteral nutrition to maintain life.

If a patient has had a surgical enterostomy procedure, the contrast agent may be administered through the opening in the abdominal wall to the specific area of the GI system (Fig. 5-15). Special care needs to be taken when imaging the patient with some types of stoma because this area can be particularly sensitive.

Computed Tomography

CT is an important modality in abdominal survey as well as in the examination of the GI system. Because CT can visualize small differences in tissue density, it clearly demonstrates abdominal organs, which are normally not apparent on conventional abdominal radiographs without the use of contrast, resulting in good visualization of structure in the upper abdomen close to the diaphragm.

On CT examination, the liver, spleen, pancreas, and kidneys appear as homogeneous soft tissue densities, making any alteration in the density resulting from pathologic conditions

FIGURE 5-15 A, Barium enema via a colostomy demonstrating enema tip within the ostomy. **B** and **C,** Spot images demonstrating administration of barium sulfate via the ostomy.

readily visible, even without contrast media. Abscesses and solid and cystic masses all have a respective range of densities between that of water and normal soft tissue densities. CT is also quite useful in the evaluation of retroperitoneal pathologies such as lymph node enlargement resulting from neoplastic disease or infection. In combination with conventional abdominal radiography, CT of the abdomen is recommended when a bowel obstruction is suspected. Finally, it has become the accepted modality for following the progress of GI malignancies and also plays a role in the diagnosis of inflammatory conditions (e.g., abscess). CT of the colon is commonly performed to evaluate neoplastic disease, diverticulitis, and appendicitis. It has the capability of locating the exact site of neoplasms and allowing the clinician to measure the size of the tumor and the presence of infiltration into surrounding tissues. It is also useful in planning radiation therapy protocols. An increase in the availability of CT dose reduction techniques is resulting in a decrease in associated radiation exposure levels.

Routine CT examination of the abdomen requires good opacification of the bowel and vascular structures because poorly opacified bowel loops may be mistaken for abdominal masses. Patients must be given an oral contrast agent approximately 45 minutes to 1 hour before abdominal CT scanning. This time allows the contrast agent to reach the distal ileum before examination. Contrast agents may also be administered rectally, depending on the anatomic structures to be imaged.

Multidetector CT (MDCT) units, in combination with oral contrast and gas distention of the colon, have the capability to perform a noninvasive endoscopic procedure called *virtual colonoscopy* (or CT colonography). This technique produces two-dimensional (2-D) and three-dimensional (3-D) images of the colon, thus enabling the radiologist and endoscopist to view anatomic landmarks and structures that may not be seen with conventional colonoscopy. This, in turn, can reduce risk and discomfort to the patient. This application is a benefit to those who may not be able to or choose not to have a traditional colonoscopy procedure, which remains the gold standard for detection of smaller polyps. Additionally, virtual colonoscopy has a high sensitivity for detection of polyps greater than 10 mm as well as lesions that may be missed with fecal blood tests, barium enemas, and sigmoidoscopy. However, it is important to note that residual stool may cause problems with accuracy of image reconstruction, potentially simulating pathology such as polyps or masses.

CT enterography is also an increasingly used technique, in which optimal visualization of the small bowel mucosa is attained through use of MDCT scanners. For these examinations, patients are given large volumes (approximately 1350 mL) of 0.1% barium sulfate prior to imaging. Additionally, for certain indications such as obscure GI bleeding, small bowel tumors, and chronic ischemia, a biphasic contrast-enhanced study may be performed. Because of the ability to acquire both intraluminal and extraluminal information of the entire GI tract in a noninvasive manner, techniques such as CT enterography and CT colonography are quickly supplanting the standard small bowel series and barium enema examinations.

Magnetic Resonance Imaging

The role of magnetic resonance imaging (MRI) in the abdomen has expanded as a result of faster sequences and shorter scan times. Evaluation of the GI tract is still limited by bowel motion; however, MRI is useful in demonstrating the presence of retroperitoneal masses impinging on the GI system. Breath-hold imaging in MRI allows the technologist to visualize abdominal organs in a matter of seconds (Fig. 5-16). A few different imaging sequences are used to differentiate between normal tissue and pathology. The most common of the imaging sequences are T1-weighted images for optimal visualization of anatomic structures and T2-weighted images for optimal visualization of diseased tissues. Three-dimensional contrast-enhanced magnetic resonance angiography (MRA) is also used in imaging of the arterial vessels of the abdomen.

For imaging of the small bowel, magnetic resonance enterography (MRE) is gradually being incorporated into routine clinical practice

FIGURE 5-16 A T2-weighted coronal breath-hold magnetic resonance image of the abdomen.

as published literature highlighting the benefits of its use are becoming more prevalent. Because of its ability to display both intraluminal and extraluminal information, similar to that of CT, MRE is often the preferred imaging modality for pediatric populations as well as pregnant women, in whom radiation exposure is of high concern. MRE has the ability to demonstrate areas of active bowel inflammation as well as complications such as bowel obstruction, fistulas, and abscesses. Furthermore, MRE sequences have the ability to depict bowel motility, which is a potential advantage when attempting to distinguish between fixed and transient segments of luminal narrowing. Subsequently, sequences can be repeated to capture various vascular phases, reassess abnormal bowel segments, or improve image quality without increasing the radiation risk to the patient. The examination is performed by having the patient ingest 1 to 2 liters (L) of a 0.1% barium suspension containing sorbitol, prior to MRE of the abdomen. Use of this agent produces high signal intensity in the bowel lumen on T2-weighted images and low signal intensity in the lumen on T1-weighted images. The "dark lumen" appearance that results with the administration of the contrast is critical for the detection of mural enhancement on postcontrast T1-weighted images, which rarely can be achieved through use of water alone.

Sonography

Sonography is occasionally useful in imaging the GI system, although successful examination is highly dependent on the skill of the operator. When water is used as a contrast agent, it can be highly successful in imaging gastric emptying, gastroesophageal reflux disease (GERD), and duodenal abnormalities. More commonly, however, it is used to image the retroperitoneum because of the flexibility of angling the transducer to image that region. The aorta, kidneys, lymph nodes, and adrenal glands are subject to a variety of abnormalities, and with ultrasound it is possible to image behind the bowel and assess for abnormalities.

Most commonly used in the evaluation of appendicitis, graded compression ultrasonography is a technique performed using a 5 or 7 megahertz (MHz) linear transducer to firmly compress the anterior abdominal wall, displacing normal bowel loops in an effort to locate a potentially inflamed appendix.

Nuclear Medicine Procedures

In nuclear medicine, GI bleed scans, which are quick, noninvasive procedures useful in demonstrating GI bleeding, direct angiographers to the site of bleeding if therapeutic intervention is to be performed. This is accomplished by labeling either using technetium-99m (Tc-99m) to label red blood cells (RBCs) or Tc-99m–labeled colloid to identify the origin of the bleed. Tc-99m is a short-lived (half-life of about 6 hours) nuclear isomer that emits β-rays, enabling its use as a contrast agent. Active bleeding sites are identified through evaluation of focal areas of the tracers that conform to the bowel anatomy, increase with time, and move with peristalsis. This study is typically performed in patients with significant hemorrhage and an unprepared bowel, in whom endoscopic evaluation is not optimal.

Gastric emptying scans are used to assess the rate food exits the stomach into the duodenum. The examination is performed by having the patient consume either a solid or liquid radiolabeled meal and then observed via a gamma camera as it passes out of the stomach. Typically, a high level of radioactivity maintained within the stomach after an extended period would indicate poor gastric emptying (Fig. 5-17). In addition, the test may also be used to monitor the response of promotility drug treatments such as that of metoclopramide or erythromycin. One drawback of the test is that it cannot differentiate between physical obstruction and gastroparesis; that is, further diagnostic studies will often need to be ordered if the patient exhibits a delay in gastric emptying.

Urea breath tests are performed on patients with gastric ulcers to identify the presence of *Helicobacter pylori*. Infection with this bacterial

FIGURE 5-17 A nuclear medicine gastric emptying scan demonstrates a marked delay in emptying of the stomach.

FIGURE 5-18 A positron emission tomography (PET) scan for staging of colon cancer demonstrates new hypermetabolic activity of metastatic disease in the liver and right hemithorax.

species is a common cause of gastric ulcers and can be treated quite effectively with antibiotic therapy. The procedure begins by having the patient drink radioactive urea. If the bacteria are present in the stomach, they will break down the urea, and the patient will release radioactive carbon dioxide. This is captured in the breath test.

Meckel scans can also be utilized in identifying ectopic gastric mucosa as in a Meckel diverticulum. This is accomplished through injection of Tc-99m pertechnetate, which is taken up by mucus-secreting cells of the gastric mucosa. Focal uptake outside of the stomach and in the small bowel would be positive for the pathologic condition.

Positron emission tomography (PET) may be used to evaluate and stage GI cancers (Fig. 5-18). PET has been proven to demonstrate approximately 20% of esophageal cancerous lesions (Fig. 5-19) undetected by CT.

Endoscopic Procedures

As noted earlier, **endoscopy** is the use of tubular fiberoptic devices to look inside the GI tract and other hollow organs or cavities of the body. As its sophistication and specificity have increased,

it is assuming a greater role in diagnosis and therapy of the GI tract. Upper endoscopy is capable of seeing down into the esophagus, stomach, duodenum (including the ampulla of Vater), and even the proximal jejunum. Colonoscopy allows retrograde visualization of the rectum as far as the terminal ileum. The small bowel is still largely out of reach through endoscopy; however, the advent of capsule endoscopy, which involves the ingestion of a small camera pill, has resulted in its increased use in the diagnosis of small bowel tumors. The capsule encases a digital camera that transmits images to a recording device worn on a belt. The capsule has a gastric transit time of approximately 1 hour and small-bowel transit time of 3 to 4 hours. This technology is indicated in diagnosis of obscure GI bleeding, which is often caused by a lesion. This technology, however, has several drawbacks such as inability to identify the precise location of pathology, inability to biopsy or treat located pathology, and lack of reimbursement by insurance companies. The only contraindication

FIGURE 5-19 A positron emission tomography (PET) scan (**A,** frontal; **B,** lateral; **C,** oblique) of a patient with known esophageal cancer ordered for staging of the disease. Hypermetabolic focal activity is demonstrated at the level of the gastroesophageal junction designating the primary tumor and in the upper thoracic spine, right lobe of the liver, and left lung suggesting metastatic disease.

FIGURE 5-20 Endoscopic image of a sigmoid colon mass in a 72-year-old woman; the mass is seen bulging into the lumen of the colon.

to performing capsule endoscopy is a bowel obstruction. Photographic views of the interior of the body provide readily diagnosable information (Figs. 5-20 and 5-21). Therapeutic applications of endoscopy are numerous. They include polyp removal, injection and thermal methods to stop hemorrhaging, sclerosing and banding of esophageal varices, lesion biopsy, sealing of tracheoesophageal fistulas, stone removal, esophageal prosthesis insertion, and laser tumor removal (both generally for palliative purposes). In addition, enteric wall stents have been used to open the lesions in nonoperative malignancies of the colon.

Abdominal Tubes and Catheters

As with the chest, a variety of tubes and catheters can be placed within particular portions of the abdomen. The technologist must be familiar with each type of tube and exercise great caution in attempting to move patients with abdominal

tubes in place. The technologist should also ask the patient's nurse or consult the chart before altering the patient's position. In addition, some abdominal tubes and catheters allow entry into body systems that are normally sterile and require special care to avoid infection.

Gastric tubes may be placed (generally through the nose) for a variety of diagnostic and therapeutic purposes. They may be indicated for aspiration of gastric contents to help control nausea and vomiting, for decompression and removal of gastric contents because of bowel dysfunction or surgery, and for nutritional support tube feedings (gastric gavage) or medication administration. The Levin tube is the most common nasogastric (NG) tube. It is a fairly small, single-lumen tube with a plain tip, and it may be visualized radiographically. Proper placement is commonly assessed through aspiration of gastric juices and listening for proper placement within the stomach via a stethoscope. If an NG tube is placed for feeding, the patient's head must remain elevated

FIGURE 5-21 Endoscopic image of diffuse colitis with a bacterial cause in this 40-year-old man, indicated by the splotchiness of the bowel mucosa.

to prevent the tube from becoming displaced, leading to aspiration of the gastric contents. If an emergent condition exists that requires large amounts of gastric contents to be aspirated quickly (gastric lavage), the Ewald tube or the Edlich tube may be used. These tubes are placed through the mouth, are wider than the Levin tube, and contain several openings that allow quicker aspiration. The Levacuator tube may also be used for evacuation of gastric contents. This is a wide, double-lumen tube placed through the patient's mouth. The larger lumen is used for gastric lavage, and the smaller lumen allows instillation of an irrigant.

An enteral tube is a small-caliber tube used to deliver a liquid diet directly to the duodenum or jejunum. It most commonly has a weighted end to hold the tube in the proper placement. The Dobhoff tube is a common radiopaque enteral tube (Fig. 5-22). Other common types of prolonged enteral tubes include the Corpak tube and the Entriflex tube.

Nasoenteric decompression tubes are used to remove gas and fluids in the prevention and treatment of abdominal distention. At one end, these tubes have a balloon or rubber bag filled with air, mercury, or water to stimulate peristalsis and facilitate passage through the pylorus into the intestinal tract. The Miller-Abbott tube is a common type of double-lumen decompression tube. It is passed through the nose, pharynx, and esophagus with the balloon uninflated. Once the end of the tube reaches the stomach, the balloon is inflated and the tube is pulled back until it stops at the cardiac sphincter. The patient is then placed on his or her right side in the semierect position, and the air is withdrawn from the balloon and replaced with mercury. Progress of the tube is assessed by taking abdominal radiographs at regular intervals. The Harris and Cantor tubes are other types of decompression tubes. Unlike the Miller-Abbott tube, however, the Cantor tube (Fig. 5-23) and the Harris tube contain a single lumen.

The Levin tube or the Foley catheter may also be surgically placed in any portion of the GI system. A gastrostomy tube, as the name indicates, is a tube placed through the wall of the

FIGURE 5-23 Radiographic appearance of the Cantor tube in this 50-year-old man with a mechanical bowel obstruction. Approximately 4 hours after placement, it has advanced into the second portion of the duodenum.

FIGURE 5-22 A, Supine abdominal radiograph demonstrating Dobhoff tube reaching to the fourth segment of the duodenum (ligament of Treitz). **B,** Semierect abdominal radiograph demonstrating Dobhoff tube placement in same patient.

stomach, whereas a duodenostomy tube or jejunostomy tube is specific to that portion of the small intestine. A percutaneous endoscopic gastrostomy tube is frequently placed endoscopically. These tubes provide a direct route for administering liquid feedings.

CONGENITAL AND HEREDITARY ANOMALIES

Esophageal Atresia

Atresia is a congenital absence or closure of a normal body orifice or tubular organ. Esophageal atresia is a rare congenital anomaly in which the esophagus fails to develop past some point, resulting in discontinuation of the esophagus (Fig. 5-24). This anomaly is caused by a defect in cell differentiation of the trachea and esophagus during the fourth to sixth week of embryonic development. The symptoms of esophageal atresia are visible soon after birth and include excessive salivation, choking, gagging, dyspnea, and cyanosis. Diagnosis of this congenital anomaly may be established by inability to pass an NG tube into the stomach. If a radiopaque NG tube is used, the terminal end of the pouch may be demonstrated radiographically with a chest radiograph without the use of a contrast agent. Immediate surgery is required to alleviate the problem, and preoperative care must be taken to prevent aspiration pneumonia. The

FIGURE 5-24 Lateral neck image following injection of barium sulfate demonstrating esophageal atresia.

infant may not receive oral feedings, and continuous suction is necessary to prevent aspiration. Under most circumstances, this increased risk of aspiration contraindicates the use of a contrast agent to visualize the extent of the atresia.

Usually, a tracheoesophageal fistula is coincident with atresia (Fig. 5-25). This consists of an atresia at the level of the fourth thoracic vertebra with a fistula—an abnormal tubelike passage from one structure to another—to the trachea (Fig. 5-26). In addition, a gastrostomy tube may be placed in the infant's stomach to prevent reflux of gastric secretions into the trachea through the fistula. Such a condition is incompatible with life for more than 2 to 3 days, but the prognosis is good if the infant is handled appropriately before surgery to prevent aspiration.

Bowel Atresia

Ileal atresia, a congenital discontinuation of the ileum, is the most frequent type of bowel atresia, followed by duodenal atresia. This anomaly manifests a few days after birth. The most common signs and symptoms of ileal atresia are abdominal distention and the inability of the infant to pass stool. Eventually, the infant regurgitates feedings. Treatment consists of surgery to resect the atretic portion of the bowel and reconnect the bowel proximal and distal to the discontinuation. In some cases, the proximal ileum may be grossly dilated, necessitating a double-barrel

FIGURE 5-25 Five types of esophageal atresia and tracheoesophageal fistulae.

FIGURE 5-26 Lateral view of the chest on a 1-day-old premature infant demonstrates distention of the distal esophagus with air and discontinuity with the trachea. Marked gastric distention is also present. Appearance is consistent with esophageal atresia and a tracheoesophageal fistula.

ileostomy. Once the lumen of the proximal ileum returns to a more normal size, the ileostomy is reversed, and bowel anastomosis can be performed.

Duodenal atresia is a congenital anomaly in which the lumen of the duodenum does not exist, resulting in complete obstruction of the GI tract at the duodenum. In some cases, the atresia may be identified before the birth of the infant with the use of sonography. Sonographic evaluation of the fetus should demonstrate a normal stomach with amniotic fluid coursing through it. Atresia is suggested on sonography if a dilated stomach is noted without other fluid collections noted in the fetal abdomen. Although rare (one in approximately 20,000 births), it is evident soon after birth when vomiting begins and the epigastrium becomes distended. A radiographic indication of duodenal atresia is the "double bubble sign."

Gaseous distention of the stomach creates one bubble, and gas in the proximal duodenum creates a second bubble (Fig. 5-27). As with esophageal atresia, oral feedings should be withheld in infants with duodenal atresia. Nasogastric decompression of the stomach is indicated to prevent vomiting and possible aspiration of the gastric contents. Treatment consists of surgery to open the duodenum for connection to the pylorus. During surgery, it is common to examine the other areas of the small bowel and the large bowel for other sites of atresia and malrotation, which often accompany duodenal atresia.

Colonic atresia is a congenital failure of development of the distal rectum and anus, which may occur to a variable extent (Fig. 5-28). A frequent complication is fistula formation to the genitourinary system (Fig. 5-29), which often can be repaired surgically. Prognosis is excellent after surgical intervention for all three types of bowel atresia.

Imperforate anus or **anal agenesis** is a congenital disorder in which anal opening to the exterior is absent. A fistula may be present between the colon and the perineum or the urethra in boys or between the colon and the vagina in girls. This condition can be demonstrated radiographically with a cross-table lateral rectum projection with the patient lying prone or by performing a fistulogram. It is corrected surgically shortly after birth and may require a temporary colostomy.

Hypertrophic Pyloric Stenosis

Hypertrophic pyloric stenosis (HPS) is a congenital anomaly of the stomach in which the pyloric canal leading out of the stomach is greatly narrowed because of hypertrophy and hyperplasia of the pyloric sphincter (Fig. 5-30). It is the most common indication for surgery in infants. Its exact cause is unknown, but it seems to be genetically related. Current literature suggests that infants born to mothers with a history of pyloric stenosis, or instances of increased gastrin secretion by the mother within the third trimester of pregnancy, may increase the probability of HPS occurring in the infant. Researchers believe the

FIGURE 5-27 A, Marked distention of the stomach and duodenal bulb with bowel gas distal to the duodenum. Visualization of the classic "double bubble sign" indicates duodenal atresia. **B,** The "double bubble sign" in a lateral projection of the same 1-day-old infant.

muscle mass is stimulated by the transforming growth factor-alpha (TGF-α) and the nerves within the muscular layer are not functioning properly. HPS occurs more frequently in whites than in blacks or Asians, four times more often in male children (1 in 200), and most often in first-born male children. HPS is typically suggested by projectile bile-free emesis in a previously healthy infant around 2 to 6 weeks of age. Affected infants often become dehydrated and fail to gain weight. It is most commonly confused with pylorospasm, which, in contrast, is an incomplete obstruction to fluid flow into the duodenal bulb resulting from spasmodic changes in pyloric muscle tone.

When the classic "olive" sign of hypertrophied pyloric muscle is palpated, the diagnosis of HPS can be made clinically, and the patient can be sent to surgery without the need for imaging examinations. Accurate measurements of pyloric muscle thickening are useful in surgical planning, even when the diagnosis is clinically evident.

When no "olive" is palpated, imaging by radiography, sonography, fluoroscopic upper GI (UGI) series, or a combination of all these modalities can be performed for initial diagnosis.

Abdominal radiography may show gastric distention with HPS. On occasion, a mass impression of the thickened pyloric muscle on an air-filled gastric antrum may be noted; however, initial radiography is usually limited to determining a strategy for further workup.

Sonography has become the standard and highly accurate method for diagnosing HPS without the need for radiation exposure. It allows imaging of the pyloric muscle and channel, and the constant imaging of an elongated, thick-walled pylorus indicative of HPS. Prolonged sonographic observation of the passage of gastric contents may be tedious but helps avoid surgery in cases simulating HPS. Measurements of pyloric channel length, pyloric diameter, and muscle thickness are often used for diagnosis. Abnormal muscle wall thicknesses can range from 4.8 +/–

FIGURE 5-30 A thin column of barium flowing from the stomach into the pylorus in this 1-month-old boy with projectile vomiting indicates hypertrophic pyloric stenosis.

FIGURE 5-28 Spot image demonstrating imperforate anus in a pediatric patient.

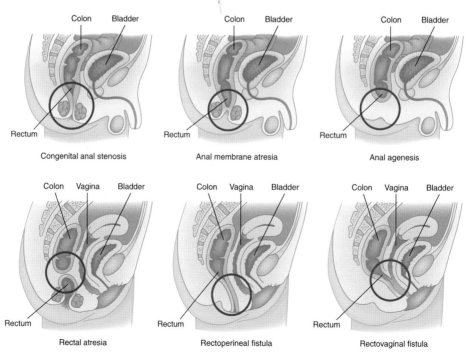

FIGURE 5-29 Anorectal stenosis and imperforate anus.

0.6 mm in HPS patients, compared with 1.8 +/– 0.4 mm in normal persons.

An upper GI study demonstrates delayed gastric emptying accompanied by the mass impression of the hypertrophied pyloric muscle on the barium-filled antrum ("shoulder sign"), the filling of the proximal pylorus ("beak sign"), or the entire elongated pylorus ("string sign") as barium trickles through the narrowed pyloric canal. However, because of delayed gastric emptying in cases of HPS, the demonstration of the beak and string signs may be difficult to detect, requiring considerable fluoroscopic time, as well as an increased radiation risk to the patient.

Scintigraphy is seldom indicated but may provide useful information about gastric emptying if other tests fail to reveal any. Furthermore, delayed images in standard positions allow scintigraphy to assess gastric transit without additional radiation exposure. Delayed gastric emptying has been defined as more than 50% retained labeled liquid within the stomach after 120 minutes in children younger than 2 years of age.

A surgical pyloromyotomy procedure is used to incise the hypertrophied muscle fibers and thus increase the opening of the pyloric channel. Affected infants generally are able to begin normal feedings within a few days after the surgical procedure. Pylorospasm is said to be the most common cause of gastric outlet obstruction in pediatrics and, unlike HPS, it is treated conservatively.

Malrotation

Aberrations in the normal process of intestinal rotation in utero may result in the anomalous position of the small bowel and the large bowel, with abnormal fixations predisposing the patient to internal herniation and volvulus. Malrotation exists when the intestines are not in their normal position (Fig. 5-31), which occurs in an equal male-to-female ratio. Varying degrees of malrotation of the intestinal tract exist, ranging from failure of fixation of the cecum in the RLQ to complete transposition of the bowel, a condition

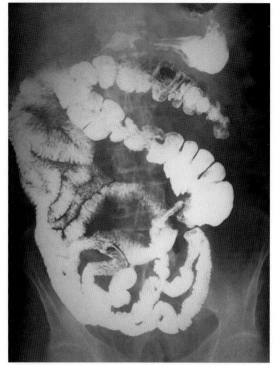

FIGURE 5-31 Malrotation of the bowel indicated by the position of the small bowel on the right side of the abdomen and the colon on the left. Note how the terminal ileum enters the cecum from the right.

in which the small bowel is on the right and the colon is on the left.

When malrotation is suspected in an infant with bilious vomiting, a UGI series should be the examination of choice and is considered the gold standard. During the examination, the focus is on following the initial column of oral contrast media through the upper GI system. Evaluation is made of any deviation in the normal route through the duodenum from right to left of midline, as well as its turn upward to the height of the duodenal bulb to the area of the ligament of Treitz. This is also referred to as the *duodenojejunal flexure*. Additionally, a UGI study may demonstrate a high greater curvature, a greater curvature crossing the esophagus, a downward-pointing pylorus, two air–fluid levels, or a lowering of the gastric fundus, all of which are suggestive of gastric torsion, commonly associated with malrotation of the bowel. A barium enema examination may also be useful in evaluating the location of the cecum, which is normally located in the RLQ of the abdomen. Such errors of fixation are often asymptomatic, but they may lead to bowel volvulus or incarceration of bowel in an internal hernia.

Sonography is useful as a complementary tool to confirm the diagnosis of malrotation, with demonstration of the position of the third part of the duodenum between the aorta and the superior mesenteric artery (SMA) in the transverse and sagittal planes. However, it is important to note that the obscuration of the entire course of the normal fluid-filled duodenum by overlying gas may limit the usefulness of sonography in the acute setting.

In some instances, the patient may have clinical signs of bowel obstruction, as discussed later in this chapter. Surgery is the choice for correction of a volvulus or bowel incarceration, with resection of the involved bowel to relieve the intestinal infarction. Complete reversal of all abdominal organs, although rare, is known as **situs inversus**.

Hirschsprung Disease (Congenital Aganglionic Megacolon)

Hirschsprung disease or **congenital aganglionic megacolon** refers to the absence of neurons (Meissner and Auerbach autonomic plexus) in the bowel wall, typically in the sigmoid colon. Occurring in approximately 1 in 5000 births, this defect is a familial disease, primarily affecting men. Although the exact cause of Hirschsprung disease is unknown, a link to inheritance of the "rearranged during transfection" (*RET*) proto-oncogene localized to chromosome 10 has been established. A malformation of the parasympathetic nervous system results in the absence of neurons in the bowel wall preventing the normal relaxation of the colon and subsequent peristalsis. This anomaly results in gross dilatation of the colon to the point of narrowing and constriction (Fig. 5-32).

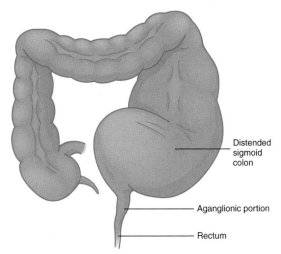

FIGURE 5-32 Congenital aganglionic megacolon.

This generally becomes apparent shortly after birth, when the affected infant passes little meconium and the abdomen becomes distended. As the patient ages, the continued effects are severe constipation and recurrent fecal impactions. It is important to diagnose this disease early because it can progress to toxic megacolon if left untreated. Toxic megacolon develops from bacterial overgrowth leading to fluid and electrolyte imbalances that could result in death.

Barium enemas demonstrate a transition from the narrow, distal rectum to a dilated proximal colon (Fig. 5-33). However, it should be noted that barium enema examination is strictly contraindicated in patients with known or suspected toxic megacolon. Initial treatment in an infant may consist of a temporary colostomy until surgical resection is possible later. In some cases, multiple surgeries may be performed during infancy to correct the anomaly.

Meckel Diverticulum

Meckel diverticulum is a congenital diverticulum of the distal ileum. This saclike anomaly is located within 6 feet of the ileocecal valve and is a remnant of a duct connecting the small bowel to the umbilicus in the fetus. Children with Meckel diverticulum often develop an ulcer in

FIGURE 5-33 Barium enema on a 6-day-old infant demonstrates a normal rectosigmoid leading to a distended large bowel consistent with Hirschsprung disease.

the adjacent bowel, and a common sign is repeated episodes of bleeding from the ulcerated site. Symptoms in adolescents and adults include cramping, vomiting, and bowel obstruction. The symptoms mimic those of appendicitis except for the location of the pain. Diagnosis of Meckel diverticulum is difficult, as it may not be visible on a radiograph of the small bowel. However, nuclear medicine Meckel scans are useful in diagnosing this anomaly by identifying ectopic gastric mucosa. This is accomplished through injection of Tc-99m pertechnetate, which is taken up by the mucus-secreting cells of the gastric mucosa. The treatment involves surgical resection of the diverticulum.

Gluten-Sensitive Enteropathy

Gluten-sensitive enteropathy, formally known as *celiac sprue* or *celiac disease*, is an autoimmune hereditary disorder involving increased sensitivity to the gliadin fraction of gluten, an agent found in wheat, barley, and rye products such as bread, which interferes with normal digestion and absorption of food through the small bowel. The gliadin acts as an antigen and combines with antibodies within the intestinal mucosa, which promotes the aggregation of K lymphocytes. These lymphocytes cause mucosal damage in combination with an increase in crypt cells within the mucosa. With such a condition, the bowel dilates, mucosal folds atrophy, and peristalsis slows or stops. Common symptoms include diarrhea, flatulence, weight loss, and abdominal distention. In addition, patients often present with nutritional deficiencies specific to the primary disease and the area of the GI system affected by the disorder.

Radiographic changes generally seen with gluten-sensitive enteropathy are segmentation of the barium column, flocculation (resembling tufts of cotton), and edematous mucosal changes (Fig. 5-34). Laboratory tests demonstrate low albumin, calcium, potassium, and sodium levels in combination with elevated alkaline phosphatase and prothrombin time. Diagnosis is usually confirmed by biopsy of the small bowel. Treatment of gluten-sensitive enteropathy consists of avoidance of substances containing gluten. Vitamin therapy is also used to ensure adequate amounts of nutrients that are not available because of malabsorption in the small bowel.

Carbohydrate Intolerance

Carbohydrate intolerance is the inability to digest certain carbohydrates, including lactose, because of an acquired lactase deficiency. This disorder affects approximately 60% of the nonwhite population and 20% to 30% of the white population. In this condition, the small bowel lacks enough of the enzyme lactase, which is used to break down lactose into simple sugars that can be absorbed. The result is that lactose stays in the bowel and acts as an osmotic agent, causing fluid to weep from the wall into the lumen of the colon, creating cramping and diarrhea. The

FIGURE 5-34 Gluten-sensitive enteropathy in a 15-year-old patient with a history of diarrhea, indicated on this small bowel study by dilated bowel loops, thickened folds, a grayish appearance of the barium (because of excess fluid in the bowel), and a delayed transit time.

diarrhea also leads to other nutritional deficiencies because the nutrients are purged before they can be absorbed through the intestinal mucosa. Lactose mixed with barium shows the barium moving quickly through the bowel and becoming diluted in the distal ileum and colon (Fig. 5-35). Patients affected by this condition avoid symptoms by abstaining from consumption of dairy products.

INFLAMMATORY DISEASES

Esophageal Strictures

Esophageal strictures may occur in varying degrees, with the symptoms displayed differing according to the amount of obstruction produced. Strictures may be secondary to the ingestion of caustic materials such as strong acids or alkalines (Fig. 5-36) or from any factor that inflames the mucosa and creates scarring. Common types of caustics include household cleansers and detergents containing sulfuric acid and sodium hydroxide. These caustic agents burn the esophagus and cause edema, swelling,

FIGURE 5-35 A, Abdominal distention, pain, and diarrhea led to this small bowel examination, diagnosed as normal for this 35-year-old patient. **B,** Mixing of lactose with barium on a repeat study led to mild bowel dilatation, rapid transit time, and dilution of barium in the distal small bowel, indicative of lactase insufficiency.

FIGURE 5-36 Longstanding esophageal stricture in a 78-year-old man caused by accidental ingestion of a caustic agent at age 3 years.

and possibly perforation. Endoscopy is usually performed to assess the damage to the esophagus, and the esophageal lesions are treated with corticosteroid therapy.

Strictures can be differentiated radiographically from normal peristalsis by their unchanging appearance; peristalsis is transitory. The mucosa of a benign stricture appears normal with a smooth contour; the contour of a malignant stricture typically appears ragged. Esophageal strictures require repeated dilation with special mercury-filled tubes of varying diameters to maintain proper patency. Common tubes for this purpose include the Hurst dilator and the Maloney dilator and pneumatic balloon dilators that are passed over a wire.

Gastroesophageal Reflux Disease

Gastroesophageal reflux disease (GERD) results from an incompetent cardiac sphincter, which allows the backward flow of gastric acid and contents into the esophagus. Reflux esophagitis is the primary cause of esophageal inflammation; however, reflux is not necessarily always abnormal. Heartburn, or symptomatic reflux, has been experienced by most people at one time or another. Furthermore, regurgitation, or gastroesophageal reflux, is common in the first 3 months of life and resolves in time. It usually has no definitive pathologic cause and is unrelated to a functional defect. It is only when the normal event lead to chronic symptoms and complications such as esophagitis, a stricture, or an esophageal ulcer that it becomes of concern.

To confirm the diagnosis of gastroesophageal reflux, esophageal manometry to determine the pressure in the upper and lower esophageal sphincters, pH monitoring of the esophagus, an acid perfusion (Bernstein) test, and esophagoscopy are performed, in addition to barium swallow and UGI procedures. Of the previously mentioned diagnostic examinations, the extended pH probe is considered the current gold standard. Imaging studies are performed primarily to prove the refluxing of gastric contents into the esophagus and to exclude any anatomic abnormalities. Depending on clinical circumstances, the degree of reflux based on number of events over a given period of time, the height of the refluxing column, the quality of the esophageal mucosa, and evidence of aspiration into the lungs are assessed and reported. It is important to note that reflux may often not be evident on a barium swallow. The associated sensitivity and specificity of UGI examinations range from 31% to 86%. The brief duration of the UGI series often results in false-negative results, whereas the frequent occurrence of nonpathologic reflux may result in false-positive results. Thus, the UGI series is not considered a useful test to reliably determine the presence or absence of GERD but more so to identify pathology such as ulcers and strictures caused by chronic irritation that may be associated with a predetermined diagnosis of GERD.

Reflux scintigraphy with Tc-99m–labeled sulfur colloid mixed with food has shown comparable sensitivity and specificity to that of barium studies in the diagnosis of GERD. Furthermore, nuclear medicine scintigraphy can be used over a prolonged time without increasing radiation exposure and at a lesser radiation dose than the UGI series. A 1-hour scintigraphic study formatted in 60-second frames provides a quantitative representation of postprandial GERD, particularly if gastric emptying is not rapid. The use of this study is typically limited to patients in whom other modalities have already identified an anatomic cause.

Sonographic diagnosis of reflux is made by noting water, which has been previously placed into the stomach, refluxing into the distal esophagus after tube removal. Because sonography typically demonstrates more episodes of reflux in comparison to a UGI series, some clinicians consider it too sensitive, and thus less specific, in diagnosing GERD. Sonography provides functional and morphologic information and therefore may be useful for identifying patients who should be referred for pH monitoring. Current literature suggests that color Doppler ultrasonography may be used in place of the more invasive pH-probe testing procedure.

Treatment includes elevating the head of the individual's bed and the patient avoiding drinks such as coffee or alcohol that stimulate acid secretion or foods such as chocolate that decrease sphincter competence. Smoking must be avoided because it also lowers sphincter competence. GERD is also treated with antacids to wash the gastric acids out of the esophagus and for pain relief and therapy with a variety of medicines such as histamine 2 blockers (H_2 blockers) to inhibit their production or prokinetic agents to enhance motility. Surgery as a treatment is the last option for those whose symptoms have failed to respond to medical therapy. It is performed using video-assisted laparoscopic techniques.

Peptic Ulcer

Normally, the GI system is protected by a mucosal barrier and epithelial cells that remove excess hydrogen ions. Mucosal blood flow also helps to remove excess acid, thus maintaining a normal

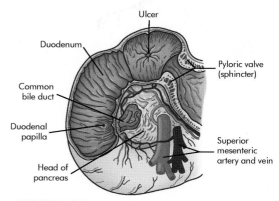

FIGURE 5-37 Common location of duodenal ulcer.

pH balance. A **peptic ulcer** is an erosion of the mucous membrane of the lower end of the esophagus, stomach, or duodenum (Fig. 5-37). The most likely site of a peptic ulcer is in the duodenal bulb and on the lesser curvature of the stomach. Duodenal ulcers are found in adults of all ages and are almost always benign. Gastric ulcers may affect individuals at any age but primarily those over 40 years of age.

Current studies suggest that peptic ulcers result from disruption of the normal mucosal defense and repair mechanisms. Nonsteroidal antiinflammatory drugs (NSAIDs) and the bacterium H. pylori alter the mucosa, making it more susceptible to the effects of acid normally residing in the GI tract. H. pylori is a gram-negative, spiral-shaped bacillus, which was identified in 1983. Researchers believe the H. pylori increases gastrin production, making the mucosa more susceptible to acid damage. NSAIDs inflame the mucosa because they are able to diffuse through the mucosa into the epithelium and damage the epithelial cells.

The main symptom of a gastric ulcer is pain, usually above the epigastrium and radiating to all parts of the abdomen. Food ingestion or antacids provide temporary relief, but the pain usually returns when the stomach is empty. In some patients, food may actually increase pain as it stimulates peristalsis, which irritates the ulcer. Symptoms of a duodenal ulcer are more consistent, and pain generally begins midmorning. The

FIGURE 5-38 A, Prone right anterior oblique projection of the duodenal bulb demonstrates a dense collection of barium in an ulcer crater, suggesting that it is on the anterior duodenal wall. **B,** Persistent collection of barium in the middle portion of the duodenal bulb indicating a superficial ulcer crater, with radiating folds extending from the ulceration. An incisura (fold) along the lower bulb margin points to the ulcer.

pain subsides with food ingestion but returns 2 to 3 hours later.

Diagnosis is made primarily via endoscopy. However, double-contrast radiographic GI studies may be performed. Intermittent healing in the midst of continuing inflammation leads to considerable scarring at the base of the ulcer. Gastric ulcers generally display as radiating, spikelike wheels of mucosal folds that run to the edge of the crater (Fig. 5-38). Seen en face, the edge of this ulcer appears round and regular (Fig. 5-39).

Ulcers are commonly treated with multidrug therapy in combination with a proton pump inhibitor. The drug regimen currently used is a combination of antibiotics and acid-blocking drugs. The most common drugs used to eradicate *H. pylori* include omeprazole or lansoprazole, clarithromycin, amoxicillin or metronidazole, and bismuth citrate or a proton pump inhibitor. Surgery is rarely performed and primarily is required only for complications of ulcers, for example, bleeding or perforation. Complications may include pneumoperitoneum or peritonitis if the ulcer perforates into the abdomen. Perforations are generally confirmed by CT evaluation or conventional erect abdominal radiography. Ulceration into an artery, which is the most common

FIGURE 5-39 A duodenal ulcer in a 25-year-old man, evidenced by a radiolucent ulcer crater resulting from the surrounding edema.

complication associated with ulcers, may produce life-threatening hemorrhage. Finally, the edema, spasm, and scarring produced by ulceration may result in bowel obstruction.

Gastroenteritis

A number of inflammatory disorders of the stomach and intestine fall into the general grouping

FIGURE 5-40 A, Air-filled, dilated small bowel loops seen on this abdominal radiograph are suggestive of an obstruction in this 30-year-old patient with abdominal pain, nausea, and vomiting. **B,** Barium readily refluxes from a barium enema into the distal ileum, demonstrating dilatation without obstruction. The dilatation was secondary to inflammation caused by gastroenteritis.

of **gastroenteritis,** inflammation of the mucosal lining of the stomach and small bowel (Fig. 5-40). Erosive gastritis appears to be a precursor to gastric ulcer formation and results from a compromised mucosal barrier within the stomach. Causes of erosive gastritis include ingestion of aspirin and other NSAIDs, alcohol, and steroids; physical stress or trauma; and viral or fungal infections. Acute gastric erosions heal rapidly once the cause is eliminated. Gastric erosions may be identified on double-contrast examinations of the stomach. Complete erosion appears as slitlike collections of barium surrounded by radiolucent halos of swollen, elevated mucosa. In some cases, scalloped or nodular antral folds may also be visualized. Antral gastritis appears to result from alcohol, smoking, and *H. pylori* infection. Radiographically, it is demonstrated by decreased distensibility of the antrum

in combination with thickened mucosal folds within the antrum, which tend to be oriented on its longitudinal axis and result in a narrowed antrum.

Ingestion of foods contaminated with *Salmonella* and other types of bacteria—most commonly, poultry, meat, dairy products, and eggs—may also result in gastroenteritis. Because of the methods used in the mass production of eggs, a dramatic increase in *Salmonella* infections occurred in the 1980s. Diarrhea results from mild mucosal ulcerations within the small bowel and the ability of the *Salmonella* bacteria to produce a secretory factor. This is a threat to the normal electrolytic balance of the body, with the diarrhea lasting 3 to 4 days. A good patient history often points out the offending agent, and treatment consists of proper fluid management and relief of nausea and vomiting.

Regional Enteritis (Crohn Disease)

Regional enteritis, also known as **Crohn disease (CD)** or **granulomatous colitis,** is a chronic IBD of unknown cause and is increasing in prevalence. Research indicates that affected individuals have a genetic predisposition for CD, with 10% to 20% of affected individuals having a positive family history. The discovery of the *NOD2/CARD15* gene on chromosome 16 has been indicated as a determinant in susceptibility to CD. Individuals with the disease are primarily affected by an unregulated intestinal immune response to various agents such as food or environmental factors, which results in crypt cell inflammation and abscesses, leading to the development of small ulcers. CD eventually affects all layers of the bowel wall. The bowel wall thickens in response to the inflammation and may form fistulas to adjacent loops of bowel, skin, or other abdominal viscera. CD typically occurs in the lower ileum but may be seen anywhere throughout the GI tract, from the mouth to the anus. The small bowel alone is affected in about a third of patients, the colon alone in 20% to 30% of patients, and combined involvement of the colon and the small bowel is seen in 40% to 50% of patients.

This disease has a bimodal distribution, with initial diagnosis being made in young adults of both sexes between the ages of 14 and 24 years as well as in older adults in their 50s and 60s, with presenting symptoms suggestive of appendicitis or acute bowel obstruction. Subsequent fibrotic scarring may give rise to mechanical obstruction of the bowel. The combination of mucosal edema and crisscrossing fine ulcerations gives the bowel a "cobblestone" appearance on the radiograph. The string sign (Fig. 5-41) is demonstrated when the terminal ileum is so diseased and stenotic that the barium mixture can only trickle through a small opening that looks like a string. Presentation of the disease in two or more areas with normal intervening bowel between is identified as "skip areas" (Fig. 5-42), thus the designation "regional" enteritis. Most cases involve both the ileum and the cecum

FIGURE 5-41 The string sign, demonstrating a diseased, stenotic terminal ileum.

(45%); however, it may be present only in the ileum (35%) or only in the colon (20%), and in rare cases, it may affect the entire small bowel. Regional enteritis is a chronic disease characterized by periods of exacerbation interspersed with periods of inactivity. In addition, these patients tend to have an increased chance of developing carcinoma of the bowel with a very poor prognosis. CD is classified as early stage, intermediate stage, or advanced stage, and the progression of the disease may be demonstrated radiographically by performing a small bowel series, enteroclysis, or a double-contrast barium enema.

The initial diagnosis of CD is based on a combination of clinical, laboratory, histologic, and imaging findings, with no single diagnostic test serving as the gold standard for reaching a diagnosis. Imaging is commonly used to distinguish CD from other conditions causing colitis through demonstration of small bowel involvement. Furthermore, imaging is also utilized to accurately assess the subtype of disease, location, and

FIGURE 5-42 A, Small bowel study demonstrating "skip areas" of normal bowel between diseased bowel in patient with regional enteritis (Crohn disease). **B,** Spot image demonstrating Crohn disease linear ulcerations. **C,** Endoscopic images of Crohn disease linear ulcerations.

severity to determine the appropriate treatment protocol. Radiology studies, traditionally, have played a smaller role in long-term surveillance of patients with known CD, but recent developments in imaging techniques hold promise for predicting disease activity and monitoring therapy.

Although abdominal radiography may often depict abnormalities in CD patients, it has a low predictive value of only 62%, making this modality a poor screening test for patients presenting with initial symptoms. Since negative findings will rarely preclude the need for further imaging studies, radiography typically is reserved for evaluating for the presence of obstruction, perforation, or toxic colon distention associated with advanced disease. Although small bowel barium studies were at one point the primary method for diagnosing CD, the introduction of capsule endoscopy is playing an increasingly larger role in making the initial diagnosis. However, a 5% incidence of capsule retention proximal to unsuspected bowel strictures often necessitates surgery for capsule removal, so imaging studies such as the small-bowel follow-through (SBFT) will often serve as a screening tool prior to capsule endoscopy examinations. When evaluating the colon for possible CD involvement, endoscopy is the preferred initial examination of the colon and is superior to barium enema in detecting early changes and initial diagnostic examination. The barium enema is typically reserved for patients with unsuccessful colonoscopies or those with contraindications such as anticoagulation therapy.

CT has traditionally been thought to only be useful in assessing extraenteric complications of CD such as fistulas or abscesses; however, the advent of CT enterography has shown promise for its use in the initial diagnosis of suspected CD. Through the use of a neutral enteric contrast to dilate the bowel loops, as well as intravenous (IV) contrast timed specifically to best display bowel wall enhancement, active disease can be identified by bowel wall thickening along with mural hyperenhancement. Furthermore, utilization of cross-sectional CT imaging provides better visualization of pelvic small bowel loops that can often be obscured by overlapping bowel during radiographic barium studies.

CT colonography (CTC) techniques are not usually indicated for the detection of CD since IV contrast is not typically administered and the blind administration of room air or carbon dioxide for colonic distention may be a contraindication in a severely inflamed colon (toxic megacolon). Furthermore, colonic cleansing, which is required for CTC, is not usually required for detecting inflammation by the enterography or enteroclysis technique.

Similarly to CT, contrast-enhanced MRI, utilizing fast imaging and MRE techniques, has the ability to optimize bowel distention and accurately display bowel wall changes in patients with early-stage CD. Additionally, specific characteristics related to bowel changes, including bowel wall thickening and mural hyperenhancement, as well as high T2 mural signal, can be visualized without the radiation concerns that are associated with CT. This is a definite benefit when considering pediatric populations, pregnant women, as well as patients receiving serial imaging.

Transabdominal sonography is capable of demonstrating the presence of CD through findings of bowel wall thickening greater than or equal to 4 to 5 mm, visualization of the "target" sign when seen in cross-section, and reduced or absent peristalsis in the affected loops. One potential drawback of this imaging approach is the high dependency on user ability, with sensitivity in diagnosing CD increasing from 75% to 87% as experience is gained by the machine operator.

Although nuclear medicine currently has little impact in the evaluation of patients with suspected CD, an increased interest in the role of Tc-99m white blood cell (WBC) imaging has been gaining ground as a possible superior imaging modality compared with contrast-based radiographic imaging. Tc-99m WBC scans seem to be ideally suited for obtaining a precise temporal snapshot of inflammatory distribution and intensity within the GI tract, in just a single examination. However, in instances in which patients present with inconspicuous signs suggestive of CD, as well as relatively normal laboratory results, a negative Tcm-99m WBC study may eliminate the need for further endoscopic investigation. In situations where patients already have a histologically confirmed diagnosis of CD, technetium hexamethyl propylene amine oxime (HMPAO)–labeled WBCs, with single proton emission computed tomography (SPECT) imaging, can be utilized to monitor chronic CD and assess disease activity. HMPAO-labeled leukoscintigraphy has several advantages over barium studies, including simultaneous examination of both the large bowel and the small bowel in a single patient encounter, lower radiation exposure, and higher patient acceptance.

Treatment of regional enteritis includes drug therapy to decrease inflammation, relieve diarrhea, and treat the infection. Bowel resection to remove the involved section of the intestine is necessary approximately 70% of the time,

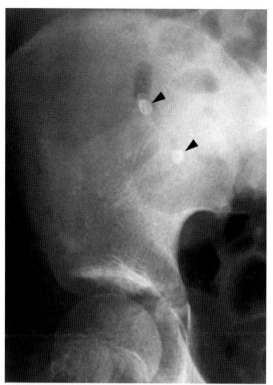

FIGURE 5-43 Fecalith within the appendix, a common cause of appendicitis.

particularly if perforation or hemorrhage is present. Recurrence of the disease in other areas of the bowel, however, is common. The disease is rarely cured, but rarely fatal.

Appendicitis

Appendicitis is an inflammation of the vermiform appendix resulting from an obstruction caused usually by a fecalith (Fig. 5-43) or rarely by a neoplasm. It is the most common abdominal surgical emergency in the United States. Appendicitis is most frequent in the late teens and 20s and has a fairly equal distribution between the sexes. Complications, usually resulting from gangrenous or perforated appendicitis, occur in approximately 3% to 5% of all cases. Delayed diagnosis and treatment of appendicitis account for much of the morbidity and mortality associated with this disease.

The obstruction leads to inflammation and distention and affects the blood supply to this portion of the bowel. Venous blood return is decreased, which, in turn, results in deoxygenation of the tissue. All of these factors leave the appendix susceptible to infection from bacteria such as *Escherichia coli*, which are normally found in the intestinal tract. Poor blood supply may also lead to gangrene, perforation, and possible rupture. Once the vermiform appendix ruptures, the infection spreads to the peritoneum, leading to general peritonitis that could result in death.

The signs and symptoms of appendicitis include initial pain in the epigastrium that moves to the RLQ and becomes persistent. Nausea and vomiting may occur as a reflex symptom because the vagus nerve supplies both the stomach and the appendix. Individuals also have low-grade fever, sudden onset of constipation, and an elevated WBC count. The elevation of WBCs helps distinguish appendicitis from other colicky abdominal disorders.

Many patients presenting with acute appendicitis may not require imaging, since the clinical presentation is often sufficient enough for a reliable diagnosis to indicate the need for surgical treatment. Conventional radiography is relatively limited in its value of diagnosing acute appendicitis. Furthermore, fluoroscopic examinations such as barium SBFT or barium enema are more often useful as a follow-up to cross-sectional imaging studies, to evaluate for other causes of RLQ pain, including small bowel obstruction, infectious ileitis, and IBD.

Currently, CT is the most accurate imaging modality for evaluating patients who do not have a clear clinical diagnosis of acute appendicitis (Fig. 5-44). The use of CT in demonstrating appendicitis has a sensitivity of 91% and specificity of 90%, with increased confidence in identifying the appendix when thinner slices and multiplanar reformatting of collected data is utilized. Both IV and rectal contrast enhancement, if utilized in adult patients, increase the accuracy of a CT assessment of RLQ pain. Sonography may be utilized as an alternative to

FIGURE 5-44 Computed tomography of abdomen and pelvis indicating appendicitis.

CT. Sonographic imaging has a sensitivity of 78% and specificity of 83% when used for diagnosing suspected appendicitis. Although CT has an overall higher accuracy, when a sonographic examination is conducted by an experienced sonographer, it is almost as effective as a CT procedure but without the risks of ionizing radiation. Thus, sonographic evaluation is preferred in children and pregnant women, especially when any questionable results are followed up by either CT or MRI (when available).

Because of slower acquisition time, higher cost, and relatively decreased availability in comparison with CT and sonography, MRI is yet to be utilized routinely for emergent diagnosis of this pathologic condition. Although nuclear medicine imaging with WBC scans can provide some useful information, its level of sensitivity and specificity is significantly inferior to that of CT, sonography, and MRI.

Surgical removal of the appendix is the most common treatment, and in cases of early surgical intervention, the mortality is low. However, complications such as abscess formation or perforation and peritonitis place the individual at a greater risk and greatly increase the recovery period.

Ulcerative Colitis

Ulcerative colitis is an inflammatory lesion of the colonic mucosa. Its cause is unknown, but it is thought to be an autoimmune disease. It is four times more common in whites, especially in Jewish persons of eastern European (Ashkenazi) descent, than in nonwhites. A familial tendency to develop this disease is believed to exist, with evidence of ulcerative colitis occurring in identical twins supporting the genetic theory of causation. Typically, it affects 15- to 25-year-olds, who develop excessive diarrhea with blood, pus, and mucus in the stool. The disease generally starts in the rectum and spreads to the sigmoid, sometimes involving the entire colon. Its clinical course is highly variable in severity and prognosis.

Inflammation of the mucosa and submucosa (reticulin fibers beneath the mucosal epithelium) causes abscesses to form in the crypt cells, separating them from their blood supply and leading to epithelial necrosis and mucosal ulceration. Gradually, the mucosa is replaced by fibrous tissue whose crevices give a rough, cobblestone appearance to the involved colon (Fig. 5-45).

Signs and symptoms include intermittent spells of bloody diarrhea and abdominal cramping. Colon strictures are a rare complication of ulcerative colitis. Another complication of ulcerative colitis is toxic colitis or megacolon, an acute dilatation of the colon from colonic paralytic ileus (Fig. 5-46). The dilated bowel is particularly susceptible to rupture; a barium enema is absolutely contraindicated. People with ulcerative colitis have a greatly increased incidence of colon cancer, especially if the entire colon is affected for over 10 years.

Sigmoidoscopy and colonoscopy are the usual means of diagnosing ulcerative colitis because 90% to 95% of the cases involve the distal colon or rectum. Barium enemas are used to support the clinical diagnosis and to assess the progression of the disease and its complications. When filled with barium, the normally smooth colon outline becomes irregular because of the ulceration present. Pseudopolyps are islands of

FIGURE 5-45 A left posterior oblique barium enema radiograph demonstrating ulcerative colitis in the proximal colon.

FIGURE 5-46 Barium enema in a 61-year-old man demonstrates toxic megacolon secondary to ulcerative colitis. Pseudopolyps are seen in the descending colon.

unaffected mucosa that become visible when surrounded by affected mucosa. Another radiographic indication of ulcerative colitis is an easily recognized loss of colon haustration and mucosal edema, which may be referred to as the "lead pipe" sign.

Certain characteristics of ulcerative colitis distinguish it from regional enteritis (CD) (Fig. 5-47). Ulcerative colitis is a disease of the mucosa of the colon, whereas regional enteritis affects all layers of the bowel wall. Also, ulcerative colitis typically begins at the anus and ascends, often results in megacolon and bowel perforations, and frequently progresses to cancer; by contrast, regional enteritis usually begins in the terminal ileum and cecum and descends through the bowel, often with skip areas. It rarely produces megacolon or bowel perforations.

Treatment of ulcerative colitis is initially medical in nature and often involves dietary restrictions. Steroid therapy is used to treat ulcerative colitis, and it may be administered either orally or rectally. Development of an obstruction or neoplasm may necessitate surgical intervention. This involves removal of the colon from cecum to sigmoid with establishment of an ileostomy or ileorectal or ileoanal anastomosis.

ESOPHAGEAL VARICES

Varicose veins are abnormally lengthened, dilated, and superficial veins; those in the esophagus are referred to as **esophageal varices**. They occur in the esophagus because of portal hypertension. Conditions that cause resistance to the normal blood flow through the liver (such as cirrhosis) cause a bypass of the normal venous drainage mechanism. Instead, blood is directed through the esophageal and gastric collateral veins. The increase in blood flow through these channels results in venous dilatation.

Esophageal varices are best demonstrated in a recumbent position because gravity causes poor visualization in the erect position. A thin barium mixture shows the varices as wormlike defects within the column of barium on the radiograph (Fig. 5-48). Use of thick barium may be

CROHN DISEASE

ULCERATIVE COLITIS

Stricture
Linear
ulceration
Fissures

Skip lesions

Small intestine

Transmural inflammation

Pseudopolyp

Continuous colonic involvement, beginning in rectum

Active disease:
superficial ulceration

AND/
OR

Inactive
disease:
atrophy

Large intestine

FIGURE 5-47 Distribution patterns of regional enteritis and ulcerative colitis.

A

B

FIGURE 5-48 A, Long, serpentine filling defects in the esophagus of a 41-year-old with chronic alcoholism, indicative of esophageal varices. **B,** Similar filling defects seen in the cardia of the stomach of the same patient, indicative of gastric varices.

counterproductive because it can cover the varices. Esophageal varices may also occasionally be visualized as a retrocardiac posterior mediastinal mass on a conventional chest radiograph obtained with the patient in the recumbent position.

Patients with esophageal varices are subject to rupture and hemorrhage, which may be massive and often fatal. Statistics show that ruptured varices have accounted for approximately one third of all deaths from cirrhosis. An erect image taken for this situation should be done with great caution because the patient's blood loss may be significant. The resultant reduced blood pressure along with the elevation may cause the patient to faint.

Treatment for esophageal varices may consist of endoscopic sclerotherapy, banding ligation, or infusion of vasopressin, a natural hormone useful in stopping hemorrhage. Compression of the varices through balloon tamponading may be occasionally used. Shunts such as transjugular intrahepatic portosystemic shunts (TIPSS), applied via interventional radiology or in surgery, may be used to help redirect liver blood flow, thus reducing portal hypertension and easing venous pressure in the esophageal and gastric collateral circulation. Sonography has been helpful in affected patients over time to access the direction of flow with TIPSS. Occasionally, the shunt may become blocked, and the shunt not functioning correctly may be a clinical concern. Doppler interrogation of the shunt with ultrasound may give quantitative analysis about the direction and magnitude of the flow of blood within the shunt.

DEGENERATIVE DISEASES

Herniation

A **hernia** is a protrusion of a loop of bowel through a small opening, usually in the abdominal wall. Popularly referred to as a *rupture*, it occurs because of an anatomic weakness. As the bowel loop herniates, it pushes the peritoneum ahead of it. An inguinal hernia, which is common

FIGURE 5-49 Moderate left inguinal hernia (*arrow*) on this computed tomography image of a 96-year-old man. Also well defined are (*1*) the femurs, showing the lesser trochanters projecting posteriorly, and (*2*) the ischial tuberosities.

in men, occurs when a bowel loop protrudes through a weakness in the inguinal ring (Fig. 5-49) and may descend downward into the scrotum. Femoral and umbilical herniations (Fig. 5-50) occur in both sexes.

If a herniated loop of bowel can be pushed back into the abdominal cavity, it is said to be *reducible*. If it becomes stuck and cannot be reduced, it is called an *incarcerated hernia*. As described previously, this can result in a bowel obstruction (Fig. 5-51). If the constriction through which the bowel loop has passed is tight enough to cut off blood supply to the bowel, it is called a *strangulated hernia*. Prompt surgical intervention is required in this case to avoid necrosis of that portion of the bowel. Bowel that has already become necrotic can generally be surgically resected.

Hiatal Hernia

A **hiatal hernia** is a weakness of the esophageal hiatus that permits some portions of the stomach to herniate into the thoracic cavity. Hiatal hernias

FIGURE 5-50 Computed tomography demonstration of a large anterior abdominal hernia containing multiple loops of small bowel and possibly some large bowel without evidence of obstruction in this 70-year-old man.

occur in about half of the population over age 50 years. In its early stages, a hiatal hernia is reducible. Chronic herniation may be associated with GERD.

A direct, or sliding, hiatal hernia occurs when a portion of the stomach and gastroesophageal junction are both situated above the diaphragm (Fig. 5-52). This type of hernia constitutes the outstanding majority (about 99%) of all hiatal hernias. A Schatzki ring is often visible with this condition (Fig. 5-53) and consists of a mucosal ring that protrudes into the lumen. Such a ring has traditionally been thought to be congenital but may be related to gastric reflux. It is, however, generally of no clinical significance unless it produces narrowing sufficient to cause dysphagia, usually less than 13 mm in diameter.

FIGURE 5-51 A, Upright abdominal view of a 3-month-old indicates multiple dilated loops of bowel with air and fluid levels present, suggesting a mechanical bowel obstruction. **B,** A prone cross-table lateral view shows the small bowel forming a beaklike projection at the point of obstruction at the internal inguinal ring in this incarcerated hernia.

A

B

FIGURE 5-52 A, Demonstration of contrast material above the hemidiaphragm on an upper gastrointestinal series of this 51-year-old woman. **B,** The esophagus narrows to the stomach, which is seen to empty passively, above the hemidiaphragm in this sliding hiatal hernia.

A far less common type of hiatal hernia is the rolling, or paraesophageal, hiatal hernia. This occurs when a portion of the stomach or adjacent viscera herniates above the diaphragm while the gastroesophageal junction remains below the diaphragm (Fig. 5-54). If all of the stomach slides above the diaphragm, an intrathoracic stomach (Fig. 5-55) results. Unlike the sliding hiatal hernia, a paraesophageal hernia is potentially life threatening because of the risk of volvulus, incarceration, or strangulation of the hernia.

Most hiatal hernias are asymptomatic, but some are accompanied by reflux. Most patients experiencing reflux complain of a full feeling in the chest, particularly after meals. Some reflux of gastric contents leads to complaints of heartburn. An upper GI examination may pinpoint the herniation. Treatment of hiatal herniation is generally conservative to minimize discomfort.

BOWEL OBSTRUCTIONS

Both the small bowel and the large bowel of the normal person are nearly always active in peristalsis. Many lesions of various types (e.g., inflammatory, degenerative) can interfere with this action and cause an obstruction of either the small bowel or the large bowel (Table 5-1). The resultant obstruction can be either a **mechanical bowel obstruction**, as occurs from a blockage of the bowel lumen, or a **paralytic ileus**, which results from a failure of peristalsis. Gradations of each exist, and both may be present at the same time. Initial diagnosis of a small bowel obstruction with conventional abdominal

FIGURE 5-53 Schatzki ring demonstrated in the case of a sliding hiatal hernia.

TABLE 5-1	Large and Small Bowel Obstruction
Cause	**Pathophysiology**
Small bowel obstruction	Adhesive secondary to previous abdominal surgeries: 50% to 70% Hernia: inguinal, ventral, or femoral: 20% to 25% Tumors: may be associated with intussusception: 10% Mesenteric ischemia: 3% to 5%
Large bowel obstruction	Colon/rectal cancer: 90% Volvulus: 4% to 5% Diverticular disease: 3% Other causes (inflammatory bowel disease, adhesions, hernia)

From Feldman, M, Friedman LS, Brandt LJ: *Sleisenger & Fordtran's gastrointestinal liver disease,* ed 7, Philadelphia, 2003, Saunders; Table 39-2 *Common causes of intestinal obstruction* protusion of the intestine through a weakness in the abdominal in McCance. From McCance KL, Huether SE: *Pathophysiology: the biologic basis for disease in adults and children,* ed 5, St. Louis, 2006, Mosby.

FIGURE 5-54 A, Paraesophageal hiatal hernia, demonstrating narrowing in the fundus. **B,** Lateral view of the same patient demonstrates the cardioesophageal junction in its normal place below the hemidiaphragm. The fundus is highlighted by radiolucency of the lung.

radiography may be difficult because of the frequency of vomiting and the use of nasogastric decompression.

General signs and symptoms of a bowel obstruction include vomiting, abdominal distention, and abdominal pain. Sequential radiographs over 12 to 24 hours help to determine the diagnosis and to locate the level of the obstruction in individuals with mechanical obstructions. Most commonly, gas confined to the small bowel with multiple air and fluid levels visible on an erect abdominal radiograph indicates a mechanical obstruction, whereas gas distributed throughout both the large bowel and the small bowel is indicative of paralytic ileus. The small bowel tends to be more distended in cases of mechanical obstruction. Physical signs are also helpful in distinguishing the type of obstruction present. Bowel sounds, the normal sounds of a bowel in motion as heard on auscultation, are absent with an ileus; they are present with a mechanical obstruction and are often hyperactive and high-pitched. Emesis

containing bile may also indicate a mechanical obstruction.

Mechanical Bowel Obstruction

A mechanical bowel obstruction (Fig. 5-56) is one in which the lumen of the bowel becomes occluded, as might occur for a variety of reasons such as hernias, tumors, volvulus, intussusceptions, or, most often postoperatively, adhesions (Fig. 5-57). A simple mechanical obstruction does not involve the blood supply to the bowel, whereas a strangulating obstruction may lead to bowel infarction. Nearly half of all strangulating mechanical bowel obstructions are caused by an incarcerated (i.e., trapped) hernia, a condition discussed earlier in this chapter as a degenerative disease. Entrapment of a hernia, usually involving the small bowel, causes impairment of blood flow and swelling of the affected tissues. The resultant edema affects arterial blood flow to the bowel and may lead to ischemic necrosis, perforation, and peritonitis. Prompt surgical

FIGURE 5-55 Intrathoracic stomach indicated by the presence of the entire stomach above the diaphragm, also with malrotation of the stomach.

FIGURE 5-56 Abdominal radiograph demonstrating a mechanical bowel obstruction, with numerous loops of dilated bowel seen within the midabdomen. The patient had an acute onset of abdominal pain, nausea, and vomiting.

intervention and reduction are required to relieve an incarcerated hernia.

A **volvulus** is a twisting of a bowel loop about its mesenteric base, usually at either the sigmoid or the ileocecal junction (Fig. 5-58). This most commonly occurs in older adults and is identifiable on a conventional abdominal radiograph as a collection of air conforming to the shape of the affected, dilated bowel. Some twists resolve spontaneously; however, bowel that is twisted more than 360 degrees requires surgical intervention. Surgical untwisting and resection are necessary to prevent necrosis and perforation of the bowel caused by a lack of blood supply.

An **intussusception** occurs when a segment of bowel, constricted by peristalsis, telescopes into a distal segment and is driven further into the distal bowel by peristalsis. Recall that the bowel is connected to the mesentery, so as the bowel telescopes into itself, the mesentery (with its rich

FIGURE 5-57 Intestinal obstructions.

FIGURE 5-58 A barium enema radiograph depicting a cecal volvulus. Note how the column of barium stops at the level of the volvulus.

blood supply) is also involved. Radiographically, the area of intussusception may appear as a "coiled spring." Intussusception is responsible for approximately 5% of all mechanical obstructions and most frequently affects the ileocecal valve (Fig. 5-59). It is more common in children and infants than in adults. Its presence in an adult generally signifies an accompanying intraluminal mass and is generally reduced surgically so that the physician can search for the cause of the intussusception and correct the condition. In children and infants, an intussusception can often be reduced by an enema, sparing a surgical intervention.

Gallstone ileus is another cause for a mechanical bowel obstruction. In this condition, a gallstone may erode from the gallbladder and create a fistula to the small bowel. This leads to an obstruction, usually when the gallstone reaches the ileocecal valve. Radiographic signs of this include air and fluid levels or air in the biliary tree (Fig. 5-60). The gallstone itself may also be visible, often in the terminal ileum, where it causes the obstruction. Small bowel obstructions

FIGURE 5-59 A, Pediatric barium enema demonstrating intussusception before resolution and **B,** after resolution (*B*).

may also result from pathologic conditions such as Crohn disease and appendicitis previously discussed in this chapter.

Diagnosis is initially based on clinical signs and symptoms including abdominal distention,

FIGURE 5-60 Abdominal radiograph demonstrating air within the biliary ductal system.

abdominal cramps, and vomiting, sometimes progressing to bloody stools. The quality of regurgitated material may provide clues as to the possible location of obstruction, with bilious vomit indicating a proximal location and yellow colostrum or vomitus with meconium (in pediatric patients) being more indicative of distal obstruction. Conventional supine and erect abdominal radiographs often confirm the diagnosis with air and fluid levels clearly visible in the erect position. Additionally, abdominal radiographs that are positive for bowel obstruction often direct the subsequent imaging workup, with findings of proximal obstruction indicating an upper GI or SBFT examination and distal obstruction being clarified with a contrast enema. These additional examinations are more comprehensive in nature, providing important information related to the specific location of a transition point in which the lumen changes from being patent to being obstructed. Whether water-soluble or barium contrast agents are best for diagnosing small bowel obstructions (SBOs) is still being debated. The major point of concern

is the potential for intravascular uptake of water-soluble contrasts, thus depleting the overall intraluminal volume, and, although rare, the potential for barium to convert a partial obstruction to a complete bowel obstruction.

The use of CT to distinguish between high-grade SBO and ileus has been reported to have a diagnostic accuracy of 90%. Furthermore, no oral contrast administration is necessary, with the fluid in the bowel providing adequate contrast. A more efficient diagnosis can be reached by negating the need for a contrast agent when ruling out high-grade SBO while minimizing the potential related complications such as vomiting or aspiration. However, CT is rather limited in its ability to diagnose low-grade SBO presentations. The incorporation of multiformat reconstructions to the imaging protocol, specifically in the coronal plane, has increased the accuracy in detecting transition zones in which the bowel obstruction originates. The use of CT enterography to detect the presence of lumen obliterating bowel abnormalities such as CD or neoplasms is another growing trend in SBO imaging. In comparison, MRI has shown promise in becoming used more frequently in diagnosing suspected low-grade SBO. Generally, mechanical obstructions require surgical intervention.

Paralytic Ileus

Paralytic ileus or **adynamic ileus** is a failure of normal peristalsis that may result from a variety of factors. The most common causes are surgery, especially that requiring manipulation of the bowel (postoperative ileus), and intraperitoneal or retroperitoneal infection. It may also be associated with bowel ischemia, certain drugs, electrolyte imbalance, or pancreatitis or may occur simply as a reaction to any stressful illness. Paralytic ileus generally lasts no longer than 3 days with proper medical treatment.

Signs and symptoms of paralytic ileus include distention of the abdomen, abdominal cramping, and vomiting. The absence of peristalsis causes the lumen of both the small and large intestines to fill with gas and fluid, with the resultant

FIGURE 5-61 Abdominal radiograph on a postoperative patient demonstrating paralytic ileus. Note the dilated bowel loops extending through the large intestine.

dilatation extending to the rectum (Fig. 5-61). Radiographically, gas is visible in the colon. Treatment for paralytic ileus generally consists of nasogastric suction and medical stimulation of the bowel to restore peristalsis. In some cases, colonoscopic decompression may be required.

NEUROGENIC DISEASES

Achalasia

Achalasia is a neuromuscular abnormality of the esophagus that results in failure of the lower esophageal sphincter of the distal esophagus to relax, leading to dysphagia. It occurs equally in men and women and most commonly affects individuals between the ages of 20 and 40 years. Clinically, these patients present with a slowly progressive dysphagia in swallowing both solids and liquids. Patients may also experience regurgitation, chest pain, and moderate weight loss.

Radiographically, the condition manifests as a dilated esophagus with little or no peristalsis. The distal esophagus itself is often described as having a "beaked" appearance (Fig. 5-62).

FIGURE 5-62 A, Erect esophageal image demonstrating achalasia at the level of the gastroesophageal junction. The distal esophagus terminates into a beaked appearance. **B,** Spot image of achalasia at gastroesophageal junction.

Because the distal esophagus opens only intermittently, when the pressure is high enough, food residue may be seen in the distal esophagus or even on a chest radiograph. Because the esophageal contents act as a water seal, the normal gastric gas bubble may be absent.

Initial treatment of achalasia is to reduce the pressure and obstruction at the cardiac sphincter. Esophageal dilatation is effective in approximately 85% of patients affected by achalasia. Medications such as nitrates and calcium channel blockers may be used to reduce the sphincter pressure and reduce the frequency of repeated dilatations. Botulinum toxin may also be injected into the sphincter to create chemical denervation, but this is effective for only 1 year. Patients not responding to dilatation and medication protocols may require surgical myotomy (cutting of the sphincter muscle fibers).

DIVERTICULAR DISEASES

Esophageal Diverticula

A **diverticulum** is a pouch or sac of variable size that occurs normally or is created by herniation of a mucous membrane through a defect in its muscular coat. Esophageal diverticula occur when mucosal outpouchings penetrate through the muscular layer of the esophagus. The two primary types of esophageal diverticula are pulsion and traction.

A pulsion diverticulum involves only the mucosa and results from a motility disorder of the esophagus that allows the mucosa to herniate outward. This type of diverticulum appears radiographically as a rounded projection with a narrow neck and occurs more frequently in the upper and lower thirds of the esophagus. A Zenker diverticulum is a pulsion type found at the pharyngoesophageal junction at the upper end of the esophagus on the posterior aspect just above the cricopharyngeal muscle (Fig. 5-63). A Killian-Jamieson diverticulum is similar to that of a Zenker diverticulum except that it originates on the lateral aspect of the esophagus. An epiphrenic diverticulum is another pulsion type, but it is found in the distal esophagus just above the hemidiaphragm (Fig. 5-64).

A traction diverticulum involves all layers of the esophagus and results from adjacent scar tissue that pulls the esophagus toward the area of involvement (Fig. 5-65). Such a diverticulum occurs more frequently in the middle third of the esophagus at the carina and appears radiographically as a triangle whose apex points toward the disease.

Usually, diverticula are asymptomatic until they reach a relatively large size, at which time complications may occur. For example, food and secretions may collect in the diverticulum and cause a mechanical obstruction of the esophagus. Such contents may also be aspirated by a recumbent patient, resulting in aspiration pneumonia. Failure to control the effects of diverticula through diet modifications may result in the need for surgical removal, depending on the amount of food retention in the diverticulum.

Colonic Diverticula

Diverticulosis, the presence of diverticula without inflammation, is seen in all parts of the colon, most frequently in the sigmoid colon, and particularly among adults over the age of 40 years (Fig. 5-66). Diverticula are associated with hypertrophy of the muscular layer of the bowel. They occur most often where the terminal branches of the mesenteric vessels pierce the bowel wall and are present in 35% to 50% of patients over age 50 years. Factors contributing to the development of diverticula include a pressure gradient between the lumen and the serosa of the bowel and areas of weakness within the bowel wall. The most common site for diverticula (95%) is the sigmoid colon, the narrowest portion of the colon, which generates the highest intrasegmental (between haustra) pressures.

Inflammation of a diverticulum, termed **diverticulitis**, occurs in approximately 10% to 20% of patients with known diverticulosis, especially in older adults. The inflammation is exacerbated by feces lodging in the diverticulum. Signs and symptoms include lower left quadrant pain and

FIGURE 5-63 A, Large Zenker diverticulum in the esophagus of a 67-year-old man with complaints of difficulty swallowing over the past 6 months. **B,** Zenker diverticulum in the same patient on a magnified view.

FIGURE 5-64 An epiphrenic diverticulum shown as a large collection of barium connected and adjacent to the lower esophagus.

FIGURE 5-65 Traction diverticulum indicated by the out-pouching of the esophagus at the level of the carina seen in an esophagram of a 47-year-old woman with a history of ulcer disease.

FIGURE 5-66 An air-contrast barium enema demonstrating diverticulosis in various projections. **A,** Right lateral decubitus projection. **B,** Posteroanterior axial sigmoid projection. **C,** Digital spot image.

tenderness, fever, and an increased WBC count. Because of these symptoms, sigmoid diverticulitis has been termed *left-sided appendicitis*. This condition may lead to bowel obstruction, perforation, and fistula formation. In some instances, no imaging may be required to make a diagnosis of acute diverticulitis, especially in patients with a history of attacks of diverticulitis who present with symptoms of recurrent disease. The growing trend is toward greater use of radiologic examinations to confirm the diagnosis and to evaluate the extent of the disease to detect possible associated complications that impact the selection of the most appropriate treatment protocol. Complications associated with acute diverticulitis include the presence abscesses, fistulas, obstructions, and perforations. Abdominal radiography is of limited value unless complications of pneumoperitoneum or obstruction are suspected. Furthermore, nuclear medicine has no role in evaluating patients presenting with LLQ pain, and MRI is primarily only utilized in pediatric patients with recurrent episodes of diverticulitis to reduce radiation exposure.

Traditionally, a barium enema examination was the primary imaging test performed when evaluating for colonic diverticulitis. Reported diagnostic sensitivity for this imaging examination ranges between 59% and 90%. Radiographic signs of diverticulitis on barium enema are limited, as diverticulitis is mainly an extramucosal process. A barium enema will only show the secondary effects of an inflamed colon and not the extraluminal abnormalities of abscesses and pericolonic inflammation that may be present. For this reason, the barium enema examination has largely been replaced by CT as the initial imaging examination and has been reserved for patients with equivocal CT findings or poor candidates for endoscopic evaluation due to their colonic narrowing.

CT has a much higher sensitivity for diagnosing colonic diverticulitis with a range of 79% to 99% (Fig. 5-67). Additionally, its ability to detect extraluminal pathology enables potential diagnosis of other disease processes that may mimic the signs and symptoms of LLQ pain. In cases of

FIGURE 5-67 Computed tomography scan of abdomen demonstrating diverticulitis.

suspected perforated colon due to cancer, in which clinical and radiographic findings mimic diverticulitis, the presentation of pericolonic lymphadenopathy adjacent to a segment of thickened colon wall indicates a diagnosis of diverticulitis over that of colon cancer.

As an alternative technique, transabdominal sonography with graded compression is reported to have a sensitivity of 77% to 98% and a specificity of 80% to 99% in diagnosing diverticulitis. However, sonographic imaging of the sigmoid portion of the colon, a relatively posterior structure, is highly dependent on body habitus in comparison with CT or MRI. The use of transvaginal sonography is often utilized in women of childbearing age to rule out conditions such as ectopic pregnancy or pelvic inflammatory disease that may mimic the signs and symptoms of diverticulitis.

Treatment of diverticulitis centers on reduction of inflammation and infection. Mild cases are treated with antibiotic therapy. Complications such as peritonitis may result if perforation of a diverticulum occurs, and these, of course, must be treated. Abscesses may often be treated via sonography or with CT-guided percutaneous drainage. Surgical resection of the bowel may be used to remove the diseased portion in more severe cases.

NEOPLASTIC DISEASES

Tumors of the Esophagus

Although benign and malignant tumors could occur anywhere in the esophagus, tumors of the lower third are the most common. Benign tumors are almost always **leiomyomas,** which are smooth muscle tumors, although these have an incidence of less than 10% that of malignant tumors of the esophagus. Many are discovered on radiographic examination for complaints not related to esophageal problems. These benign lesions present as intramural defects in the barium-outlined esophageal wall (Fig. 5-68). The exact location of a leiomyoma, which appears as a homogeneous soft tissue mass, may be determined on CT. Treatment of a leiomyoma consists of surgical removal through a thoracic or abdominal incision that avoids esophageal resection.

Cancers of the esophagus constitute approximately 7% of cancers of the GI system but carry a poor prognosis, with an overall 5-year survival rate of less than 10%. Squamous cell carcinomas most commonly arise in the body of the esophagus; those at the gastroesophageal junction are typically **adenocarcinomas.** These two types of esophageal cancers have different clinical and radiographic features. Diagnosis is made by endoscopic biopsy of the lesion. Regardless of the type of esophageal cancer, however, CT of the neck, chest, and abdomen is helpful to stage the spread of the disease by demonstrating tumor size, lymph node involvement, and metastases. Endoscopic ultrasonography, although highly accurate in detecting disease, is less available in many medical institutions.

Chronic irritation of the esophagus is thought to be a predisposing factor to squamous cell carcinomas, with such irritation caused by particular agents, including reflux, alcohol, and smoking, and disorders such as achalasia and esophageal diverticula. The chronic presence of irritation to

FIGURE 5-68 Sharply defined filling defect in the distal esophagus indicative of a benign, esophageal leiomyoma.

the esophageal mucosa leads to Barrett (dysplastic) epithelium, with mutation of the *TP53* gene being an early event in the development of Barrett adenocarcinoma. The primary symptom of esophageal cancer is dysphagia. However, dysphagia may not become significant until the tumor has narrowed the lumen to 50% to 75% of its normal circumference, allowing metastatic spread to the adjacent lymph nodes and mediastinal structures before diagnosis. Surgery is used as a treatment, with the goal to excise the tumor and regional metastasis. Chemotherapy, radiation therapy, or both may be used as an adjunct to surgical intervention. The rapid spread of esophageal cancer, however, requires the goal to be palliation in many cases. The radiographic appearance of a malignant squamous cell tumor may include mucosal destruction, ulceration,

FIGURE 5-69 A computed tomography scan with contrast demonstrates an increased thickening of the esophageal wall and distortion of the lumen (*arrow*), compatible with a gastroesophageal junction malignancy. Also seen are (*1*) a large metastatic lesion in the superior portion of the liver and (*2*) the aorta.

Tumors of the Stomach

Benign tumors account for fewer than 10% of all stomach tumors. Those that are clinically significant are quite rare. Most stomach tumors are malignant, and the outstanding preponderance (about 95%) of these are adenocarcinomas. Alterations in the tumor-suppressor *p53* gene, as well as cell cycle regulators, cell adhesion molecules, and DNA repair genes, all contribute in part to the development of gastric adenocarcinomas. The incidence of gastric cancer varies strikingly by geographic area, race, diet, heredity, and sex. For example, the rate is nearly five times greater in Japan than in the United States. The survival rate associated with gastric carcinoma depends on the stage of the disease. If the neoplasm is limited to the stomach mucosa, the 5-year survival rate is as high as 71%; however, advanced stages carry a poor prognosis, with overall 5-year survival rates less than 4%.

Current research indicates that the presence of *H. pylori* results in a threefold to sixfold increase in the risk of gastric adenocarcinoma. Most gastric carcinomas develop in the pyloric and antrum regions, particularly along the lesser curvature, although they may occur anywhere (Fig. 5-70). Gastric carcinomas may also be polypoid with a plaquelike, lobulated appearance. Most gastric carcinomas are diagnosed at an advanced stage because early stomach cancers do not have specific symptoms. They invade other structures by a variety of routes. These tumors metastasize fairly readily outside the stomach to involve the omentum, liver, pancreas, and colon. Liver involvement creates the possibility of discharge into the bloodstream and dispersal throughout the body. Because of the abundance of lymphatics in the stomach, approximately 75% to 85% of these patients also demonstrate metastases via the lymphatic system.

Patients who complain of persistent GI pain should have a thorough workup. The most appropriate primary diagnostic procedure is an upper GI endoscopy with biopsy. Endoscopy is often followed by a fluoroscopic UGI series. Symptoms of gastric tumors are often vague but

narrowing, and a sharp demarcation between normal tissue and the malignant tumor.

As mentioned earlier, adenocarcinomas usually occur in the lower esophagus around the gastroesophageal junction. Many believe these begin as primary gastric carcinomas that invade the lower esophagus. Others believe that a direct link exists between a disorder termed *Barrett esophagus* and the development of adenocarcinoma of the esophagus. Barrett esophagus involves progressive columnar metaplasia of the distal esophagus as a result of chronic gastroesophageal reflux. More than 90% of adenocarcinomas of the esophagus have been found to arise from the mucosa. Similar to squamous carcinomas, adenocarcinomas spread via the lymph nodes; however, unlike squamous carcinomas, they also spread below the diaphragm. Metastasis to mediastinal structures and hematogenous spread to the liver, lung, and bone occur readily (Fig. 5-69). Radiographically, early adenocarcinomas appear as plaquelike lesions or as sessile polyps, and advanced tumors appear as infiltrating lesions with irregular narrowing of the lumen with abrupt, asymmetric borders.

FIGURE 5-70 Adenocarcinoma of the stomach in a 66-year-old woman, resulting in gastric outlet obstruction. Note the area of narrowing and the abrupt transition between normal stomach and the acutely narrowed area.

include bleeding, vomiting, loss of appetite, weight loss, and early satiety. Tumors are radiographically indicated by a relative rigidity of peristalsis and filling defects on compression. Filling defects manifest as areas of total or relative radiolucency within the barium column. Polypoid tumors are clearly visible on CT examination. By identifying lymphatic involvement and extragastric spread of the cancer, CT is also useful in the staging of gastric cancers.

Surgical removal of gastric cancer has been the only successful treatment; a subtotal gastrectomy is the usual procedure. Resection of the stomach to attach to the jejunum via a gastrojejunostomy usually accompanies this procedure. Radiation therapy and chemotherapy treatments for stomach carcinoma have been less effective.

Small Bowel Neoplasms

Small bowel tumors represent fewer than 5% of all benign and malignant GI neoplasms; however, this may be an underestimate because of limitations in current imaging modalities for the small bowel. The incidence of malignancy for this small amount is about 50%. The low overall incidence is surprising, considering that the small bowel constitutes 75% of the entire GI tract, with an enormous mucosal surface. Also, it is in constant contact with enteric carcinogenic substances. Reasons for this low incidence of tumors are not entirely known or understood. Most small bowel cancers occur in the duodenum and proximal jejunum.

One predisposing factor for small bowel neoplasms seems to be the degree of polyposis in other areas of the GI tract, a condition frequently determined by heredity. Another predisposing factor is Kaposi sarcoma, most common in patients with acquired immunodeficiency syndrome (AIDS). Up to 60% of these patients have GI involvement, with the tumors arising anywhere in the stomach, small bowel, or distal colon. In addition, patients who have CD also have an increased risk for developing adenocarcinoma of the small bowel. Intermittent abdominal pain, sometimes described as cramps, is the most common symptom. Endoscopy with biopsy is the most common means of identifying small bowel neoplasms, but small bowel barium studies may assist in the diagnosis. Surgical resection is the primary means of treating small bowel neoplasms, both benign and malignant.

Colonic Polyps

Colonic polyps are small masses of tissue arising from the bowel wall to project inward into the lumen (Fig. 5-71). An adenomatous polyp is a tumor of benign neoplastic epithelium that may undergo dysplastic changes to become malignant. It consists of a saccular projection into the bowel lumen and is either sessile, that is, attached directly to the bowel wall with a wide base, or pedunculated, that is, attached by a narrow stalk (Fig. 5-72). Polyps are more frequently noted in the left colon, and particularly in the rectosigmoid areas. Other types of polyps are inflammatory, hyperplastic, and juvenile.

Although most polyps are asymptomatic, all should be removed, especially adenomatous polyps, which pose a greater risk of malignancy (Fig. 5-73). Those over 2 cm in size have a

FIGURE 5-71 Filling defect in the transverse colon near the splenic flexure indicates a polyp projecting into the lumen. A barium-filled diverticulum is seen immediately above it in this patient, who had blood in his stools.

Adenomatous polyp

Focal atypia (cancer in situ)

Focal cancer (malignant adenoma)

Focal cancer invading stalk with some "benign" polyp still in body

Invasive cancer containing piece of polyp

Polypoid invasive cancer without polyp remnant

Ulcerated invasive cancer without polyp remnant

FIGURE 5-73 Adenomatous polyp transformation.

FIGURE 5-72 Pedunculated polyp seen attached to the wall of the sigmoid colon by a long stalk on an air-contrast barium enema.

malignancy rate of over 50%. Most never reach this size, however. The complications of polyps include ulceration from chronic irritation or bowel obstruction from inflammation. Most cancers of the colon and rectum arise from previously benign polyps. Patients with polyps may have rectal bleeding, constipation, diarrhea, or flatulence, but most are asymptomatic. Radiographically an air-contrast barium enema is the examination of choice, with the polyps manifesting as rounded filling defects or contour defects in the barium shadow. Although pedunculated polyps are easily recognized and often considered benign, size is a better indicator of malignancy versus benignancy, as noted. At times, it is difficult to discriminate between fecal matter and a polyp. In general, fecal matter is mobile, whereas a polyp stays fixed to the stalk. Proctosigmoidoscopy and colonoscopy are critical in the evaluation and removal of polyps. Patients with polyps are monitored closely after discovery and are often treated with aspirin and cyclooxygenase 2 (COX-2) inhibitors to prevent new polyp formation.

Colon Cancer

Colorectal cancers are the third most common tumors in the United States and the most common GI cancer. Additionally, carcinoma of the colon is the third most common cause of mortality from cancer. The incidence of colon cancer rises significantly after age 40 years and doubles with each decade, reaching a peak at about age 75 years. In the United States, adults have a 1 in 20 chance of developing colorectal cancer in their lifetime and a 1 in 40 chance of dying from this disease. Predisposing factors include a family history of familial polyposis and ulcerative colitis. Colon cancer tends to cluster in families, with the risk of the disease in people with one affected first-degree relative being two to three times higher than in the general population. The *APC* gene, which is responsible for the colon cancer subset of adenomatous polyposis, has been mapped to chromosome 5, and mutations of the gene are found in at least 85% of all colon tumors. Hereditary nonpolyposis colorectal cancer, which accounts for as many as 5% of all colorectal cancer cases, has also been tied to mutations to as many as six different genes. Furthermore, allelic deletion on chromosomes 5, 17, and 18 is believed to be responsible for promoting the transition from normal to malignant colonic mucosa. Environmental factors also seem to correlate with colorectal cancer, as countries with higher intakes of sugar and animal fats (e.g., the United States) have a higher incidence than compared with countries (e.g., Western Asia, Central America, and Africa) with a higher fiber intake.

Recent guidelines have divided colorectal cancer risk levels into three categories. The first category is of those with an average risk, including patients 50 years of age or older. The second category is of moderate risk, and includes those with a first-degree relative with a history of adenoma or carcinoma, or a personal history of similar pathology. Finally, the third category is of those with high risk, and includes hereditary syndromes such as hereditary nonpolyposis colorectal cancer (HNPCC) and familial polyposis, or patients with a personal history of ulcerative colitis or CD.

Adenocarcinoma is the most common type of colorectal cancer and is derived from the glandular epithelium of the colon. It begins as a benign adenoma that undergoes a slow malignant transformation. Although the transformation may take up to 7 years to complete, all polypoid lesions larger than 1 cm should be removed from the colon. Adenocarcinoma is characterized by infiltration of the colon wall, as opposed to being a bulky, intraluminal mass.

Although the incidence of proximal colon cancers is increasing, nearly 50% still occur below the mid-descending colon. Most of these (70%) occur in the rectosigmoid area and are detectable by flexible sigmoidoscopy. Right colon lesions differ considerably from left colon lesions in terms of symptoms produced. Lesions in the right colon, on the one hand, may produce no early symptoms, often becoming quite large, ulcerating, and even bleeding without significant symptoms. They also tend to penetrate and extend into surrounding tissues without causing obstruction. Patients often present initially with anemia and blood in their stools. Left colon lesions, in contrast, present more often with obstruction and bleeding, largely because of a smaller lumen and an annular (ringlike) growth pattern.

Detection of colorectal cancer, when localized, is associated with a 5-year survival rate of approximately 80%. The evaluation of colon cancer includes fecal blood testing, proctosigmoidoscopy, colonoscopy, barium enema, CT, transrectal ultrasonography (TRUS), and PET imaging. The use of clinical fecal occult blood testing (FOBT) has demonstrated a 15% to 33% reduction in mortality rates. Additionally, use of screening sigmoidoscopy examinations may decrease colorectal cancer mortality rates by two thirds for cancers within reach of the scope.

When proximal GI lesions are suspected, a colonoscopy may be ordered. Colonoscopy currently is considered to be the most sensitive and specific test for detecting colorectal polyps and cancers because of its ability to obtain abnormal tissue as biopsy specimen for histologic identification of dysplasia. The primary benefits unique to the use of endoscopic imaging are the ability to directly visualize the luminal mucosal lining and availability of biopsy upon identification of abnormal tissue. CTC may be useful to screen for colorectal cancer when a fibrostenotic stricture in the colon prevents traditional colonoscopy techniques from evaluating proximally to the diseased colon.

Double-contrast barium enema (DCBE) has been noted to produce more accurate diagnoses compared with the limited single-contrast study because of the enhanced display of subtle mucosal abnormalities otherwise masked by a dense barium column. Although appropriate for colorectal cancer screening, DCBE is typically utilized when CT is unavailable. One benefit of DCBE over diagnostic colonoscopy is the dramatic reduction in the number of bowel perforations, 1 out of 25,000 versus 1 out of 2000, respectively. The radiographic appearance of adenocarcinoma has led to its designation as the "napkin-ring" carcinoma or the "apple-core" lesion, as the edges of the lesion tend to overhang and form acute angles with the bowel wall (Fig. 5-74). Although it may be difficult to distinguish between carcinoma and an inflammatory lesion (e.g., regional enteritis or ulcerative colitis), a carcinoma generally has a more clear-cut transition between the malignant mucosa and the normal mucosa. In addition, the length of bowel involved is usually shorter with carcinoma than with an inflammatory lesion.

Compared with CT, MRI is quickly gaining ground as an equal and even superior method for detecting rectal neoplasms and associated liver metastases. Prior imaging with MRI required the use of endorectal coils to attain optimal cancer staging information, which was limited to the length of the endorectal coil length. However, with the move to higher strength 3.0 T magnets,

FIGURE 5-74 The "apple core" lesion of the rectosigmoid colon consistent with adenocarcinoma, with characteristic appearance of abrupt change from normal to abnormal colon and shelflike appearance of overhanging edges caused by the mass.

most colon cancer imaging can now be performed with only the phased array coils, although such a technique may still have limited use in patients who are obese. Additionally, MRI has the ability to depict the layers of the rectal wall and assess the depth of neoplastic bowel wall penetration, and with an accuracy of 86% in predicting the circumferential margin of cancer involvement, surgeons can more reliably reduce the area of resected tissue. Diffusion-weighted imaging (DWI) techniques have shown to be more sensitive and specific compared with standard contrast-enhanced MRI with gadolinium and are believed to be superior for tumor detection and characterization when monitoring tumor response to treatment. The use of magnetic resonance colonography (MRC) techniques has the benefit over CT of not involving ionizing radiation. However, the spatial resolution of MRC is currently less than that of CT, decreasing its overall accuracy. In recent MRC research studies, evidence has shown that "dark lumen" imaging (utilizing water as a negative contrast) has proven to be more effective in identifying colorectal cancer compared with "bright lumen" imaging (utilizing gadolinium as a positive contrast agent).

TRUS is currently the standard imaging procedure for staging superficial rectal carcinomas. Similar to MRI, TRUS helps distinguish between the layers within the rectal wall and has displayed an accuracy of up to 97% in detecting the depth of tumor penetration and perirectal spread. In its ability to detect local lymph node involvement, again, TRUS is comparable with MRI with an overall accuracy of 62% to 83%. It should be noted that studies comparing the use of frontal ultrasound probe types and radial ultrasound probe types found the frontal probe to have a higher overall accuracy in staging rectal cancer. Additionally, techniques utilizing sonographic imaging of the colon dilated with water have been established; however, experience with this technique is extremely limited, and the procedure is currently not recommended for colorectal cancer screening.

It is important to note that imaging modalities, including CTC, barium enema, and MRI, are usually not appropriate for colorectal cancer screening in high-risk patients with hereditary nonpolyposis colorectal cancer and IBD. These patients are almost always examined by using colonoscopy.

PET alone or combined with CT has been shown to alter treatment protocols in almost a third of patients with advanced primary rectal cancer. PET with CT is particularly accurate in identifying hepatic and peritoneal metastases compared with CT alone. In fact, a relatively new concept of PET with CTC has been reported to be significantly more accurate in GI cancer staging compared with CTC alone. PET has a potential role in restaging colorectal cancer after

chemoradiotherapy by measuring the pretreatment and posttreatment standard uptake volume (SUV). Limitations of PET include decreased sensitivity in detecting small colonic lesions 5 to 10 mm in diameter and decreased 18F-fluorodeoxyglucose (FDG) uptake by mucinous tumors.

Without treatment, cancer spreads by invasion of local tissue via the lymphatics to the mesenteric nodes and on to the liver (Fig. 5-75) and lungs. Fortunately, the lesion does not metastasize early, leading to a good prognosis. The primary means of treatment are surgical excision of the primary tumor and its margins and resection of the bowel, if possible. A colostomy may be required, depending on the site of the tumor. Radiation therapy or chemotherapy is generally given before and after surgery for rectal cancers, especially in those with lymph nodes positive for metastasis. For inoperable tumors, radiation therapy is given to reduce the tumor size and its resultant complications (e.g., obstruction) and also to provide pain relief. Chemotherapy is given when the cancer has metastasized.

FIGURE 5-75 Computed tomography demonstration of extensive metastatic disease from the colon to both lobes of the liver, ranging from punctate to up to 5 cm in this 50-year-old woman.

PATHOLOGY SUMMARY

The Gastrointestinal System

Pathology	Imaging Modalities of Choice	Additive or Subtractive Pathology
Esophageal atresia	Radiography	None
Bowel atresia	Radiography in infant, sonography in fetus	None
Hypertrophic pyloric stenosis	Sonography abdomen, radiography, UGI	None
Malrotation	CT abdomen and pelvis with contrast, small bowel and BaE, sonography	None
Hirschsprung disease	BaE	None
Meckel diverticulum	Nuclear medicine Meckel scan	None
Gluten-sensitive enteropathy	UGI, small bowel, BaE	None
Carbohydrate intolerance	UGI mixed with lactose	None
Esophageal strictures	Ba swallow and endoscopy	None
GERD	Endoscopy, Ba swallow, UGI, nuclear medicine reflux scintigraphy, abdominal sonography	None
Peptic ulcer	Endoscopy, double-contrast UGI, nuclear medicine urea breath test	None
Regional enteritis (Crohn disease)	CT enterography (abdomen and pelvis with contrast), MRI enterography (abdomen and pelvis with contrast), routine CT abdomen and pelvis with contrast, small bowel and double-contrast BaE	None
Appendicitis	CT abdomen and pelvis with contrast, RUQ abdominal sonography, abdomen radiography	None
Ulcerative colitis	Sigmoidoscopy and colonoscopy	None
Esophageal varices	Ba swallow	None
Bowel obstruction	CT abdomen and pelvis with contrast, MRI abdomen and pelvis with contrast, supine and erect abdominal radiography	Subtractive
Achalasia	Ba swallow	Additive if food is present
Diverticular disease	CT abdomen and pelvis with contrast, MRI abdomen and pelvis with or without contrast, double-contrast Ba studies, TRUS, transabdominal graded compression sonography	None
Polyps	Colonoscopy and double-contrast BaE	None
Neoplastic disease of the GI system	CT colonography, colonoscopy, double-contrast BaE, CT	None

Ba, Barium; *BaE,* barium enema; *CT,* computed tomography; *GERD,* gastroesophageal reflux disease; *GI,* gastrointestinal; MRI, magnetic resonance imaging; *TRUS,* transabdominal graded compression sonography; *UGI,* upper gastrointestinal study.

REVIEW QUESTIONS

1. Esophageal atresia is classified as a(n) _____ condition of the gastrointestinal (GI) system.
   a. Congenital
   b. Degenerative
   c. Inflammatory
   d. Neurologic

2. An outpouching of the bowel wall caused by a weakening in its muscular layer is a(n):
   a. Atresia
   b. Carcinoma
   c. Diverticulum
   d. Polyp

3. The radiographic string sign is associated with:
   a. Achalasia
   b. Adenocarcinoma
   c. Regional enteritis
   d. Ulcerative colitis

4. Celiac disease is a type of:
   a. Atresia
   b. Herniation
   c. Malabsorption syndrome
   d. Ulcerative colitis

5. The appearance of a Schatzki ring is associated with a(n) _____ hernia.
   a. Inguinal
   b. Rolling
   c. Sliding
   d. Umbilical

6. A congenital, neurogenic disease of the GI system characterized by an absence of neurons in the bowel wall is:
   a. Achalasia
   b. Diverticulosis
   c. Hirschsprung disease
   d. Toxic megacolon

7. The fewest GI tumors, both benign and malignant, occur in the:
   a. Colon
   b. Esophagus
   c. Large bowel
   d. Small bowel

8. Which of the following statements are true of colon cancer?
   1. The majority of adenocarcinomas of the colon occur in the rectosigmoid area.
   2. The appearance of the "apple core" lesion is indicative of colon cancer.
   3. Adenomatous polyps may develop into adenocarcinoma of the colon.
   a. 1 and 2
   b. 1 and 3
   c. 2 and 3
   d. 1, 2, and 3

9. A twisting of bowel about its mesenteric base best refers to a(n):
   a. Ascites
   b. Intussusception
   c. Incarcerated hernia
   d. Volvulus

10. The condition in which a gallstone erodes from the gallbladder and creates a fistula to the small bowel is:
    a. Gallstone ileus
    b. Intussusception
    c. Incarcerated hernia
    d. Volvulus

11. Describe the differences, both clinical and radiographic, between a mechanical bowel obstruction and paralytic ileus.

12. Explain the connection between colonic polyps and the development of colorectal cancer.

13. Describe the role of computed tomography (CT) in the staging of various GI cancers.

14. Explain the physiologic alteration that causes esophageal varices, and describe the radiographic appearance of this disorder.

15. Compare and contrast the various gastric tubes in terms of their uses and radiographic appearance.

6

Hepatobiliary System

On completion of Chapter 6, the reader should be able to do the following:

- Describe the anatomic components of the hepatobiliary system and state how they are visualized radiographically.
- Discuss the role of other imaging modalities in imaging of the hepatobiliary system, particularly sonography, magnetic resonance imaging, and computed tomography.
- Characterize a given condition as inflammatory or neoplastic.
- Identify the pathogenesis of the pathologies cited and the typical treatments for them.
- Describe, in general, the radiographic appearance of each of the given pathologies.

OUTLINE

Anatomy and Physiology
  Liver
  Biliary Tree
  Gallbladder
  Pancreas
Imaging Considerations
  Radiography
  Contrast Studies
  Diagnostic Medical
    Sonography
  Computed Tomography
  Nuclear Medicine
    Procedures

Magnetic Resonance
  Imaging
Inflammatory Diseases
  Alcohol-Induced Liver
    Disease
  Fatty Liver Disease
  Cirrhosis
  Viral Hepatitis
  Cholelithiasis
  Cholecystitis
  Pancreatitis
  Jaundice

Neoplastic Diseases
  Hepatocellular
    Adenoma
  Hemangioma
  Hepatocellular Carcinoma
    (Hepatoma)
  Metastatic Liver
    Disease
  Carcinoma of the
    Gallbladder
  Carcinoma of the
    Pancreas

KEY TERMS

Ascites
Carcinoma of the gallbladder
Cholecystitis
Cirrhosis
Fatty liver disease
Gallstone ileus

Hemangioma
Hepatitis
Hepatocellular adenoma
Hepatocellular carcinoma
Hepatomegaly
Jaundice

Medical jaundice
Metastatic liver disease
Pancreatic cancer
Pancreatitis

Pseudocyst
Steatosis
Surgical jaundice

ANATOMY AND PHYSIOLOGY

The hepatobiliary system is composed of the liver, gallbladder, and biliary tree (Fig. 6-1). The pancreas is closely related and shares a portion of the biliary ductal system, hence its inclusion here.

Liver

The liver is the largest organ in the body and is sheltered by the ribs in the right upper quadrant (RUQ) of the abdomen. It is kept in position by peritoneal ligaments and intraabdominal pressure from the muscles of the abdominal wall. The functions of the liver are multiple: metabolism of substances delivered via its portal circulation; synthesis of substances, including those concerned with blood clotting, storage of vitamin B, and other materials; and detoxification and excretion of various substances.

The liver has a double supply of blood, coming from the hepatic artery and the portal vein. The hepatic artery usually originates from the celiac axis and takes oxygenated blood to the liver. The portal vein is formed by the union of the superior mesenteric and splenic veins. It is located within the liver and serves to return venous blood from the abdominal viscera to the inferior vena cava (IVC). Any interference with blood flow, which may occur with liver disease, results in consequences elsewhere in the abdominal viscera and spleen.

Biliary Tree

A system of ducts acts to drain bile produced in the liver into the duodenum (Fig. 6-2). Bile from the liver's two main lobes is drained by the right

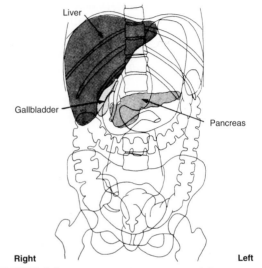

FIGURE 6-1 The hepatobiliary system and the pancreas.

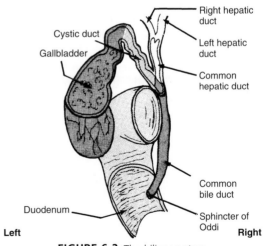

FIGURE 6-2 The biliary system.

and left hepatic ducts. These unite to form the common hepatic duct, which is joined usually in its midportion by the cystic duct from the gallbladder. Together, the cystic duct and the common hepatic duct form the common bile duct.

The common bile duct descends posterior to the descending duodenum to enter at its posteromedial aspect. Before its entrance into the duodenum, the common bile duct may be joined by the pancreatic duct from the head of the pancreas. The short part of the common bile duct, after joining the pancreatic duct, is known as the *hepatopancreatic ampulla* or, more commonly, the *ampulla of Vater.*

The flow of both bile and pancreatic juice into the duodenum is regulated by the hepatopancreatic sphincter, more commonly known as the *sphincter of Oddi.* The release of bile into the duodenum is triggered by cholecystokinin, a hormone released by the presence of fatty foods in the stomach. The purpose of bile is to emulsify fats so that they may be absorbed.

Gallbladder

The gallbladder, a digestive organ, is a pear-shaped sac located on the undersurface on the right lobe of the liver. Normally, the walls are quite thin, but they often thicken in the presence of inflammation. The sole function of the gallbladder is to store and concentrate bile that has been produced in the liver. The gallbladder receives bile from the liver via the hepatic duct and empties bile into the duodenum to aid the digestion and absorption of fats in the gastrointestinal (GI) system.

Pancreas

The pancreas is an elongated, flat organ that obliquely crosses the left side of the abdomen behind the stomach; it is a powerful digestive organ. Its functions are both exocrine and endocrine. Exocrine function is concerned with production of the three digestive enzymes trypsin, amylase, and lipase. Trypsin assists in the digestion of proteins. Amylase helps to break down large molecules of starch into smaller molecules of maltose, which eventually are broken down into glucose and stored in the liver. Lipase assists in breaking down lipids into fatty acids and glycerol. These are discharged through the pancreatic duct into the duodenum. The endocrine portion of the pancreas consists of multiple clusters of specialized cells, which are termed the *islets of Langerhans.* The specialized cells are classified as α-cells and β-cells. The function of β-cells is to produce insulin, and α-cells produce glucagon, both of which are discharged directly into the blood from the pancreas. Insulin and glucagon regulate carbohydrate metabolism. Insulin's role in this function includes making and storing glucose in the liver and in muscle tissue throughout the body and enabling the body to burn the stored glucose. When the blood flowing from the pancreas to the liver through the portal vein is hyperglycemic, insulin is released into the bloodstream via the portal vein. Glucagon acts in a similar manner, but it functions to increase the glucose level in blood. If the blood released into the portal vein is hypoglycemic, glucagon stimulates the liver to break down glycogen into glucose, thus increasing the glucose level in the bloodstream.

IMAGING CONSIDERATIONS

Radiography

A conventional abdominal radiograph may contain information about the hepatobiliary system through the demonstration of faint calcifications that might otherwise be obscured by contrast media. A plain radiograph of the gallbladder may demonstrate radiopaque gallstones composed of a mixture of cholesterol, bile pigment (bilirubin), and calcium salts or milk of calcium, which is a semiliquid sludge composed of calcium carbonate mixed with bile in the gallbladder. The hazy radiopacity results from a settling of bile as a result of an obstruction at the neck of the gallbladder, or it may develop in patients who have been fasting or have been on hyperalimentation.

Gas may occasionally be seen in the wall or lumen of the gallbladder because of the presence of gas-forming organisms in the gallbladder walls. This is more often seen in patients with poorly controlled diabetes because of poor blood supply to the organ. Gas visualized in the biliary tree may also be a result of a spontaneous fistula, as might be seen in gallstone ileus, or postoperative biliary anastomosis.

Contrast Studies

Percutaneous Transhepatic Cholangiography.
Percutaneous transhepatic cholangiography (PTC) is used to visualize the biliary tree and involves insertion of a needle into the biliary tree by puncture directly through the wall of the abdomen. With the use of a flexible, 22-gauge, skinny needle (Chiba), this procedure is safe and fairly easy to perform. The subsequent injection of iodinated contrast medium (Fig. 6-3) is useful in distinguishing **medical jaundice**, caused by hepatocellular dysfunction, from **surgical jaundice**, which results from biliary obstruction. Also, the examination is useful for detecting the presence of calculi or a tumor in the distal common bile duct. It has a high success rate in imaging the biliary ductal system, is less expensive than an endoscopic retrograde cholangiopancreatogram, and has a low complication rate of approximately 3.5%. It also may be immediately followed by a therapeutic procedure such as a biliary drainage, stone removal or crushing via contact lithotripsy or laser fragmentation, stent placement, or biopsy. This procedure is preferred in the evaluation of proximal obstructions involving the hepatic duct bifurcation, which is difficult to image with the retrograde approach via an endoscopic retrograde cholangiopancreatogram (see next section).

Endoscopic Retrograde Cholangiopancreatogram.
The endoscopic retrograde cholangiopancreatogram (ERCP), an imaging procedure performed by a gastroenterologist, is a means of visualizing the biliary system and main pancreatic duct, which provides drainage for the pancreatic enzymes into both the digestive tract and the common bile duct. A fiberoptic endoscope is passed through the duodenal C-loop to visualize the hepatopancreatic ampulla (ampulla of Vater). A thin catheter is then directed into the orifice of the common bile duct or pancreatic duct, followed by an injection of contrast medium (Fig. 6-4). In many cases, the ERCP is preferred over the PTC and is often preceded with a sonographic examination or computed tomography (CT) investigation of the pancreas. Although an ERCP is more expensive than PTC, it is often used to visualize nondilated ducts, distal obstructions, bleeding disorders, and the pancreas. The complication rate (2% to 3%) is similar to that of

FIGURE 6-3 Demonstration of the biliary system via a percutaneous transhepatic cholangiogram.

FIGURE 6-4 An endoscopic retrograde cholangiopancreatogram showing abrupt termination of the pancreatic duct about 4 cm from its opening.

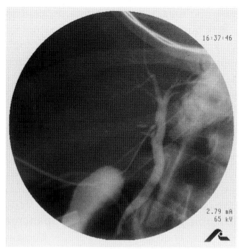

FIGURE 6-5 A digital image of an operative cholangiogram taken during surgery.

FIGURE 6-6 A sagittal sonographic view of the gallbladder demonstrating stones.

PTC and also offers the ability to perform therapeutic procedures such as sphincterotomy, stone extractions, stent placement, and biliary dilatation. Cytology and biopsy may also be performed.

Operative Cholangiography. Operative cholangiography is performed during surgery at the time of a cholecystectomy to detect biliary calculi and the need for common bile duct exploration (Fig. 6-5). A needle is placed directly into the cystic duct or common bile duct by the surgeon, and a small volume (6 milliliters [mL]) of iodinated contrast material is injected, followed by radiography. A second injection of 5 mL is made, followed by radiography a second time. The resulting images are reviewed for possible areas of concern before the surgery is completed. It is imperative that no air bubbles be injected into the ductal system with the contrast agent during this procedure because they can mimic stones.

T-Tube Cholangiography. T-tube cholangiography is used after a cholecystectomy to demonstrate patency of the common bile duct and to check for calculi. With a T-shaped tube already inserted surgically into the common bile duct, iodinated contrast medium is injected to verify removal of all calculi. The radiologist must take care not to inject air bubbles because they may give the radiographic appearance of radiolucent calculi.

Diagnostic Medical Sonography

Real-time diagnostic medical sonography is now the modality of choice for evaluating the gallbladder (Fig. 6-6) and biliary tree. This procedure is noninvasive, and the gallbladder can be imaged in almost all fasting patients regardless of the body habitus or clinical condition of the patient. When sonography is performed by a skilled sonographer, it has been proven to be almost 100% accurate in detecting gallstones, which are demonstrated as echogenic areas within the echo-free gallbladder. Thickening of the gallbladder wall is also easily identified. Sonography is also an excellent tool for determining the presence of common bile duct obstruction, evaluation of the intrahepatic biliary ductal system, and identification of abscesses. The liver may be evaluated by sonography because of its ideal location in the RUQ and broad contact with the abdominal wall. Hepatic lesions of 1 cm or greater are easily identified, with cystic lesions appearing echo-free and solid masses appearing echogenic, allowing excellent guidance for aspiration and biopsy of these lesions.

Doppler sonography enhances the diagnostic capabilities of sonography to allow for clear analysis of the circulatory dynamics, including portal blood flow and hepatic artery thrombosis following liver transplantation. Doppler sonography can also differentiate between vessels and biliary ducts based on flow characteristics.

Computed Tomography

The role of CT in the hepatobiliary system is similar to its role in the GI tract. It is the accepted modality for following malignancies and assessing masses, particularly of the gallbladder, liver, and pancreas. It is also helpful in evaluating complications of cholecystitis such as perforations and abscess formations. The use of spiral or helical CT ensures that the entire liver is imaged in one breath, eliminating respiratory artifacts and in many cases demonstrating the liver parenchyma and associated structures better than sonography. In addition to the excellent contrast resolution offered by CT, the use of large-bolus intravenous (IV) iodinated contrast media injections during dynamic CT examination has also improved evaluations of the hepatobiliary ductal system and blood flow via three-phase imaging of the liver to capture the arterial and portal venous blood flow (Fig. 6-7). If a biliary obstruction is not visible on sonographic examination, CT is generally used to identify the location and extent of the obstruction because it is not limited by patient size or the presence of bowel gas. Lacerations of the liver and resultant abdominal bleeding are readily detected on CT (Fig. 6-8), as are metastatic lesions within the liver. CT also demonstrates good visualization of pancreatic tumors and pseudocysts. In addition, CT-guided biopsy procedures for the liver (Fig. 6-9), pancreas, and kidney allow for analysis and drainage and offer significant advantages over conventional surgical biopsy and drainage.

Nuclear Medicine Procedures

Single photon emission computed tomography (SPECT) examinations permit excellent detection of hepatobiliary lesions, especially those located deep within the liver parenchyma. SPECT provides a noninvasive method of evaluating hepatic function as well as hepatic and splenic perfusion. Because nuclear medicine imaging provides information regarding physiologic function, combining SPECT and CT can often provide information about both anatomic changes and physiologic function, thus enhancing the ability to diagnose pathologies earlier than using any one modality alone. Labeling of white blood cells (WBCs) with radioactive indium is useful in locating sites of infection for treatment.

Cholescintigraphy performed in nuclear medicine is very useful to confirm cholecystitis and for distinguishing acute cholecystitis from chronic cholecystitis (Fig. 6-10). Radioactive technetium is cleared from blood plasma into bile, demonstrating the physiologic function of the liver, excretion into the biliary ductal system, and visualization of the gallbladder about 1 hour after injection. Delayed visualization or nonvisualization of the gallbladder indicates pathology. In addition, it is a noninvasive method of evaluating biliary drainage, hepatobiliary leaks following trauma or surgery, and segmental obstruction.

Magnetic Resonance Imaging

The role of magnetic resonance imaging (MRI) of the hepatobiliary system has improved greatly as a result of shorter scan times, which allow the acquisition of several images of the abdomen in a single breath. MRI is often used in conjunction with CT to evaluate pathologies and anomalies of the peritoneum, especially the liver and pancreas. MRI may also be used to identify retroperitoneal bleeds following trauma (Fig. 6-11). Contrast-enhanced three-dimensional dynamic scans of the liver imaged at timed intervals help to differentiate certain tumors from hemangiomas.

Magnetic resonance cholangiopancreatography (MRCP) is an imaging procedure that uses magnetic resonance to visualize the gallbladder and biliary system. MRCP is noninvasive and does not require the use of a contrast agent (Fig. 6-12). A heavily T2-weighted sequence is used to suppress the tissues around the biliary system, allowing the gallbladder and bile ducts to appear bright and enabling visualization of stones or

FIGURE 6-7 A and **B,** Three-phase computed tomography (CT) of the liver following a bolus injection of intravenous contrast, demonstrating the arterial circulation. **C** and **D,** Three-phase CT of the liver, delayed images demonstrating the portal venous flow.

other obstructions. MRCP usually accompanies other imaging sequences of the liver, but it takes only about 15 seconds to acquire an image.

The American College of Radiology (ACR) provides a highly researched scheme for determining which of the diagnostic imaging studies is best suited for specific clinical conditions. For patients who present with RUQ pain that may

be attributed to the biliary system, sonography of the abdomen is the highest rated imaging examination. CT of the abdomen (with and without contrast), cholescintigraphy, and MRI of the abdomen (with or without contrast) are also recommended and may be appropriate for obtaining the diagnosis. Additionally, if the patient is suspected of having inflammation of

FIGURE 6-8 Computed tomography of this 39-year-old woman after a car accident reveals large lacerations of the liver.

FIGURE 6-10 Nuclear medicine hepatobiliary scan demonstrates ready ejection of the radionuclide from the gallbladder through sequential images into the duodenum.

FIGURE 6-9 Computed tomography of needle biopsy in this 87-year-old woman clearly demonstrates the needle in the liver.

FIGURE 6-11 T2 TruFisp axial magnetic resonance image of the abdomen demonstrating a retroperitoneal hemorrhage.

the gallbladder (cholecystitis), a percutaneous cholecystotomy may be appropriate for patients in the intensive care unit, who are likely considered nonsurgical candidates.

INFLAMMATORY DISEASES

Alcohol-Induced Liver Disease

Alcohol is a known toxin, which, when metabolized by the liver, causes cellular damage; alcohol abuse has long been associated with liver disease.

Approximately two million Americans have alcohol-induced liver disease, ranging from alcoholic fatty liver to alcoholic cirrhosis of the liver. Alcohol cannot be stored in the human body, and therefore, the liver must convert it, through oxidation, to alcohol dehydrogenase, acetaldehyde, and acetate, all of which reduce cellular function. This leads to interference with carbohydrate and lipid metabolism. Oxidation also results in reduced gluconeogenesis and increased fatty acid synthesis associated with alcohol metabolism. Chronic alcohol abuse often leads to **fatty liver,**

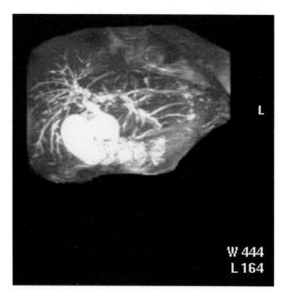

FIGURE 6-12 Magnetic resonance imaging is capable of imaging the biliary system without the use of contrast agents.

FIGURE 6-13 Computed tomography shows fatty liver infiltration.

followed by hepatitis, cirrhosis, hepatocellular carcinoma, or all of these diseases. Fatty liver is the most frequent early response to alcohol abuse. Changes in liver function result in a buildup of lipids such as triglycerides, which are deposited in the liver cells. This condition is usually asymptomatic; however, patients may have **hepatomegaly**. Fatty infiltration may be demonstrated by using CT or sonography, but CT is currently the examination of choice. CT demonstrates the fatty deposits as hypodense areas throughout the liver (Fig. 6-13). Inflammation often follows fatty changes within the liver, leading to **alcoholic hepatitis**. At this stage, many patients present with jaundice. This inflammation is diffuse throughout the liver cells and culminates in liver necrosis. This disease may be fatal, progressing quickly to liver failure; or if the individual survives the hepatitis, the condition progresses to alcoholic cirrhosis of the liver, which is an end-stage disease.

Fatty Liver Disease

Factors other than alcohol abuse may also lead to fatty infiltrates within the liver. Obese individuals with type 2 diabetes mellitus, metabolic syndrome, hyperlipidemia, or all of these diseases are at an increased risk of developing nonalcoholic fatty liver disease (NAFLD). This pathology develops as lipids accumulate within the hepatocytes forming free radicals. At some point, the liver cannot rid itself of the excessive triglycerides. This results in an excess of fatty acids within the liver, which leads to fatty infiltration of the liver, termed *steatosis*, and fatty liver disease. In the early stages, NAFLD is often asymptomatic, and diagnosis requires biopsy of liver tissue. Although the disease progresses slowly, it may advance to cirrhosis of the liver if left untreated. Management includes implementation of weight loss programs and exercise programs as treatment for insulin resistance and associated metabolic disturbances.

Cirrhosis

Cirrhosis is a chronic liver condition in which the liver parenchyma and architecture are destroyed, fibrous tissue is laid down, and regenerative nodules are formed. In its early stages, it is usually asymptomatic, as it may take months or even years before damage becomes apparent. Cirrhosis affects the entire liver and is considered an end-stage condition resulting from liver damage caused by chronic alcohol abuse, drugs, autoimmune disorders, metabolic and genetic disease, chronic hepatitis, cardiac problems, and chronic biliary tract obstruction. In 2007, chronic liver disease leading to cirrhosis of the liver ranked as the fifth leading cause of death among Native Americans, the sixth leading cause of death among Hispanics, the twelfth leading cause of death among whites, and the fifteenth leading cause of death among blacks. In the United States, it is the seventh leading cause of death in individuals aged 35 to 44 years and the fourth leading cause of death in individuals between the ages of 45 and 65 years.

The scarring and formation of regenerative nodules associated with cirrhosis result in serious complications. The functional impairments caused by cirrhosis are impaired liver function caused by hepatocyte damage, generally resulting in jaundice, and portal hypertension. Because of interference of portal blood flow through the liver, portal hypertension may lead to development of collateral venous connections to the venae cavae (Fig. 6-14). Most commonly, such connections involve the esophageal veins, which dilate to become esophageal varices, as described in the preceding chapter. These are best evaluated with endoscopy but may be seen on an esophagram. Also, the patient with cirrhosis has a tendency to bleed because the liver is unable to make the necessary clotting factors found in plasma or as a result of an esophageal variceal rupture. Such hemorrhaging may be, in fact, the first indication of portal hypertension.

Ascites, the accumulation of fluid within the peritoneal cavity (Fig. 6-15), is also seen as a result of portal hypertension and the leakage of excessive fluids from the portal capillaries. Much of this excess fluid is composed of hepatic lymph weeping from the liver surface. It is associated with approximately 50% of deaths from cirrhosis. Ascites may also result from chronic hepatitis, congestive heart failure, renal failure, and certain cancers. Abdominal sonography is commonly used in the detection or confirmation of ascites. Diagnostic and therapeutic paracentesis may be conducted with sonographic guidance to locate a site that will allow fluid to be removed

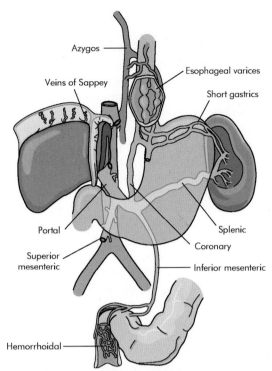

FIGURE 6-14 Varices related to portal hypertension.

FIGURE 6-15 Cirrhosis of the liver as indicated on this computed tomography scan showing a shrunken liver with significant ascites around it within the abdomen.

and to avoid damage to the floating bowel loops. A diagnostic paracentesis involves removal of 50 to 100 mL of peritoneal fluid for analysis. Patients with ascites generally complain of non-specific abdominal pain and dyspnea. Medical treatment of ascites includes bed rest, dietary restrictions of sodium, use of diuretics to avoid excess fluid accumulation, and treatment of the underlying cause.

It is important for the radiographer to be aware of the clinical diagnosis of ascites because the fluid accumulation makes it difficult to adequately penetrate the abdomen. An increase in exposure factors is necessary to obtain a diagnostic-quality radiograph. Radiographically, large amounts of ascitic fluid give the abdomen a dense, gray, ground-glass appearance. When the patient is in the supine position, fluid accumulates in the pelvis and ascends to either side of the bladder to give it a dog-eared appearance. Gradually, the margins of the liver, spleen, kidneys, and psoas muscles become indistinct as the volume of fluid increases. Loops of bowel filled with gas float centrally, and a lateral decubitus radiograph demonstrates the fluid descending and the gas-filled loops of bowel floating on top.

Conventional radiographic signs of cirrhosis are few and not specific. Morphologic changes in the liver from cirrhosis may cause displacement of other abdominal organs such as the stomach, duodenum, colon, gallbladder, and kidney. CT is the primary modality for evaluating the complications arising from cirrhosis. Fatty infiltration of the liver is well visualized by CT. The most characteristic finding in cirrhosis is an increase in the ratio of the caudate lobe and the right lobe. This occurs with cirrhosis because of atrophy of the right lobe and medial segment of the left lobe and hypertrophy of the caudate lobe and the lateral segment of the left lobe. Because of its dual arterial blood supply, the caudate lobe of the liver is usually spared in cirrhosis. Studies show that individuals with cirrhosis have an increased risk of developing hepatic carcinoma, so CT is also of value in assessing the presence of complications of cirrhosis such as ascites and hepatocellular carcinoma.

Diagnostic medical sonography is helpful in identifying liver cirrhosis and enlargement of the liver and spleen. Doppler is used to detect portal hypertension and evaluate portosystemic collateral circulation. It is used to measure the vessel size of the portal vein, which ranges from 0.64 to 1 cm in a normal adult. A portal vein larger than 1.3 cm in diameter is indicative of portal hypertension. In addition, the portal vein should distend with deep inspiration, but in patients with portal hypertension the vein lacks distensibility. Doppler integration of the portal vein allows tracing of the flow of blood within the vessel. Normal portal vein flow is toward the liver; however, with portal hypertension, the flow is shunted away from the liver because of the diseased liver's inability to accept the flow of blood. As a result, the splenic vein tries to handle this resistance by diverting the flow toward the spleen. In many cases, affected persons develop splenic varices from the increased flow from the portal vein. Sonographic evaluation of venous structures such as the superior mesenteric and splenic veins adds additional information for the clinician. However, final diagnosis of cirrhosis is generally accomplished by biopsy of liver tissue, often performed under sonographic guidance.

Treatment of cirrhosis depends on the extent of liver damage and the involvement of other organs (e.g., the esophagus and stomach). The primary goal of treatment is to eliminate the underlying causes of the disease and to treat its complications. Surgical treatment of portal hypertension may be achieved by diverting blood from the portocollateral system into the lower-pressure systemic circulation. This is accomplished by placing a shunt, eliminating the chance of variceal bleeding. A distal splenorenal shunt, in which the splenic vein is divided, with the distal portion anastomosed to the left renal vein, is most commonly used. If the patient is not a candidate for this type of shunt, a total shunt, either portocaval or mesocaval, must be placed. A palliative procedure, the transjugular intrahepatic portosystemic shunt (TIPSS), may also be used to divert the pressure of portal hypertension. The TIPSS procedure is commonly performed in the cardiovascular interventional area of a radiology department. A catheter is placed in the right internal jugular vein and pushed through the right atrium into the IVC. The needle end of the catheter is inserted into the closest portal vein in the liver, commonly the right portal vein. Through use of angioplasty, the tract is enlarged such that a shunt can be placed to reroute the flow of portal blood through the liver and into the IVC. Sonography is invaluable for assessing the long-term effect of this shunt. Typically, Doppler tracings are taken at the portal end, the midshunt, and the hepatic vein end of the shunt to ensure that flow through it allows the flow of blood to proceed through the liver to the IVC. However, all of these shunts have a tendency to thrombose, requiring patency to be assessed by angiography, CT, or sonography. The prognosis for patients with associated complications of cirrhosis such as ascites is poor, but advances in liver transplantation have changed the long-term outcome for many patients.

Lesions in the liver that have been identified on sonography, MRI, or CT are highly recommended to be further evaluated with MRI of the abdomen, with and without contrast, to conclusively differentiate between benign and malignant lesions. If the patient is unable to tolerate MRI contrast, CT of the abdomen is the next modality recommended to delineate the liver lesion in question.

If abdominal ascites is suspected in a patient with acute abdominal pain, the use of helical CT is highly recommended to document the presence of free fluid in the abdomen, as it is sensitive and very cost-effective in evaluating the patient with acute abdominal pain.

Viral Hepatitis

Hepatitis is a relatively common liver condition, with an estimated 70,000 cases reported annually in the United States. At least six types of viral agents that cause acute inflammation of the liver have been identified (Table 6-1). This inflammation interferes with the liver's ability to excrete bilirubin, the orange or yellowish pigment in bile. Clinical evidence of the disease includes nausea, vomiting, discomfort, and tenderness over the liver area, and laboratory results indicate a disturbance in liver function. Additional signs and symptoms include fatigue, anorexia, photophobia, and general malaise. Jaundice may also develop within 1 or 2 weeks because of the disturbance of bilirubin excretion. If the liver inflammation lasts 6 months or more, the condition is classified as chronic.

Hepatitis A virus (HAV) is a single-stranded ribonucleic acid (RNA) picornavirus. It is excreted in the GI tract in fecal matter and is spread by contact with an infected individual, normally through ingestion of contaminated food such as raw shellfish or through contaminated water. It is the most common form of hepatitis and is highly contagious. The incubation period of the disease is relatively short (15 to 50 days), and its course is usually mild. HAV infection does not lead to chronic hepatitis or cirrhosis of the liver.

Hepatitis B virus (HBV) is transmitted parenterally through infected serum or blood products. Its incubation period is much longer (50 to 160 days), and its effects are more severe than those of HAV. The etiologic makeup of HBV is very complex, consisting of a viral core of deoxyribonucleic acid (DNA), which replicates within the cells of the liver. The viral core is covered with a surface coat. HBV may result in an asymptomatic carrier state, acute hepatitis, chronic hepatitis, cirrhosis, and hepatocellular carcinoma. Three distinct antigen–antibody systems have been shown to have a link to HBV. These include hepatitis B surface antigen (HBsAg), which appears in the incubation stage and is the first indication of HBV infection; hepatitis B core antigen (HBcAg), which is found in liver tissue but not in serum; and hepatitis B extracellular antigen (HbeAg), which reflects active viral replication. Most health care workers are now required to receive HBV vaccination. Vaccination has dramatically reduced the incidence of infection, and the vaccines are safe with very few side effects.

TABLE 6-1	Characteristics of Viral Hepatitis					
Characteristic	Hepatitis A	Hepatitis B	Hepatitis D	Hepatitis C	Hepatitis E	Hepatitis G
Size of virus	27 nanometer (nm) DNA virus	47 nm DNA virus	36 nm RNA virus, defective with HbsAg coat	30–60 nm RNA virus	32 nm RNA virus	30–60 nm RNA virus
Incubation period	30 days	60–180 days	30–180 days	35–60 days	15–60 days	Unknown
Route of transmission	Fecal–oral, parenteral, sexual	Parenteral, sexual	Parenteral, ? fecal–oral, sexual	Parenteral	Fecal–oral	Parenteral, sexual
Onset	Acute with fever	Insidious	Insidious	Insidious	Acute	Unknown
Carrier state	Negative	Positive	Positive	Positive	Negative	Positive
Severity	Mild	Severe; may be prolonged or chronic	Severe	Mild to severe	Severe in pregnant women	Unknown
Chronic hepatitis	No	Yes	Yes	Yes	No	Unknown
Age-group affected	Children and young adults	Any	Any	Any	Children and young adults	Any
Prophylaxis	Hygiene, immune serum globulin HAV vaccine	Hygiene, HBV vaccine	Hygiene, HBV vaccine	Hygiene, screening blood, interferon-alpha	Hygiene, safe water	

DNA, Deoxyribonucleic acid; *HAV,* hepatitis A virus; *HbsAg,* hepatitis B surface antigen; *HBV,* hepatitis B virus; *RNA,* ribonucleic acid.
From McCance KL, Huether SE, Brashers VL, & Rote NS, *Pathophysiology: The biologic basis for disease in adults and children,* 6 ed, Mosby Elsevier, St. Louis, MO.

Hepatitis C virus (HCV) is caused by a parenterally transmitted RNA virus. Type C accounts for 80% of the cases of hepatitis that develop after blood transfusions. A routine test for anti-HCV antibody has been developed, so transmission via transfused blood has been significantly decreased. HCV may cause either acute or chronic hepatitis, with 10% to 20% of affected patients eventually developing cirrhosis of the liver.

Hepatitis D virus (HDV) is caused by an RNA virus and occurs only concurrently with acute or chronic HBV. It cannot occur alone. Hepatitis E virus (HEV) is also an RNA viral agent. It is most commonly responsible for outbreaks of waterborne epidemic acute hepatitis in developing countries. Although the infection may be severe, it does not progress to a chronic state. Hepatitis

G virus (HGV), which has been recently isolated, may also be transmitted via blood products and may cause chronic hepatitis.

The diagnosis of viral hepatitis is usually made through laboratory testing because the disease is carried in the bloodstream during the acute phase. Evidence of hepatitis may be seen on radiographs of the abdomen that demonstrate *hepatomegaly* (enlargement of the liver), although this is a nonspecific finding. Cellular necrosis may be confirmed through nuclear medicine scanning of the liver, CT, or liver biopsy. Sonography is also useful in distinguishing the characteristics of the liver.

HAV is usually mild; the majority of patients recover without complications. Treatment generally consists of bed rest and medication for nausea and vomiting. In a healthy individual, the liver regenerates after hepatitis damage, and complete recovery is gained. Patients with type B, type C, type D, and type G generally go on to develop chronic hepatitis. In some, the disease may progress to liver failure.

Percutaneous liver biopsy is the gold standard for determining the type of disease that may be present in the liver. This is a recommended diagnostic step when the liver appears irregular on sonography, CT, or MRI. A pathologist examines the liver specimen and makes the final diagnosis and the type of disease that is present in the sample provided.

Cholelithiasis

Cholelithiasis (gallstones) is fairly common, with at least 20% of all persons in the United States developing them by the age of 65 years. Women are more likely than men to have them. Their occurrence is also more common in people with diabetes, those who are obese, older adults, and individuals who eat primarily a diet high in saturated fat, sugar, and sodium and low in fiber and nutrient density (Western diet). Heredity plays a role in the development of gallstones. Although most commonly found in the gallbladder, gallstones can be located anywhere in the biliary tree. Symptoms associated with cholelithiasis may be vague, including bloating, nausea, and pain in the right upper quadrant. Sludge may develop within the gallbladder and may be identified sonographically. Sometimes sludge develops in patients who have been fasting or who have been on hyperalimentation and is a normal variant from underusage of the bile in the gallbladder; in other cases, sludge may be a precursor to development of gallstones.

The characteristics of gallstones are quite varied. They may occur as a single stone or as multiple stones. About 80% of all stones are composed of a mixture of cholesterol, bile pigment (bilirubin), and calcium salts. The remaining 20% are composed of pure cholesterol or a calcium–bilirubin mixture. Most stones are radiolucent because only approximately 10% of all stones contain enough calcium to be

FIGURE 6-16 A sagittal sonographic image of a dilated gallbladder containing stones.

radiopaque. Those that are radiopaque may be difficult to distinguish from renal stones, but oblique radiographs help separate the two structures (kidney and gallbladder) from each other, demonstrating the gallbladder anterior to the kidney. As noted before, sonography readily demonstrates the presence of cholelithiasis (Fig. 6-16). The best image is obtained when the gallbladder is distended and filled with bile, so patients should fast 8 hours before sonographic examination. The three major sonographic criteria for gallstones include an echogenic focus, acoustic shadowing below the stone, and gravitational dependence. Gallstones may be the size of a pinhead to that of a large marble. The small stones tend to travel into the biliary tree and may result in obstruction. Obstruction of the bile duct causes pain and jaundice and may result in cholangitis.

It is highly recommended that patients who do not have fever, have normal WBC counts, and have gallstones as demonstrated by sonograms undergo cholescintigraphy, CT of the abdomen (with or without contrast), and MRI of the abdomen (with or without contrast) to ensure that other forms of biliary disease are not present.

Surgical removal of the gallbladder (cholecystectomy) is usually the treatment of choice, with more than 500,000 such procedures performed annually in the United States. Since its introduction in 1988, laparoscopic cholecystectomy has replaced many traditional open cholecystectomies. This technique allows a less traumatic entry, excision, and removal of the gallbladder, resulting in shortened hospitalization and reduced costs. Radiographers are commonly called to the operating environment to image injections of contrast medium into the exposed biliary duct to determine if all stones have been removed. If additional stones are suspected but not visualized, a T-tube may be inserted to allow for later study, as noted earlier.

Cholecystitis

Cholecystitis is an acute inflammation of the gallbladder. It is characterized clinically by a sudden onset of pain, fever, nausea, and vomiting. It is common in individuals with chronically symptomatic cholelithiasis. Its diagnosis is clinically suspected and supported through a sonographic examination or radionuclide cholescintigraphy. A radiopharmaceutical composed of technetium-99m (^{99m}Tc) in combination with diisopropyliminodiacetic acid (DISIDA) allows visualization of the biliary ductal system and results in a highly sensitive examination with consistently reliable results. Nonvisualization of the gallbladder is a good indicator of acute cholecystitis. Repeated attacks of acute cholecystitis cause damage to the gallbladder, thickening of the walls (Fig. 6-17), and decreased function.

FIGURE 6-17 Sonogram demonstrating a thickened wall of the gallbladder, often indicative of cholecystitis.

Complications of untreated gallbladder disease include infarction and a possible gangrenous state, prompting rupture of the walls. Perforation of the gallbladder occurs in approximately 5% to 15% of all patients with acute cholecystitis and can be diagnosed in several ways. Cholescintigraphy provides the best images of perforation; however, stones may be visible outside the gallbladder on conventional abdominal radiographs, CT images, or sonographic images. Sonography and CT often also demonstrate a nonspecific pericholecystic fluid collection. If a rupture does occur, bile peritonitis may result and require immediate treatment.

Occasionally, a stone may erode through the wall of the gallbladder in cases of chronic cholecystitis and create a fistula to the bowel, most frequently the duodenum. If the stone becomes impacted in the small bowel and causes an obstruction, the condition is referred to as **gallstone ileus**. Gallstone ileus is characterized by air in the biliary ductal system, clearly visible on a conventional abdominal radiograph. The radiopaque gallstone may also be visible within the bowel surrounded by intestinal gas. Surgical removal of the stone is necessary to relieve the obstruction. Treatment of chronic cholecystitis also includes laparoscopic removal of the inflamed gallbladder.

Pancreatitis

Inflammation of the pancreatic tissue is known as **pancreatitis**. It is one of the most complex and clinically challenging disorders of the abdomen and is classified as acute or chronic, according to clinical, morphologic, and histologic criteria. Acute pancreatitis resolves without impairing the histologic makeup of the pancreas and most often results from biliary tract disease. However, chronic pancreatitis does impair the histologic makeup of the pancreas, resulting in irreversible changes in pancreatic function. Its causes include excessive and chronic alcohol consumption, obstruction of the hepatopancreatic ampulla by a gallstone or tumor, and even the injection of contrast media during ERCP. Once activated by

FIGURE 6-18 Pancreatitis with demonstration of a 5-cm pseudocyst in the head as seen on computed tomography.

FIGURE 6-19 Transverse sonographic image of the pancreas.

any of these causes, trypsin, the pancreatic enzyme that is normally excreted through the ducts into the duodenum, begins to autodigest the organ itself. This has serious consequences and carries a high mortality rate. Hemorrhagic pancreatitis is a complication of pancreatitis and consists of erosion into local tissues and blood vessels, with subsequent hemorrhaging into the retroperitoneal space. A **pseudocyst** is a fluid collection caused by pancreatitis. It is readily visualized by sonographic or CT examination (Fig. 6-18).

Symptoms of pancreatitis vary from mild abdominal pain, nausea, and vomiting to severe pain and shock. Radiographic indications of pancreatitis are subtle and previously centered on displacement of the duodenal C-loop or the stomach by the diseased pancreas or calcified stones within the pancreatic or biliary ducts. However, CT has made a major contribution to the diagnosis and staging of acute pancreatitis. It adequately demonstrates not only the pancreas itself but also the retroperitoneum, the ligaments, the mesenteries, and the omenta. The infected pancreas is usually enlarged, with a shaggy and irregular contour. In advanced cases, fluid collections are demonstrated within the pancreas and within the retroperitoneum. ERCP is of value in determining the reasons for acute recurrent pancreatitis, chronic pancreatitis, or the

complications associated with pancreatitis. Because pancreatic disease is often asymptomatic in the early stages of disease, sonography is good for assessing the texture and size of the organ. The pancreas is routinely imaged as part of the RUQ sonogram. In most sonographic examinations, the head and body of the pancreas can be measured and compared with normal values for the age of the patient. Pancreatitis is suggested on a sonogram by the decreased echo texture and an associated enlargement in the size of the organ (Fig. 6-19). In addition, recent advances in MRI allow for noninvasive, contrast-free imaging of the biliary tree. Laboratory testing is the most common way to diagnose pancreatitis, through evaluation of serum and occasionally the urine amylase level.

Sonography and CT of the abdomen with contrast are equally recommended by the ACR for diagnosis of acute pancreatitis. MRI of the abdomen (with and without contrast) is appropriate if the aforementioned imaging modalities are not available.

Management of patients with pancreatitis consists of a pain-relieving drug in mild cases and maintaining proper fluid levels to prevent shock, a frequent occurrence in acute pancreatitis. Proper dietary restrictions (e.g., abstinence from alcohol) are also important. The role of surgery in chronic pancreatitis remains controversial with regard to the effectiveness of results. The prognosis is excellent in patients with mild pancreatic inflammation and edema. However, a swollen pancreas, with extravasation of fluid within the retroperitoneum or pancreatic necrosis as demonstrated by CT, results in a more severe prognosis. Although most CT examinations are performed with the use of IV contrast agents, research has shown that use of contrast agents during the onset of acute pancreatitis may cause necrosis in areas with poor blood supply. Pancreatic necrosis increases mortality and the incidence of infection, so patients should be well hydrated before a contrast-enhanced CT examination is performed. Chronic pancreatitis also increases the risk for pancreatic cancer, so most patients are continuously monitored for malignancy.

FIGURE 6-20 A sagittal sonographic image demonstrating a stone (*arrow*) lodged in the distal portion of the common bile duct close to the ampulla of Vater (*A*) resulting in dilation and obstruction of the common bile duct.

Jaundice

Jaundice, a yellowish discoloration of the skin and whites of the eyes, is not a disease itself but rather a sign of disease. The accumulation of excess bile pigments (i.e., bilirubin) in the body tissues "stains" the skin and eyes this yellowish color. Normally, bile and its pigments are secreted into the bowel and eliminated. Bilirubin is a type of bile pigment that is produced when hemoglobin breaks down. Normal serum bilirubin levels are equal to or less than 1 mg per 100 mL but must exceed 3 mg per 100 mL to be visible to the observer.

Medical (nonobstructive) jaundice occurs because of hemolytic disease, in which too many red blood cells (RBCs) are destroyed or because of liver damage from cirrhosis or hepatitis. Its most common appearance is transient in the first few days after birth, when more bile pigments are released than can be handled. A liver that is damaged from disease simply cannot excrete the bilirubin in a normal fashion, and it enters the bloodstream.

Surgical (obstructive) jaundice occurs when the biliary system is obstructed and prevents bile from entering the duodenum. A common cause of this obstruction is blockage of the common bile duct caused by stones or masses. The longer

the obstruction persists, the more likely it is that complications (e.g., liver injury, infection, or bleeding) will arise.

The jaundiced patient often undergoes a sonographic examination of the liver, biliary tree, and pancreas to determine if the jaundice is obstructive (Fig. 6-20) or nonobstructive. The common bile duct is readily identified; generally, a normal size implies nonobstructive jaundice, and a dilated common bile duct suggests an obstruction. A variety of other methods may be used to diagnose the cause of jaundice, including ERCP, MRCP, and CT. A sonographic or CT-directed needle biopsy may be used if an intrahepatic cause of the hepatitis is suspected. Treatment of jaundice centers on the diagnosis and treatment of its underlying cause. In the case of obstructive jaundice, surgical excision of the obstructing body may be necessary. Endoscopic removal of common duct stones is frequently done, and endoscopy also offers the opportunity to stent or bypass a tumor.

NEOPLASTIC DISEASES

Hepatocellular Adenoma

Hepatocellular adenoma is a benign tumor of the liver. Most tumors are asymptomatic, but the incidence of this disease has increased over the past few years. Hepatocellular adenomas occur most often in women using oral contraceptives, which play a role in the development of these benign lesions. In terms of imaging, both CT and sonography are useful in demonstrating hepatic lesions.

Hemangioma

A **hemangioma** is the most common tumor of the liver. It is a benign neoplasm composed of newly formed blood vessels, and these neoplasms may form in other places within the body. For instance, a port-wine stain on the face (a superficial purplish red birthmark) is an example of a hemangioma elsewhere in the body. Hemangiomas are generally well-circumscribed, solitary tumors. They may range in size from microscopic to 20 cm. They are more common in women than in men, especially in postmenopausal women.

Normally, the texture of the liver is homogeneous on sonographic evaluation, but an area of increased echogenicity may occasionally be demonstrated. When this appears as a solitary, round lesion, the diagnosis is usually a hemangioma. These lesions generally do not become malignant; however, sonography may be used to assess the lesion if it is suspected that it has changed in size or character. In most cases, a hemangioma is insignificant, but it may manifest symptoms such as RUQ pain as a result of tissue displacement or bleeding. Diagnosis may be complicated when it occurs with a known malignancy because its characteristics may be difficult to distinguish from metastasis. Nuclear medicine scans using labeled RBCs that are attracted to the highly vascular tumor are virtually diagnostic in assessing the presence of a hemangioma. These scans demonstrate the tumor as a defect in the early phases and display prolonged and persistent uptake on delayed scans. A CT of the liver following an injection of IV contrast medium demonstrates the hemangioma with peripheral enhancement. MRI demonstrates marked hyperintensity on T2-weighted images, which corresponds with fibrosis within the tumor. After an

FIGURE 6-21 An axial magnetic resonance imaging slice through the liver reveals a hemangioma.

IV injection of a gadolinium contrast agent, peripheral enhancement of the hemangioma occurs in early scans, followed by filling in of the tumor (Fig. 6-21), similar to the appearance on an enhanced CT examination.

A study completed on focal nodules in the liver and comparing the use of sonography, CT, and MRI found that MRI had a diagnostic advantage. MRI appears to have a higher sensitivity and specificity, especially when MRI contrast is administered, and provides physiologic information regarding the mass.

Hepatocellular Carcinoma (Hepatoma)

Hepatocellular carcinoma, a primary neoplasm of the liver, accounts for approximately 3% of all cancers in the United States. An association between cirrhosis and hepatocellular carcinoma exists, with chronic hepatitis B or C and alcoholism associated with each. Thus, the incidence of this neoplasm is on the rise because of an increase in chronic hepatitis B and C infections in the United States. Most primary hepatomas originate in the liver parenchyma, creating a large central mass with smaller satellite nodules. Although vascular invasion is common, death occurs from

FIGURE 6-22 Large, heterogeneous lesion in the liver consistent with hepatoma.

FIGURE 6-23 Computed tomography scan of the liver demonstrating metastatic spread from bronchogenic carcinoma (*arrows*).

liver failure, often without extension of the cancer outside the liver.

Hepatocellular carcinoma is suspected in patients with cirrhosis who experience an unexpected deterioration and in patients with increased jaundice, abdominal pain, weight loss, an RUQ mass, ascites, or a rapid increase in liver size. Plain abdominal radiographs may demonstrate hepatomegaly. Sonography and CT are often used to reveal the extent of the tumor (Fig. 6-22). Arteriography may demonstrate the increased vascularity associated with a carcinoma. A definitive diagnosis requires a liver biopsy, generally under sonographic guidance.

Surgical resection of the hepatocellular carcinoma represents the only possibility for cure. Hepatomas that are diffuse or have multiple nodules generally preclude surgery. The general lack of radiosensitivity of these tumors makes radiotherapy ineffective. Patients treated with chemotherapy demonstrate tumor shrinkage and an addition of a few months to their lives. The disease, however, is generally fatal except in those who have had successful resection of a single liver mass.

The ACR highly recommends resection of the tumor and possible liver transplantation as the best treatment for patients with hepatocellular carcinoma. Transarterial embolization may also be an appropriate treatment for lesions that are solid and are at least 5 cm in size. Selective

radiation therapy treatments that are directed internally are also possible, depending on the extent of the disease and whether it has invaded the portal vein.

Metastatic Liver Disease

Metastatic liver lesions are much more common than primary carcinoma because of the liver's role in filtering blood. The liver is a common site for metastasis from other primary sites such as the colon, pancreas, stomach, lung, and breast (Fig. 6-23). Primary cancers located in the abdomen, especially those drained by the portal venous system, often metastasize to the liver (Fig. 6-24). Sonography is most commonly used to screen patients for **metastatic liver disease;** however, CT and MRI also allow an accurate diagnosis. Again, liver biopsy, often under sonographic guidance, provides the definitive diagnosis.

The recommended treatment for metastatic liver disease is to use a combination of intramuscular injection of long-acting octreotide (a somatostatin analogue) and transarterial embolization,

FIGURE 6-24 Computed tomography scan after duodenal cancer resection in a 21-year-old woman demonstrates local recurrence and metastases to the liver on its lateral border in this slice.

especially if the medication fails to decrease the tumor size. Selective radiation therapy treatments that are directed internally may also be used if the patient continues to be symptomatic and medication fails to provide some relief.

Carcinoma of the Gallbladder

Carcinoma of the gallbladder occurs infrequently, but most neoplasms within the gallbladder are malignant. Most primary carcinomas of the gallbladder, approximately 85%, are adenocarcinomas, with the remaining 15% being anaplastic or squamous cell cancers. Carcinoma of the gallbladder is more common in women and older adults, with gallstones present in about 75% of all cases. The symptoms are nonspecific, including RUQ pain, jaundice, and weight loss. Another risk factor associated with the development of gallbladder carcinoma is a "porcelain" gallbladder, which results from chronic cholecystitis (Fig. 6-25). Approximately 22% of patients with porcelain gallbladders develop carcinoma.

The best methods for imaging gallbladder carcinoma include CT and sonography. Radiographically, the appearance of the carcinoma may vary. It may appear as a mass replacing the gallbladder or as a polypoid mass within the gallbladder, or the appearance may be as subtle as focal thickening of the gallbladder wall. Clinically and radiographically, this cancer may be

FIGURE 6-25 A "porcelain" gallbladder in a 70-year-old man with a history of recurrent indigestion.

FIGURE 6-26 Gallbladder carcinoma resulting in metastasis to surrounding structures, as seen on this computed tomography scan of a 23-year-old man. The gallbladder (*arrow*) is surrounded by metastasis, with significant metastasis into the pancreas area and right kidney.

difficult to differentiate from cholecystitis with pericholecystic fluid accumulation or an abscess. Unfortunately, the prognosis with gallbladder carcinoma is often poor because metastases to the liver usually occur before the primary disease is diagnosed (Fig. 6-26). It may spread via direct invasion of the liver, via intraductal tumor extension, or via the lymphatic system to regional lymph nodes. Approximately 88% of patients die within 1 year of diagnosis, and the 5-year survival rate following diagnosis is only 4%.

Carcinoma of the Pancreas

Pancreatic cancer is usually rapidly fatal and is the fifth most common cause of cancer-related death in the United States. Its diagnosis is difficult because of the location of the pancreas and the lack of symptoms before extensive local spread. Even with advances in CT and sonography, the prognosis is poor. In most cases, the tumor is well advanced before the diagnosis is made. Its incidence is greater in men than in women and in blacks than in whites. A clear-cut association with cigarette smoking has been demonstrated, and other risk factors include alcoholism, chronic pancreatitis, diabetes mellitus, and a family history of adenocarcinoma. Most tumors (approximately 90%) arise as epithelial tumors of the duct (adenocarcinoma) and cause pancreatic obstruction (Fig. 6-27). In addition, the majority (60% to 70%) of these neoplasms arise in the head of the pancreas, followed by the body (10% to 15%), and then the tail (5% to 10%). The rich supply of nerves to the pancreas results in pain as a prominent feature of this carcinoma. The tumor infiltrates and replaces normal tissue without significant hemorrhage, necrosis, or

FIGURE 6-27 Pancreatic carcinoma in the head of the pancreas, as indicated by atrophy of the pancreatic body and tail. Numbers shown are for density sampling, with 10, 20, and 30 in the pancreas.

calcification. Signs and symptoms are nonspecific and include pain, weight loss, jaundice, fatigue, nausea, vomiting, and diabetes.

Carcinomas of the pancreatic head may be visible on barium studies of the stomach and small bowel because the head of the pancreas lies within the duodenal C-loop. Carcinomas of the body and tail may affect the duodenojejunal junction and cause distortion on a barium-filled small-bowel study. When sonography is used to evaluate the biliary tree, the sequence of images begins with the right and left branches of the common hepatic duct within the liver and ends with the common bile duct to its termination at the hepatopancreatic ampulla. Tumors of the pancreatic head cause enlargement and may result in compression of the duodenum. With the compression of the duodenum, the hepatopancreatic ampulla is also compressed, causing a dilation of the distal common bile duct. Sonographic images of a common bile duct that begins coursing normally but increases in size distally to more than 1 cm in diameter should suggest the possibility of a pancreatic head mass. The ACR highly recommends CT of the abdomen, with and without contrast, as the best method of imaging the pancreas, the most common finding being a mass deforming the pancreas. The use of sonography and MRI, with and without contrast, is also recommended for patients who have been experiencing weight loss, fatigue, anorexia, and symptoms for more than 3 months. However, in most cases, by the time the mass is visible on the CT image, the tumor is not resectable because of its size. If the lesion is not resectable, a percutaneous needle aspiration under CT guidance is performed to obtain a biopsy of the tissue. In cases where the tumor is resectable, CT helps stage the disease. Radical surgery as a treatment mode is about the only hope for cure, but it carries a high mortality rate. Radiation therapy is difficult because of the proximity of the pancreas to highly radiosensitive structures such as the spinal cord, and chemotherapy also produces poor results. The prognosis for pancreatic carcinoma is very poor, demonstrating a 5-year survival rate of only 2%.

PATHOLOGY SUMMARY
The Hepatobiliary System

Pathology	Imaging Modalities of Choice	Additive or Subtractive Pathology
Fatty infiltration	CT and sonography	Subtractive
Cirrhosis	CT	Both
Ascites	CT and sonography	Additive
Hepatitis	CT, MRI, nuclear medicine, and sonography	None
Cholecystitis	Sonography and CT	None
Cholelithiasis	Sonography and CT	Calcified stones, additive
Pancreatitis	CT, ERCP, and sonography	None
Hemangioma	CT, nuclear medicine, angiography, and sonography	None
Hepatoma	CT and nuclear medicine	Additive
Hepatocellular adenoma	CT and sonography	Additive
Hepatocellular carcinoma	CT, MRI, and sonography	Subtractive
Metastatic disease of the liver	CT, MRI, and sonography	Subtractive
Carcinoma of the gallbladder	CT and sonography	None
Carcinoma of the pancreas	CT and sonography	Additive

CT, Computed tomography; *ERCP,* endoscopic retrograde cholangiopancreatography; *MRI,* magnetic resonance imaging.

REVIEW QUESTIONS

1. Bile drains from the liver's right and left hepatic ducts directly into the:
   a. Common bile duct
   b. Common hepatic duct
   c. Cystic duct
   d. Duodenum
2. The noninvasive modality of choice that does not employ ionizing radiation for visualization of gallbladder disease is:
   a. Computed tomography
   b. Diagnostic medical sonography
   c. Nuclear medicine
   d. All of the above
3. Impairment of normal liver function might result in:
   a. Cirrhosis
   b. Jaundice
   c. Milk of calcium
   d. Viral hepatitis

4. Patients with liver cirrhosis have a tendency to develop:
   1. Ascites
   2. Esophageal varices
   3. Jaundice
   a. 1 and 2
   b. 1 and 3
   c. 2 and 3
   d. 1, 2, and 3
5. Which types of viral hepatitis may be transmitted via blood or blood products?
   a. A
   b. B
   c. C
   d. E
   e. Both a and d
   f. Both b and c
6. Liver conditions commonly associated with alcohol abuse include:
   a. Biliary obstruction
   b. Cholelithiasis
   c. Cirrhosis
   d. Hemangioma

7. The yellowish discoloration of the skin associated with jaundice is caused by:
   a. Accumulation of milk of calcium
   b. Transmission of infected fecal material
   c. Paralysis of small-bowel wall
   d. Presence of bilirubin in blood
   e. None of the above

8. Gallstone ileus refers to impaction of a gallstone in the:
   a. Biliary tree
   b. Gallbladder
   c. Liver
   d. Small bowel

9. The diagnostic imaging modalities of choice for following the progress of a liver malignancy are:
   1. Computed tomography
   2. Radiography
   3. Sonography
   a. 1 and 2
   b. 1 and 3
   c. 2 and 3
   d. 1, 2, and 3

10. A malignant liver tumor is a:
    a. Hepatitis
    b. Hemangioma
    c. Hepatocellular carcinoma
    d. Jaundice

11. Compare and contrast medical versus surgical jaundice.

12. Explain the process by which alcoholism results in fatty infiltration of the liver.

13. What are the advantages of imaging the biliary ductal system antegrade with percutaneous transhepatic cholangiogram (PTC) versus retrograde with endoscopic retrograde cholangiopancreatogram (ERCP)? What are the disadvantages of PTC?

14. Explain why cancers of the gallbladder and pancreas carry a poor prognosis.

15. Describe the physiologic cause of esophageal varices in conjunction with cirrhosis of the liver.

7

Urinary System

LEARNING OBJECTIVES

On completion of Chapter 7, the reader should be able to do the following:

- Describe the anatomic components of the urinary system and their functions.
- Discuss the role of other modalities in imaging the urinary system, particularly sonography and computed tomography.
- Discuss common congenital anomalies of the urinary system.
- Characterize a given condition as inflammatory or neoplastic.
- Identify the pathogenesis of the pathologies cited and the typical treatments for them.
- Describe, in general, the radiographic appearance of each of the given pathologies.

OUTLINE

KEY TERMS

Acute glomerulonephritis
Adenocarcinoma
Bladder carcinoma
Bladder diverticula

Bladder trabeculae
Bright disease
Crossed ectopy
Cryoablation

Cystitis
Ectopic kidney
Foley catheter
Horseshoe kidney
Hydronephrosis
Hyperplasia
Hypoplasia
Malrotation
Medullary sponge kidney
Nephroblastoma
Nephroptosis
Nephrosclerosis
Nephrostomy tube
Neurogenic bladder
Polycystic kidney disease
Pyelonephritis
Pyuria

Radiofrequency ablations
Renal agenesis
Renal calculi
Renal colic
Renal cyst
Renal failure
Staghorn calculus
Supernumerary kidney
Suprapubic catheter
Uremia
Ureteral diverticula
Ureteral stents
Ureterocele
Urethral valves
Urinary meatus
Urinary tract infection
Vesicoureteral reflux

ANATOMY AND PHYSIOLOGY

The urinary system consists of two kidneys, two ureters, a urinary bladder, and a urethra (Fig. 7-1). The urinary system forms urine to remove waste from the bloodstream for excretion. The kidneys are the site where urine is formed and excreted through the remarkable processes of filtration and reabsorption, involving up to 180 liters (L) of blood per day. Urine formed by this process amounts to approximately 1 to 1.5 L per day and passes from the kidneys to the bladder through the ureters. Stored in the bladder, it is eventually excreted through the urethra.

The kidneys are retroperitoneal, normally located between the twelfth thoracic vertebra and the third lumbar vertebra. The right kidney lies slightly lower because of the presence of the liver superiorly. The notch located on the medial surface of each kidney is the hilus, the area where structures enter and leave the kidney. These structures include the renal artery and vein, lymphatics, and a nerve plexus. Microscopically, the nephron is the functional unit of the kidney responsible for forming and excreting urine (Fig. 7-2). The nephron unit is composed of the

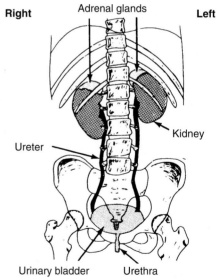

FIGURE 7-1 The urinary system.

glomerulus, Bowman capsule, and numerous convoluted tubules. Blood flowing through the glomerulus, a ball-like cluster of specialized capillaries, is filtered and cleaned of impurities. Fluid moves out of the glomerulus into Bowman capsules and through the various convoluted tubules,

FIGURE 7-2 The microscopic structure of a nephron.

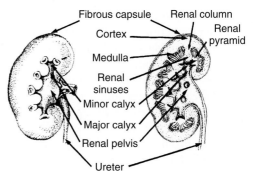

FIGURE 7-3 The structure of a kidney.

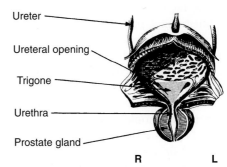

FIGURE 7-4 An anterior cutaway view of the bladder.

resulting in the production of urine. The nephron unit terminates into a collecting tubule, which forms a tube opening at the renal papilla into a minor calyx. Minor calyces terminate in the major calyces, which, in turn, terminate at the renal pelvis (Fig. 7-3).

The ureters extend from the kidneys to the urinary bladder and are approximately 10 inches in length (Fig. 7-4). They normally enter the bladder obliquely in the posterolateral portion of the bladder, equidistant from the urethral orifice in a triangular fashion. A number of variations of this exist. The function of the ureters is to drain the urine from the kidneys to the bladder.

The bladder is located posterior to the symphysis pubis. It serves as a reservoir for urine before urine is expelled from the body. The bladder is very muscular and capable of distension. Valves located at the junction of the ureters and bladder prevent the backflow of urine.

The urethra is a tube leading from the urinary bladder to the exterior of the body. The female urethra is approximately 1 to $1\frac{1}{2}$ inches in length, whereas the male urethra is approximately 8 inches in length. In men, the urethra passes through the prostate gland and also serves as a part of the reproductive system by receiving seminal fluid via the ejaculatory ducts, which open into the urethra from the prostate. The male urethra is classified by three separate portions: (1) the prostatic portion, (2) the membranous portion, and (3) the cavernous portion. The urethra opens to the exterior of the body via the **urinary meatus**.

IMAGING CONSIDERATIONS

Urinary disorders may be suggested by abnormal laboratory or clinical findings. Clinical findings include frequent urination, polyuria, oliguria, dysuria, or obstructive symptoms. The urine may also have an abnormal color, resulting from a variety of factors. Kidney pain is generally located in the flank or back around the level of the twelfth thoracic vertebra, whereas bladder pain resulting from cystitis is usually limited to the urinary bladder. Patient renal function should be assessed before administering intravenous contrast agents in radiology. The most common laboratory tests conducted include serum creatinine, blood urea nitrogen (BUN), and glomerular filtration rate (GFR). In a normal adult, serum creatinine production and excretion are constant. Creatinine is a waste product derived from a breakdown of a compound normally found in muscle tissue. BUN levels are influenced by urine flow and the production and metabolism of urea. BUN designates the ability of the urinary system to break down nitrogenous compounds from proteins to produce urea nitrogen. Individuals with significant kidney function impairment often have raised blood levels of creatinine, urea nitrogen, or both because the glomerulus cannot adequately filter substances, the tubular system is not functioning properly, or both. The GFR may be estimated (eGFR) by using the serum creatinine value in combination with the patient's age, race, and gender. Normally, the GFR should be 90 milliliters per minute per 1.73 meters cubed (mL/min/1.73 m^2) or greater. Intravenous contrast agents should not be used in patients with a BUN greater than 50 milligrams per deciliter (mg/dL) or a serum creatinine greater than 3 mg/dL. The exact GFR threshold contraindicating the administration of intravenous (IV) contrast medium has not been established at this time.

KUB RADIOGRAPHY

KUB (kidney, ureter, bladder) radiography is useful in demonstrating the size and location of the kidneys. These organs may be visible radiographically because of the perirenal fat capsule that surrounds them. The kidneys are generally well fixed to the abdominal wall and are seen to move with respiratory effort. As mentioned earlier, the right kidney is usually located inferior to the left kidney because of the presence of the liver. Men's kidneys are generally larger than those of women. The kidneys lie in an oblique plane within the abdomen and tend to parallel the borders of the psoas muscle shadows. Evaluation of the kidneys using only a KUB image is limited because the kidney shadows may often be obscured by bowel content and are difficult to visualize because of the inherent low subject contrast in the abdomen. However, KUB

FIGURE 7-5 A preliminary or scout image before injection of intravenous contrast for an intravenous urogram. The image demonstrates the renal and psoas major muscle shadows.

radiography is the usual beginning for intravenous urography (IVU), sometimes referred to as intravenous pyelography (IVP) (Fig. 7-5). In this case, its primary purposes are to (1) determine if adequate bowel preparation has been accomplished and (2) visualize radiopaque calculi of the KUB that may otherwise be hidden by the presence of contrast media. The radiologist also examines areas unrelated to the urinary tract because they may hold clues to the diagnosis and may also assist in differentiating between gastrointestinal (GI) and genitourinary disorders.

Intravenous Urography

One procedure used to assess the urinary system is the IVU (or IVP). The indications for performing IVU include suspected urinary tract obstruction, abnormal urinary sediment (especially hematuria), systemic hypertension, or, frequently in men, symptoms of prostatism. Although few serious adverse effects typically accompany the injection of urographic contrast agents, current research indicates an increased risk of mortality in white female older adults because of renal failure and anaphylaxis. The risk of adverse reactions to an iodinated contrast agent increases because of a variety of factors, including a history of previous contrast reactions; asthma or other allergies; heart disease; dehydration; preexisting kidney disease; treatment with β-blockers, NSAIDs, or interleukin-2 (IL-2); a history of other pathologic diseases such as sickle cell anemia, polycythemia, and myeloma; or all of these factors. The use of nonionic, low-osmolar contrast agents significantly reduces minor and moderate reactions. These contrast agents still contain iodine, but the molecular makeup prevents them from disassociating into ions (nonionic) in the bloodstream, thus reducing the risk of an anaphylactic reaction. Visualization of the urinary system depends on the concentration of contrast material filtered by the kidneys and present in the collecting system; therefore, the patient must have fairly normal physiologic function for diagnostic images to be obtained. Other imaging techniques such as sonography and computed tomography (CT) should be considered in patients with compromised renal function.

Many IVU routines allow for an image to be taken within 30 seconds to 1 minute after contrast medium injection. Because the contrast agents for most IVU examinations are injected by hand, the timing generally begins on completion of the bolus injection and will vary from institution to institution. This is termed the *nephrogram phase* and may be used to demonstrate the contrast agent in the nephrons before it reaches the renal calyces. Ready visualization of the renal parenchyma allows for an inspection of the renal outline. Indentations or bulges may indicate the presence of disease. The nephrogram image is also used to check for normal kidney position, which may be altered by congenital malposition, ptosis, or the presence of a retroperitoneal mass.

Although the numbers and types of images obtained may vary from one institution to

FIGURE 7-6 A 15-minute postinjection image during intravenous urography demonstrating the normal collecting system.

another, a series of collecting system sequence images are the final part of IVU (Fig. 7-6). The renal pelvis, calyces, ureters, and bladder are examined for any abnormalities. The calyces should be evenly distributed and reasonably symmetric. Usually, they appear as buttercup-shaped projections surrounding the renal papillae. Calyceal dilatation may be demonstrated as a result of acute or chronic urinary tract obstruction, obstructive uropathy, or reflux. Dilatation secondary to destruction of the renal pyramids is less common.

Because of the peristaltic activity of ureters, only part of their length in a collecting system sequence may be demonstrated (Fig. 7-7). Nonopaque ureteral calculi sometimes cause filling defects and an obstructive dilatation of the ureter. The majority of all urinary tract calculi are found at the vesicoureteral junction. Any pronounced deviation of the ureter suggests the presence of a retroperitoneal mass. Various filling defects may be demonstrated in the contrast agent–filled

FIGURE 7-7 A right posterior oblique projection after contrast injection for intravenous urography demonstrating the correct entrance of the ureters into the posterior bladder wall.

FIGURE 7-8 A postvoid image after an intravenous urography examination.

ureter during IVU, including tumors, blood clots, and nonopaque calculi. Common bladder defects visualized during IVU include urinary catheter balloons, normal uterus and colon, and extrinsic deformities such as uterine or sigmoid colon tumors. A "postvoid" image usually completes an IVU procedure and allows assessment of the bladder function (Fig. 7-8).

Cystography

Cystography is a common radiographic examination for studying the lower urinary tract. This involves insertion of a urinary catheter into the urethra and retrograde filling of the bladder with iodinated water-soluble contrast material (Fig. 7-9). A frequent indication for this procedure is to identify **vesicoureteral reflux** (VUR). In the normal bladder, increased pressure as the bladder fills effectively shuts down any chance of reflux. Bladder infection, however, may render

FIGURE 7-9 A normal cystogram without reflux as seen in this oblique projection of the bladder in a 56-year-old woman.

the ureteral "valve" incompetent, refluxing the infection into the kidney. Cystography may also be used to study congenital bladder anomalies, tumors, diverticula (Fig. 7-10), calculi, bladder rupture, or neurogenic bladder. Voiding (micturition) cystography is sometimes used in conjunction with retrograde cystography to allow study of the urethra on voiding. Urethrography may be accomplished using the antegrade approach, as with voiding cystourethrography, or retrograde when cystography is not necessary. The antegrade approach is used to study the posterior urethra, especially in the male patient, and the retrograde approach is helpful in studying the anterior urethra (Fig. 7-11). The usual intent of voiding cystography is to allow study of a urethral stricture (Fig. 7-12).

Retrograde Pyelography

Retrograde pyelography requires the placement of a catheter into the ureteric orifice in a retrograde fashion. This is usually performed by a urologist during cystoscopy to allow injection of contrast medium directly into the urinary tract to outline the renal collecting system. The approach is termed *retrograde* because the contrast agent is injected through the ureter into the affected kidney, opposite the normal direction of urine flow. Indications for this study may include

FIGURE 7-10 Bladder diverticula in an 88-year-old man demonstrate the presence of numerous calculi within them.

FIGURE 7-12 A voiding cystourethrogram demonstrates a urethral diverticula. The mucosal margin of the prostatic urethra is ragged as a result of scarring after transurethral resection.

FIGURE 7-11 Retrograde urethrography procedure demonstrating a urethral stricture in a male patient. The location of the stricture is confirmed by its consistent appearance on all three images.

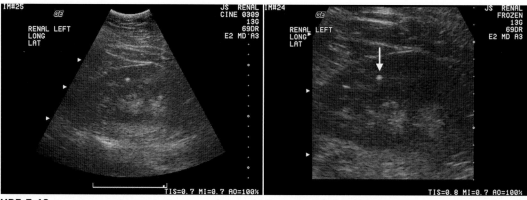

FIGURE 7-13 A sonogram demonstrating a renal stone in the cortex of the kidney.

hematuria of unknown cause, hydronephrosis, and, in cases of a nonfunctioning kidney, the determination of further information about possible obstruction.

Sonography

Sonography is a noninvasive method of imaging both functioning and nonfunctioning kidneys. Because sonography can clearly demonstrate the parenchymal structure of the kidney and the renal pelvis without the use of contrast agents, it is becoming the primary method of visualizing the kidneys and evaluating most renal disorders. It is useful in evaluating kidney stones (Fig. 7-13), calcifications, hydronephrosis (Fig. 7-14), abscesses, renal masses, and renal cysts and to assess renal size, atrophy, or both. Sonography is the modality of choice for evaluating individuals after kidney transplantation. Doppler techniques are helpful in assessing blood flow in the renal arteries and veins for both transplant recipients and individuals with suspected renal artery stenosis. Sonography is also used to visualize abnormalities of the urinary system present in the fetus.

Computed Tomography

CT is an excellent modality for imaging the kidneys because it can detect small differences in tissue densities within the body. Kidneys can be

FIGURE 7-14 A sonogram confirming hydronephrosis of the kidney and proper placement of a ureteral stent to assist in allowing the kidney to drain properly into the urinary bladder.

visualized on CT with or without the use of a contrast agent. Abdominal CT is particularly important in determining the nature of renal masses, either solid or cystic, which may not be visible on a KUB radiograph because of the presence of gas in the bowel. CT evaluation of the urinary system generally requires the use of an IV contrast agent to differentiate renal cysts from solid masses and to evaluate the extent of the lesion (Fig. 7-15). Because most institutions use an automatic injector in CT, scanning may begin when the bolus of contrast medium is injected or shortly after injection, and a delay is programmed into the scanner to allow the contrast medium to reach the bladder before the pelvis is imaged.

FIGURE 7-15 A computed tomography image of a complex cystic structure of the left kidney after contrast injection during the nephrogram phase.

FIGURE 7-16 A computed tomography image demonstrating a calcification in the left kidney indicative of a renal stone without the use of a contrast agent.

CT is also useful for looking for sites of obstruction caused by **renal calculi** or retroperitoneal masses, which may distort the urinary tract; assessing renal infection or trauma; and staging tumors of the lymph nodes. A CT renal stone study is considered the imaging modality of choice by the American College of Radiology (ACR) when patients present with an acute onset of flank pain or other symptoms suggest the presence of renal calculi. Because CT displays excellent contrast resolution, stones are identified more easily than with conventional radiography, but without the use of an intravenous contrast agent (Fig. 7-16). In addition, pelvic CT is the imaging modality of choice for the evaluation of bladder tumors or masses.

Renal Angiography

Renal angiography is one of the most invasive imaging procedures performed on the urinary system. It is usually indicated to further evaluate a renal mass suspected of being malignant, to embolize blood flow to a renal mass, or to assess renal artery stenosis that may cause hypertension, as well as to assess other vascular disorders such as aneurysms or congenital anomalies. It is also performed on kidney donors before surgical removal of the kidney to serve as a "road map" of vascular anatomy for the surgeon. In renal angiography, a catheter is introduced peripherally, most commonly into the femoral artery. The catheter tip may be placed into the specific renal artery of interest or into the abdominal aorta just superior to the renal arteries. The contrast agent is injected via the catheter to image the vasculature of the kidney or kidneys.

Magnetic Resonance Imaging

The role of magnetic resonance imaging (MRI) has greatly improved as a result of breath-hold imaging sequences and bolus injections of gadolinium contrast agents. Abdominal MRI is useful in follow-up studies in patients with known renal cell carcinoma or invasive bladder cancers and adrenal masses. Additionally, magnetic resonance angiography (MRA) is now highly recommended by the ACR in the diagnosis of renovascular hypertension (Fig. 7-17). Contrast-enhanced three-dimensional MRA obtains coronal images of the renal arteries in as little as 20 seconds. The images can then be rotated for better visualization. MRA is also an excellent modality for demonstrating other vascular anomalies such as thrombosis, aneurysms, and arteriovenous malformations (AVMs). Because it allows for imaging of the urinary system in all three planes, it is also used in conjunction with CT for the evaluation of renal masses and their extensions. In cases of renal cyst evaluation, MRI is capable of differentiating between fluid accumulation from hemorrhage and infection. Pelvic MRI is used to readily demonstrate the seminal vesicles and prostate gland in men as well as masses within the urinary bladder. Because of its ability to clearly image soft tissue, pelvic MRI allows thorough evaluation of invasive cancers within the urinary bladder.

FIGURE 7-17 A contrast-enhanced three-dimensional magnetic resonance angiography image of the renal arteries demonstrating normal renal artery patency.

Interventional Procedures and Techniques

Percutaneous nephrostography is an antegrade study in which the contrast medium is injected directly into the renal pelvis. It involves posterolateral insertion of a needle or catheter into the renal pelvis using medical sonography, fluoroscopy, or sometimes a combination of both modalities (Fig. 7-18). The nephrostomy tube may be left in place to provide drainage of an obstructed kidney or to allow retrieval of the calculus with a basket catheter. Sometimes the procedure is used to relieve obstruction in patients for whom immediate surgery is not possible.

Extracorporeal shock wave lithotripsy (SWL) is a method used to locate and treat renal calculi. After the location of the stone is determined radiographically, fluoroscopy or sonography aids in alignment of a high-frequency shock wave directed at the stone. If the treatment is successful, the stone disintegrates into fragments and is excreted via urination, thus helping the patient avoid surgery and a much lengthier recovery period (Fig. 7-19).

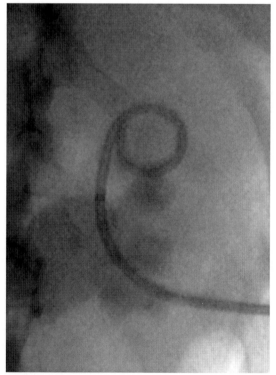

FIGURE 7-18 Placement of a right percutaneous renal drainage tube under fluoroscopic guidance.

FIGURE 7-19 A, Scout film taken before lithotripsy demonstrates a large, solid renal stone in the right kidney. **B,** Two months after lithotripsy, the stone is clearly seen to be fragmented and beginning to descend the right ureter. A stent has been placed in the right ureter to aid in draining urine. **C,** A film taken 2 months later demonstrates further movement of stone fragments down the ureter. The stent is still in place.

Percutaneous renal biopsy or drainage may be performed under fluoroscopy, sonography, or CT guidance. Biopsies help in the evaluation of the histologic origin of renal masses. Percutaneous drainage may be used to aspirate renal cysts or abscesses.

Percutaneous radiofrequency ablation and percutaneous cryoablation is a minimally invasive alternative treatment for patients who are poor candidates for a major surgery. Percutaneous ablative therapy is a successful treatment option for patients with renal cell carcinoma because these procedures not only preserve renal function but also decrease postoperative morbidity and recovery time. Percutaneous radiofrequency ablation involves insertion of a probe into the tumor site and induction of a high electrical current that heats up the tumor and eventually destroys it. The process of cryoablative therapy is the exact opposite. Probes are inserted into the tumor and high pressure argon and nitrogen gases are circulated throughout the probes. This allows the core temperature of the tumor to reach as low as −190 degrees Celsius, causing ice crystallization, which necrotizes the tumor. With this procedure, the tumor goes through multiple freeze-and-thaw cycles.

Urinary Tubes and Catheters

When certain types of pathologies such as tumors or stone formation inhibit the normal flow of urine through the urinary system, several types of tubes may be used to allow drainage of urine. A **nephrostomy tube** connects the renal pelvis to the outside of the body (see Fig. 7-18). It is inserted percutaneously through the renal cortex and medulla into the renal pelvis to allow urine to drain outside of the body directly from the renal pelvis. Special care must be taken, as patients are readily prone to infections because of the direct opening into the urinary system.

Ureteral stents may also be placed in cases of ureteral obstruction. Unlike nephrostomy tubes, ureteral stents do not connect the urinary system to the outside of the patient's body (Fig. 7-20). **Ureteral stents** are placed surgically or via

FIGURE 7-20 An abdominal radiograph demonstrating bilateral renal calculi with a left ureteral stent properly placed to allow drainage of urine into the urinary bladder.

cystoscopy, with the upper portion of the stent in the renal pelvis and the lower portion within the urinary bladder. The stent maintains patency of the diseased ureter and enables urine to flow normally. These stents are visible on plain abdominal radiographs and on CT scans of the abdomen (Fig. 7-21).

Urinary catheterization is performed to obtain urine specimens, relieve urinary retention, monitor renal function, and manage urinary incontinence. A **Foley catheter** is the most common indwelling urinary catheter. It is placed within the urinary bladder using sterile technique. Once the catheter is placed through the urethra and the urinary sphincter, a small balloon is inflated to keep the catheter in place within the urinary bladder. This catheter is generally connected to a bag that collects urine as it flows through the catheter to the outside of the body. Care must be taken to ensure that the catheter is not displaced during a

FIGURE 7-21 An abdominal computed tomography scan demonstrating a right percutaneous nephrostomy placement and ureteral stent.

FIGURE 7-22 An intravenous urogram demonstrating agenesis of the left kidney accompanied by a large, functioning right kidney.

radiographic procedure, and at all times the urine collection bag must be placed at a level lower than that of the patient's bladder to prevent the reflux of urine back into the bladder, which could result in a **urinary tract infection** (UTI). A Foley catheter must be placed in the patient before cystography or cystourethrography is performed to allow installation of contrast material into the bladder. Again, the importance of proper sterile technique cannot be overemphasized. For patients such as those with quadriplegia who require long-term catheterization, a **suprapubic catheter** may be used instead of a Foley catheter.

CONGENITAL AND HEREDITARY DISEASES

Anomalies of the kidneys and ureters are caused by errors in development. They can be classified as anomalies of number, size and form, fusion, and position. About 10% of all persons have some sort of congenital malformation of the urinary system, and these congenital anomalies often result in impaired renal function leading to infection and stone formation. At least half of those with kidney anomalies have malformations elsewhere in the urinary system or in other systems, most commonly the reproductive system, which may result in sexual dysfunction

or infertility. Surgical correction may be required for complications associated with the anomaly.

Number and Size Anomalies of the Kidney

In an embryo, the urinary system develops in three stages with the formation of the kidneys beginning from growth of the ureteric duct and the development of metanephric tissue. If proper growth does not occur, the kidney does not form in the normal manner. **Renal agenesis** or **aplasia** is a relatively rare anomaly occurring in approximately 1 in 1000 live births and is more common in males than females. This anomaly can be detected by prenatal sonography, and it generally manifests as absence of a kidney on one side (unilaterally) and an associated unusually large kidney on the other side (Fig. 7-22). This condition is known as *compensatory hypertrophy*. In instances of unilateral renal agenesis, more frequently the left kidney is absent. The single hypertrophic kidney is more subject to trauma because of its enlarged size. In an individual with only one kidney, protection against disease is very important. The absence of both kidneys, termed *Potter syndrome* or *bilateral agenesis,* is more common in males and is incompatible with life. Almost half of the infants with this problem are stillborn and those who are born alive die within the first 4 hours of birth.

A **supernumerary kidney,** which is also relatively rare, involves the presence of a third, small, rudimentary kidney. It has no parenchymal attachment to a kidney, and in about half the cases, the supernumerary kidney drains from an independent renal pelvis into the ureter on that side. It often becomes symptomatic as a result of infection.

Hypoplasia is a rare anomaly of size involving a kidney that is developed less than normally in size but contains normal nephrons (Fig. 7-23). Usually, hypoplasia is associated with hyperplasia of the other kidney. It requires renal arteriography to differentiate congenital hypertrophic changes from atrophy caused by acquired vascular disease (Fig. 7-24). The clinical significance of hypoplasia depends on the volume of the functioning kidney; however, hypertension often accompanies this anomaly. **Hyperplasia** is the opposite condition; it involves overdevelopment of a kidney. Again, this is often associated with renal agenesis or hypoplasia of the other kidney.

Fusion Anomalies of the Kidney

Fusion anomalies of the kidneys are often distinguishable on plain radiographs. **Horseshoe kidney,** the most common fusion anomaly, is a condition affecting approximately 0.25% of the population in the United States, with men affected twice as frequently as women. In this condition, the lower poles of the kidneys are joined across the midline by a band of soft tissue, causing a rotation anomaly on one side or both sides. The ureters exit the kidneys anteriorly instead of medially, and the lower pole calyces point medially rather than laterally (Fig. 7-25). Kidney function is generally unimpaired in this condition; however, if obstruction is present because of the abnormal location of the ureters, pyeloplastic surgery may be required. The lower bridge frequently lies on a sacral promontory, where it is susceptible to trauma and may be palpated as an abdominal mass.

FIGURE 7-23 The normal vasculature of this small kidney demonstrates renal hypoplasia.

FIGURE 7-24 An abdominal computed tomography image of an atrophic right kidney.

FIGURE 7-25 Horseshoe kidney with apparent obstruction on the computed tomography scan of a 72-year-old woman.

FIGURE 7-26 A retrograde pyelogram demonstrates the left ureter crossing midline to connect with the lower pelvis of an anomalous right kidney, as consistent with crossed fused renal ectopy.

In **crossed ectopy**, one kidney lies across the midline and is fused with the other kidney (Fig. 7-26). This is the second most common fusion anomaly. Both kidneys demonstrate various anomalies of position, shape, fusion, and rotation with crossed ectopy. The crossed kidney generally lies inferior to the uncrossed one, and its ureter crosses the midline to enter the bladder on the proper side. Its drainage may be impaired by malposition of its ureter within the renal pelvis, which may require surgical repair with pyeloplasty.

Position Anomalies of the Kidney

Anomalies of position are relatively common. **Malrotation** consists of incomplete or excessive rotation of the kidneys as they ascend from the pelvis in utero. This is generally of little clinical significance unless an obstruction is created. An **ectopic kidney** is one that is out of its normal position, a condition found in approximately 1 in 800 urologic examinations. Most patients are asymptomatic throughout their lives; however, the incidence of ureteropelvic junction obstruction or VUR is increasing. Ectopic kidneys are usually lower than normal, often in a pelvic

location (Fig. 7-27) or a sacral location. In rare cases, the ectopic kidney may be in an intrathoracic location. In severe cases of ectopy, surgical intervention may be necessary. In some lean and athletic persons, the kidney is mobile and may drop toward the pelvis when the person is in the erect position. This is termed *kidney prolapse* or **nephroptosis.** Nephroptosis is distinguished from a pelvic kidney by the length of the ureter; if the ureter is short, it is a congenital pelvic kidney.

Renal Pelvis and Ureter Anomalies

Renal pelvis and ureter anomalies are frequent. They may be unilateral or bilateral, and they have a tendency to be asymmetric. Such anomalies may occur as a double renal pelvis, either in isolation or in combination with a double ureter (Figs. 7-28 and 7-29). The problem with these and other upper urinary tract anomalies is that they may impair renal drainage, predisposing the patient to infection and calculi formation.

FIGURE 7-27 An ectopic kidney, indicated by a urogram taken at the end of angiography, demonstrates the left kidney with a shortened ureter in the left pelvis.

FIGURE 7-29 A duplicated right collecting system emptying into a loop of bowel. The urinary bladder has been surgically removed because of bladder carcinoma and replaced with a loop of small intestines.

FIGURE 7-28 A congenital double ureter is clearly seen on the left side.

Lower Urinary Tract Anomalies

A simple **ureterocele** is a cystlike dilatation of a ureter near its opening into the bladder. Ureteroceles usually result from congenital stenosis of the ureteral orifice. Radiographically, a ureterocele appears as a filling defect in the bladder with a characteristic "cobra head" appearance. A ureterocele that appears with ureteral duplication is an "ectopic" ureterocele; it often causes substantial obstruction, primarily of the upper pole, and kidney infection and may lead to **renal failure**. Treatment in this situation involves endoscopic or open surgical repair to allow for increased flow of urine into the bladder.

Ureteral diverticula are probably a congenital anomaly and may actually represent a dilated, branched ureteric remnant. The appearance of ureteral diverticula is the same as that of any other diverticula and is best demonstrated by retrograde urography (Fig. 7-30). **Bladder**

FIGURE 7-30 The left ureteric diverticula, visible as double densities superimposed on the posterior bladder, is seen on this intravenous urogram of a female patient with recurrent urinary tract infections.

FIGURE 7-31 Bladder diverticula visible on the bladder's left margin in this cystogram.

FIGURE 7-32 Large, trabeculated bladder and large tortuous ureters and renal pelves seen on this cystogram of a 15-year-old boy, consistent with bladder outflow obstruction secondary to congenital posterior urethral valves.

diverticula (Fig. 7-31) may occur as a congenital anomaly or be caused by chronic bladder obstruction and resultant infection. They usually occur in middle-aged men and may be diagnosed via cystography or cystoscopy. In severe cases, the bladder may have to be surgically reconstructed. **Urethral valves** are mucosal folds that protrude into the posterior (prostatic) urethra as a congenital condition. These may cause significant obstruction to urine flow (Fig. 7-32). Such "valves" occur in men, are usually discovered during infancy or early childhood, and are commonly diagnosed by using voiding cystourethrography. The condition is corrected by endoscopic surgery at an early age to prevent renal damage.

Polycystic Kidney Disease

Polycystic kidney disease (PKD) is a congenital, familial kidney disorder that may be classified as either autosomal recessive or autosomal dominant. This anomaly results from mutations of the *PKD-1* and *PKD-2* genes and occurs in 1 in 1000 live births. Innumerable tiny cysts within the nephron unit are present at birth and may be discovered with in utero ultrasonography. Autosomal recessive PKD is a rare condition causing childhood cystic disease and ultimately resulting in childhood renal failure. Without a family history of autosomal recessive PKD, diagnosis is often difficult. Sonography plays an important role in demonstrating renal and hepatic cysts and is also used for obtaining a tissue sample via percutaneous biopsy.

Autosomal dominant PKD is often asymptomatic in childhood, although it may be visible sonographically. The cysts gradually enlarge as the patient ages, and clinical symptoms become apparent in adulthood. It is the cause of approximately 10% of end-stage renal disease in adults. This enlargement compresses and eventually destroys normal tissues. The late presentation of the condition occurs because the cysts are initially very small and do not cause problems until tissue destruction becomes significant. Symptoms include lower back pain, UTIs, and stone formation. In addition, approximately 30% to 35% of affected individuals have cysts in the liver, which do not affect liver function, and 50% are diagnosed with renal hypertension.

The diagnosis of multiple cysts is readily confirmed with ultrasonography, which reveals multiple echo-free areas in both kidneys, or with CT evaluation demonstrating a moth-eaten appearance of the functional renal tissue. Both ultrasonography and CT have the advantage of demonstrating the disease in its early stages, before it may be visible on conventional radiographs. IVU images of PKD show bilateral enlargement of the kidneys with poorly visualized outlines (from the presence of cysts) and calyceal stretching and distortion (Fig. 7-33). Over half the individuals with PKD eventually develop uremia in their mid to late 50s and require dialysis or kidney transplantation. Therapy for this condition consists of good management of UTI, basic fluid and electrolyte management, hypertension management, avoidance of physical activities that could cause trauma to the abdomen, and management of pain caused by the occasional rupture of a cyst.

Medullary Sponge Kidney

Medullary sponge kidney involves congenital dilatation of the renal tubules leading to urinary

FIGURE 7-33 Polycystic kidney disease visible as multiple masses in the kidneys in this computed tomography scan of a 64-year-old man.

stasis and increased levels of calcium phosphate (nephrocalcinosis). The diagnosis is not usually made until the fourth or fifth decade of life, when infective complications emerge. The only visible abnormality is the dilatation of the medullary and papillary portions of the collecting ducts, usually bilaterally (Fig. 7-34). Calculi are contained in about 60% of symptomatic patients, and infection and intrarenal obstruction are common. IVU reveals linear markings in the papillae or cystic collections of contrast medium in the enlarged collecting ducts. However, this anomaly is often difficult to differentiate from renal cystic disease, tuberculosis, or other disorders resulting in nephrocalcinosis (deposits of calcium phosphates in the renal tubules). Diagnostic sonography is generally unable to demonstrate the cysts, as they are very small and generally lie deep within the medulla of the kidney. Therapy for this condition consists of treatment of infection and, if possible, resolution of nephrolithiasis with lithotripsy.

INFLAMMATORY DISEASES

Urinary Tract Infection

UTIs are the most common of all bacterial infections. They occur in individuals of all ages and both genders. They are more common in boys

2 0F

FIGURE 7-34 Medullary sponge kidney demonstrated by large bilateral papillae and dilated tubules visible within the papillae in this 20-year-old woman with recurrent cystitis.

during infancy, generally resulting from a congenital anomaly. The incidence increases in girls around the age of 10 years, and by the age of 20 years, women are twice as likely to develop UTI as men. Up to 35% of all women experience UTI at least once in their lifetime. A quantitative urine culture is essential in the treatment approach for UTI because the causes are broad. In most cases of UTI, the infecting organism is a gram-negative bacillus that invades the urinary system by an ascending route through the urethra to the bladder and to the kidney. Some authors believe that the offending bacteria ascend during micturition, possibly related to a turbulent stream or reflux on completion of voiding. Research also suggests that compared with women who are not sexually active, those who are sexually active tend to experience UTIs more frequently, especially when they use a diaphragm and spermicide as forms of birth control. It is believed that the spermicide inhibits the normal flora of the vagina and allows overgrowth of *Escherichia coli*. The only clearly demonstrated mechanism, however, is by instrumentation of the urethra and bladder by cystoscopy, urologic surgery, or Foley catheter placement. Antibiotics are used to clear the bacterial infection.

Pyelonephritis

Acute **pyelonephritis**, considered the most common renal disease, is a bacterial infection of the calyces and renal pelvis. Any stagnation or obstruction to urine flow in any part of the urinary tract predisposes the patient to kidney infection. The microorganisms involved are generally *E. coli, Proteus,* or *Pseudomonas*, which reach the kidney by ascending the ureters or via the bloodstream. Acute pyelonephritis is rare in men with a normal urinary tract but is common in women, especially pregnant women after urinary catheterization or as the increased size of the uterus compresses the ureter and decreases urinary clearance of bacteria. Pyelonephritis is a problem for women who have had recurrent UTIs and as a result have *E. coli* bacteria (80%) that have progressed up the ureter and infected portions of the kidney. Patients with acute pyelonephritis have fever, flank pain, and general malaise. Urinalysis demonstrates **pyuria**, the presence of pus (white cells) created by the body's reaction to the infection. Reactions include renal inflammation and edema in combination with purulent urine. Abscesses may form in the kidneys and create a flow of pus into the collecting tubules. Diagnosis of the condition

FIGURE 7-35 A, The right kidney is small and has a scarred surface, as seen on this intravenous urogram of a 25-year-old woman with recurrent urinary tract infections. **B,** Selective renal angiography demonstrates a thinned cortex caused by scarring and bunching of the renal vessels, as consistent with chronic pyelonephritis.

is usually made on the basis of laboratory results, as radiographic findings are often nonspecific. In most cases, IVU is normal even during an acute attack. The calyces may be blunted, and collecting structures may be less well visualized because of interstitial edema. Treatment consists of administering antibiotics to eliminate the infectious bacteria.

Recurrent or persistent infection of the kidneys, such as that caused by chronic reflux of infected urine from the bladder into the renal pelvis, may result in chronic pyelonephritis. It generally has no relation to acute pyelonephritis and is seen sometimes in patients with a major anatomic abnormality (e.g., an obstruction) or more commonly in children with VUR. Chronic pyelonephritis is often bilateral and leads to destruction and scarring of the renal tissue, with marked dilatation of the calyces. The eventual result is an overall reduction in kidney size, readily seen on IVU (Fig. 7-35, A). The renal pyramids atrophy, giving the calyces a clubbed

appearance. Scars may also be seen and appear as indentations of the renal cortex on the kidney outline in the nephrogram phase (see Fig. 7-35, B). Chronic pyelonephritis may be caused by a congenital duplication of ureters that allows a chronic reflux of urine, by an obstruction of the urinary tract, or by a neurogenic bladder. Hypertension may result from chronic pyelonephritis. Sonography is useful in assessing and grading medical renal disease, including pyelonephritis and renal hypertension. One of the subjective sonographic techniques includes comparing the echogenicity of the kidney with that of the liver because the liver has a homogeneous sonographic texture. For a normal grading, the cortical area of the kidney should be less echogenic than the liver (Fig. 7-36). As the disease breaks down the cortical tissue, the echogenicity becomes equal to that of the liver. In the final phases of renal disease, the kidney exhibits greater echogenicity than the liver. Treatment of pyelonephritis in a chronic stage centers on control of hypertension,

FIGURE 7-36 A diagnostic medical sonogram demonstrating the echogenic texture of a normal kidney.

removal of any cause for obstruction, and use of antibiotics to control infection.

Acute Glomerulonephritis

An antigen–antibody reaction in the glomeruli causes an inflammatory reaction of the renal parenchyma known as **acute glomerulonephritis** or **Bright disease**. This inflammation begins in the cortex of the kidney and in the tiny arcuate arteries that infuse the glomeruli. The major characteristic of the glomeruli is that they allow for extraordinarily high levels of water and small solutes to flow through the system. Although the kidney has an incredible capacity to cleanse blood, glomeruli can be damaged by vascular pressure, metabolic diseases such as diabetes, and immune disorders such as systemic lupus erythematosus. Acute glomerulonephritis is an immunologic reaction that may follow streptococcal infection of the upper respiratory tract or the middle ear. It differs from acute pyelonephritis, which primarily affects the interstitial tissue rather than the nephrons. Often a renal biopsy procedure is conducted to get a sample of the glomeruli to ascertain the level of disease or erosion within them. CT or sonographic guidance helps the physician obtain samples of renal tissue and send them to the laboratory for inspection. The biopsy samples allow the pathologist to look for the level of disease or erosion. A

granular pattern develops within the glomeruli from deposits of antigens and the resulting antibodies. These microscopic deposits in the glomerulus are the gold standard for diagnosing glomerulonephritis. This condition occurs mainly in children after streptococcal infection, with most patients recovering completely. Radiographically, the kidneys appear larger, particularly during the nephrogram phase of IVU, because of edematous accumulation. Treatment may include diuretic therapy to reduce the edema and its resultant pressure on the glomeruli, as well as antiinflammatory medications and steroid therapy. Renal dialysis may be used for severe, chronic cases.

Cystitis

Cystitis, which is an acute or chronic inflammation of the bladder, is a fairly common infection that is generally caused by bacteria such as *E. coli* and *Staphylococcus saprophyticus*. Cystitis is more prevalent in women than in men because the short urethra in women allows bacteria easier access into the bladder. The bladder lining's natural resistance to inflammation, however, serves as a protective mechanism. Inflammation and congestion of the bladder mucosa cause the patient to experience burning pain on urination or the urge to urinate frequently. Although cystitis is not a serious infection, it may cause further problems by spreading into the upper urinary passages, including the renal pelvis and the kidney.

VUR, the backward flow of urine out of the bladder and into the ureters, may be seen in cases of cystitis. In the normal urinary tract, VUR is prevented by compression of the bladder musculature on the ureters during micturition. Failure of this valve mechanism usually results from a shortening of the intravesical portion of the ureter caused by abnormal embryologic development, leading to ureteric orifices that are displaced laterally. As this portion of the ureter lengthens with growth, this type of VUR may disappear completely with age. Congenital VUR is also seen in duplication of collecting systems

FIGURE 7-37 Left ureteral reflux visualized during intravenous urography. The patient has a pelvic fracture.

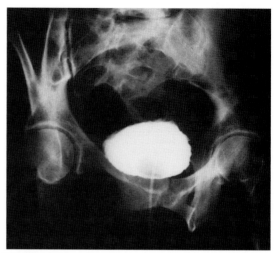

FIGURE 7-38 Mildly trabeculated bladder as seen in this 34-year-old woman with a small-capacity bladder.

and ureters with reflux into an ectopically placed ureter serving the upper pole of the kidney. VUR may also result from a **neurogenic bladder**, a bladder dysfunction caused by interference with the nerve impulses concerned with urination. Cystography may demonstrate the presence of reflux (Fig. 7-37) and grade its severity. It may show a roughening of the normally smooth bladder wall, a radiographic appearance referred to as **bladder trabeculae** (Fig. 7-38). Treatment of cystitis includes antibiotic therapy and an abundance of fluids. Prevention of pyelonephritis is paramount.

URINARY SYSTEM CALCIFICATIONS

With the exception of the gallbladder, more calculi are found in the urinary tract than anywhere else in the body. Renal calculi are stones that develop from urine and precipitate crystalline materials, especially calcium and its salts. If the body's normal equilibrium is upset, these products may precipitate out of the solution. Factors that cause this precipitation include metabolic disorders such as hyperparathyroidism, excessive intake of calcium, and a metabolic rate that causes high urine concentration. Chronic UTI is also related to stone formation.

Men develop calculi more often than women do, especially after age 30 years. Nearly all urinary tract calculi are calcified to some extent; however, approximately 5% of stones do not calcify (Fig. 7-39). These are generally made of pure uric acid and present a more difficult diagnosis to the physician because they are one of several filling defects, including blood clots and tumors. Most stones are formed in the calyces or renal pelvis. A **staghorn calculus** is a large calculus that assumes the shape of the pelvicalyceal junction (Fig. 7-40). Because of the calcium content in renal calculi, most are visible on abdominal radiography, IVU, or retrograde pyelography. Sonography (Fig. 7-41) and noncontrast CT of the abdomen (Fig. 7-42) are often used to demonstrate stones. In many institutions, a CT stone study is the first modality of choice because it does not require contrast administration. It is an excellent method for differentiating abdominal or flank pain caused by renal calculi versus appendicitis or an abdominal aortic

FIGURE 7-39 Smooth, oval, noncalcified filling defect seen in the right renal pelvis, suggestive of a radiolucent uric acid stone in this 40-year-old woman with hematuria.

FIGURE 7-40 An abdominal radiograph without intravenous contrast demonstrating a large staghorn calculus.

FIGURE 7-41 Large calculi seen on this ultrasonogram of the kidney of a young woman. Note the absence of sound transmission beyond the stone as indicated by the dark pathway beneath it.

FIGURE 7-42 Abdominal computed tomography stone study without contrast enhancement demonstrating a right renal stone without hydronephrosis.

aneurysm. In addition, it can be used to detect the location of the stone and the degree of obstruction present.

Stones tend to be asymptomatic until they begin to descend or cause an obstruction. Renal stones generally do not have a smooth texture and often have multiple jagged edges, causing pain as they move through the ureter. The most common site for a calculus to lodge and create an obstruction is the ureterovesical junction (Fig. 7-43). Obstructions may also occur in the ureter at the pelvic brim. Movement of stones or acute obstruction results in severe, intermittent pain, which is known as **renal colic**. So as the stone moves along the course of the ureter toward the flank or genital regions, it is highlighted by sudden, periodic (paroxysmal) attacks, between which a constant low-grade pain is felt. Renal calculi may also cause bleeding (hematuria), fever, chills, frequent urination, and secondary infection. The physician is generally able to distinguish between biliary colic and renal colic because biliary colic usually causes referred pain to the subscapular area or the epigastrium. The probability for recurrent calculus formation is increased by as much as 50% in individuals who develop an initial renal stone; therefore, many patients are placed on a prophylactic regimen such as diuretics, potassium alkali, and increased fluid intake to help reduce their chance of developing further stones.

In most instances, the first treatment is to wait for the stone to pass normally through the urinary system in combination with the administration of antibiotics for the presence of any infection. If the stone is not passed, either lithotripsy of the stone or surgical excision of the cause of obstruction is necessary. SWL is often used to crush calculi less than 2 cm in diameter located in the renal pelvis or ureter. A percutaneous nephrolithotomy may be used to remove larger renal calculi, and ureteroscopy is necessary to remove larger stones within the ureter. Depending on the size of the stone, it may be removed with a special basket catheter, or it may be crushed into smaller pieces by using laser or pneumatic lithotripsy. All of these methods use fluoroscopic guidance.

In addition to the kidneys, other sites of calcification in the urinary tract include the wall of the bladder and, in men, the prostate gland. Calcification of the bladder wall is very rare and is usually caused by calcium deposition in a tumor extrinsic to the bladder, such as a tumor in the ovary or the rectum. Rarely, it may also be on the surface of a bladder tumor. Bladder calculi often cause suprapubic pain. Prostatic calcification appears as numerous flecks of calcium of varying size below the bladder. It does not, however, correlate with either prostatic hypertrophy or carcinoma and usually is of no real significance.

Urinary tract calcifications are sometimes difficult to distinguish from other abnormal calcifications such as gallstones, vascular calcifications, and calcified costal cartilages. To be in the kidney, the calcification must remain within the outline of the kidney on both frontal and oblique projections. In the case of gallstones, oblique projections of the abdomen help demonstrate whether the calculus in question is anterior to the kidney. The pancreas may also demonstrate calcification that usually conforms to its shape (Fig. 7-44).

DEGENERATIVE DISEASES

Nephrosclerosis

Nephrosclerosis involves intimal thickening of predominantly the small vessels of the kidney. It may occur as part of the normal aging process

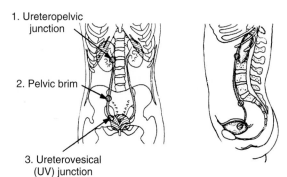

1. Ureteropelvic junction

2. Pelvic brim

3. Ureterovesical (UV) junction

FIGURE 7-43 The three points at which kidney stones usually become lodged.

FIGURE 7-44 Pancreatic calcification as indicated by the masses of calcium in the left-upper quadrant that conform neatly to the shape of the pancreas.

FIGURE 7-45 Pelvic computed tomography without contrast enhancement demonstrating the position of a transplanted kidney in the left pelvis.

as well as in younger patients in association with hypertension and diabetes. Reduced blood flow caused by arteriosclerosis of the renal vasculature causes atrophy of the renal parenchyma. Local infarction may occur, appearing as an irregularity of the cortical margin, usually an indentation. The collecting system of the affected kidney is usually normal, but the kidney itself is decreased in size. Laboratory tests will also demonstrate a gradual increase in BUN and creatinine levels. Other conditions that cause the kidneys to appear smaller than normal include hypoplasia, atrophy after obstruction, and ischemia from large vessel obstruction. Treatment of nephrosclerosis consists of managing the associated hypertension, administration of diuretic agents, and use of proper dietary restrictions (e.g., low-sodium diet).

Renal Failure

Although it can arise acutely, renal failure usually represents the end result of a chronic process such as chronic glomerulonephritis or PKD that gradually results in diminished kidney function. The kidney's normal regulatory and excretory functions become impaired because of loss of glomerular filtration and subsequent deterioration of the renal parenchyma. **Uremia**, which is characteristic of renal failure, consists of retention of urea in blood. Although not toxic in itself, urea is normally excreted by the kidneys. Its blood level correlates with retention of other waste products and is thus a measure of the severity of renal failure. Common laboratory findings include a progressive increase in serum creatinine and BUN. Medical imaging may be requested to locate the cause in cases of acute renal failure. This includes abdominal radiography to rule out urinary calculi and medical sonography or abdominal CT to assess hydronephrosis and kidney size. Renal angiography or radionuclide renal scanning may also be indicated when clinical evaluation suggests a vascular anomaly. A renal biopsy may be necessary if the cause cannot be identified by other, less invasive means.

The gradual deterioration of renal function brings with it a host of changes in other body systems. The patient experiences moderate anemia, hypertension, heart arrhythmia, congestive heart failure, and other problems related to the body's severe electrolyte and acid–base imbalances. Treatment consists of dialysis and possible transplantation (Fig. 7-45).

Hydronephrosis

Hydronephrosis is an obstructive disorder of the urinary system that causes dilatation of the renal pelvis and calyces with urine. In case of longstanding hydronephrosis, the resultant increase in intrarenal pressure causes ischemia, parenchymal atrophy, and loss of renal function. Although the most common cause of hydronephrosis is a calculus (Fig. 7-46), it may also occur as a congenital defect or because of a blockage of the system by a tumor, stricture, blood clot, or inflammation (Fig. 7-47). Patients with hydronephrosis often complain of pain in their flanks, and their urine may demonstrate blood or pus. The long-term changes of hydronephrosis are reversible if the cause of obstruction is relieved early in the process. As in most urinary system pathologies, abdominal sonography is the initial examination of choice because the kidneys do not have to be functioning properly and intravenous contrast agents are not necessary for the kidneys to be visualized on sonography (Fig. 7-48). Additional information regarding increased vascular resistance can be obtained by using Doppler ultrasonography. Abdominal CT (Fig. 7-49)

FIGURE 7-46 A large hydronephrosis of the right kidney easily identified with computed tomography without the use of a contrast agent.

FIGURE 7-48 A sonogram of the kidney demonstrating hydronephrosis.

FIGURE 7-47 Gross bilateral hydronephrosis as caused by pyelonephritis in this 64-year-old man.

FIGURE 7-49 Hydronephrosis of the right kidney demonstrated without contrast enhancement.

allows diagnosis of obstruction more than 90% of the time and is the most highly recommended imaging modality when an obstruction is suspected.

NEOPLASTIC DISEASES

Masses can cause filling defects in the urinary tract, becoming visible when they stretch and displace the collecting system or form an evident mass. Almost all solitary masses are either malignant tumors or simple cysts.

Profuse hematuria resulting from a blood clot also causes a filling defect. The diagnosis of the condition depends on the radiologist's awareness of a history of hematuria. Distinguishing between a blood clot and a tumor is difficult for the physician. However, blood clots tend to have a smooth outline and show change on repeat examinations after treatment.

Renal Cysts

Renal cysts are an acquired abnormality common in adults. It is estimated that more than half the people at age 50 years have renal cysts. Simple cysts may be solitary or multiple and bilateral. They are usually asymptomatic and do not impair renal function, but they may cause symptoms from rupture, hemorrhage, infection, or obstruction. Their pathogenesis is unknown, but obstruction of nephrons by an acquired disease may have a relationship. They are commonly found in a lower pole of the kidney and are readily demonstrated with CT (Fig. 7-50), MRI (Fig. 7-51), and sonography.

Radiographically, cysts have sharply defined margins and show calyceal spreading, but they can be distinguished from tumors by nephrotomography, in which a cyst shows an absence of a nephrogram phase after contrast medium injection. In contrast, tumors, the majority of which have vascularity, may show irregular opacification during the nephrogram phase. Treatment, if needed, consists of aspiration of the cyst contents. Most cysts are asymptomatic, and no treatment is needed.

FIGURE 7-50 A small, simple cyst on the right kidney demonstrated by an abdominal computed tomography scan without contrast enhancement.

FIGURE 7-51 A T2 TruFisp weighted magnetic resonance imaging scan of the abdomen demonstrating a renal cyst of the left kidney.

Renal Cell Carcinoma

The most common malignant tumor of the kidney is renal cell carcinoma (RCC), an adenocarcinoma arising from the proximal convoluted tubule. It occurs two to three times more frequently in men than in women, with an increased incidence after age 50 years, and accounts for approximately 2% of adult cancer-related deaths. Its cause is unknown, but chronic inflammation from obstruction, cigarette smoking, obesity, and hypertension are thought to contribute to the development of renal carcinoma. The affected patient often first reports hematuria but may also experience flank pain, fever, or a palpable mass. RCC may be an incidental finding on abdominal sonography or abdominal CT.

CT is most useful in demonstrating the density of the renal carcinoma and its degree of metastasis, including extension to adjacent areas and lymph nodes, as well as venous involvement (Fig. 7-52). The ACR recommends abdominal CT with and without contrast or abdominal MRI with and without contrast, for staging and follow-up of renal cell carcinomas (Fig. 7-53). Confirmation of a mass may also be accomplished with IVU. Radiographically, the space-occupying lesion may be evident and may distort, stretch, and displace the kidney's collecting system, as visualized on IVU.

If the carcinoma is caught early, surgical excision of the kidney in combination with chemotherapy provides a significant cure rate. The use of radiofrequency ablation and cryoablation therapies in interventional radiology is increasing as an alternative to nephrectomy is some patients. In addition, targeted immunotherapy such as interferon and interleukin-2 is also currently being tested. The tendency of adenocarcinoma to metastasize early from the kidneys poses a serious threat. Staging of the tumor is critical (Table

FIGURE 7-52 Computed tomography demonstrating a large metastatic lesion in the left kidney of this 25-year-old man with renal adenocarcinoma.

FIGURE 7-53 A, An axial T2 TruFisp magnetic resonance imaging of the abdomen demonstrates a mass involving a large portion of the left kidney. **B,** Axial T1-weighted postcontrast image shows the same mass, consistent with renal cell carcinoma. Note the internal necrosis (*arrows*).

TABLE 7-1	Staging of Renal Cell Carcinoma

Stage	Metastasis
I	Tumor confined within kidney capsule ≤7 cm in size
II	Invasion through renal capsule and renal vein but within surrounding fascia ≥7 cm in size
III	Involvement of adrenal glands and vena cava and one nearby lymph node:
	T3a–T3c, N0, M0: The main tumor has reached the adrenal gland, the fatty tissue around the kidney, the renal vein, the large vein (vena cava) leading from the kidney to the heart, or all of these. It has not spread beyond Gerota fascia. No spread to lymph nodes or distant organs has occurred.
	T1a–T3c, N1, M0: The main tumor may be any size and may be located outside the kidney, but it has not spread beyond Gerota fascia. The cancer has spread to one nearby lymph node but has not spread to distant lymph nodes or other organs.
IV	Distant metastases (e.g., liver and lung) and more than one lymph node:
	T4, N0–N1, M0: The main tumor has invaded beyond Gerota fascia. It has spread to no more than one nearby lymph node. It has not spread to distant lymph nodes or other organs.
	Any T, N2, M0: The main tumor may be any size and may be located outside the kidney. The cancer has spread to more than one nearby lymph node but has not spread to distant lymph nodes or other organs.
	Any T, any N, M1: The main tumor can be any size and may be located outside the kidney. It may or may not have spread to nearby lymph nodes. It has spread to distant lymph nodes, other organs, or both.

T, Tumor; *N*, node; *M*, metastasis.
Data from American Cancer Society. Available at http://www.cancer.org/cancer/kidneycancer/detailedguide/kidney-cancer-adult-staging.

7-1), as survival is highly dependent on the tumor grade, cell type, and the extent of metastasis. The most common sites of metastasis are the lungs, brain, liver, and bone. Because pulmonary metastases are common, chest radiography should be performed immediately on discovering a renal carcinoma.

Nephroblastoma (Wilms Tumor)

Nephroblastoma is a malignant renal tumor found in approximately 500 children per year. It is an embryonal tumor that is almost invariably diagnosed before 5 years of age. It is associated with the deletion or inactivation of the *WT1* or *WTX* (X chromosome) tumor suppressor gene and may be inherited or sporadic in origin. Wilms tumor is more common in blacks than in whites and Asians, and slightly more common in girls than in boys. Children with nephroblastoma

often have no symptoms but may have the tumor discovered by a parent or physician who feels a large, palpable abdominal mass. The relative firmness and immobility help distinguish Wilms tumor from hydronephrosis and renal cysts. Diagnostic sonography is also used extensively to differentiate a cystic mass from a solid mass. On urography, the kidneys appear quite enlarged, with marked calyceal spreading—an indication nearly diagnostic of the condition when seen in children. Abdominal CT is the modality of choice for assessing the extent and spread of the tumor (Figs. 7-54, *A* and *B*, and 7-55) and has replaced IVU because CT can demonstrate spread to the lymphatics, liver, and contralateral kidney.

Staging of the tumor is very important (Table 7-2), as the cure rate is very high (95%) for stage I to stage III disease. Left untreated, widespread metastases to the lungs, liver, adrenal glands, and bone occur. Early surgical excision, combined

A

B

FIGURE 7-54 Computed tomography examination of a 3-year-old male with Wilms tumor of the left kidney, stage IV, demonstrates a large growth on the axial (*A*) and coronal (*B*) images.

with radiation therapy and chemotherapy, is the most effective treatment.

Bladder Carcinoma

Bladder carcinoma is usually seen three times more often in men than in women, particularly after age 60 years. Its cause is clearly related to cigarette smoking and certain industrial chemicals. Bladder carcinoma may be classified as urothelial carcinoma, formerly known as *transitional cell carcinoma* (most frequent), *squamous cell carcinoma* (usually resulting from chronic irritation), or *adenocarcinoma*. Painless hematuria is

FIGURE 7-55 A computed tomography image demonstrates a huge, noncalcified mass arising from the left kidney, as seen in Wilms tumor.

TABLE 7-2	Staging of Wilms Tumor
Stage	**Tumor Characteristics**
Stage I (40% to 45%)	Tumor limited to the kidney, completely resected
Stage II (20% to 25%)	Tumor ascending beyond the kidney or into vessels of renal sinus, but appearing to be totally resected
Stage III (20% to 25%)	Residual nonhematogenous tumor confined to the abdomen, positive lymph node in renal hila
Stage IV (10%)	Hematogenous metastases (e.g., lung, liver, bone, brain)
Stage V (5%)	Bilateral disease either at diagnosis or later, but need to stage each kidney

Note: Staging system of the Third National Wilms Tumor Study Group (NWTS-3).
Data from American Cancer Association. Available at http://www.cancer.org/cancer/wilmstumor/detailedguide/wilms-tumor-staging.

FIGURE 7-56 Urothelial carcinoma of the bladder, seen as a space-occupying lesion on this right posterior oblique view of the bladder on a cystogram of a 67-year-old man.

FIGURE 7-57 Large bladder carcinoma in this 65-year-old man as seen on computed tomography.

the main symptom. Tumors are generally small and located in the area of the trigone. IVU or cystography may reveal a filling defect in the bladder (Fig. 7-56), but it is often difficult to distinguish among tumor, stone, and blood clot. Therefore, cystoscopy is the method of choice for investigation of bladder carcinoma, and diagnosis is made via biopsy or resection. CT (Figs. 7-57 and 7-58), sonography, and MRI are useful in staging the disease once the diagnosis is confirmed.

Treatment depends on the invasiveness of the tumor. Superficial tumors may be treated with transurethral resection or ablation, in combination with chemotherapy and immunotherapy, while invasive tumors require resection or total cystectomy with adjuvant chemotherapy, radiation therapy, or a combination of both, depending on the amount of involvement and extent of metastasis. Radiation therapy may also be used for palliative care. In the case of total cystectomy, the distal ureters are generally attached into a loop of the bowel (Fig. 7-59), most frequently the ileum. With bladder carcinoma, distant metastases usually develop late.

FIGURE 7-58 Pelvic computed tomography examination demonstrates an extensive mass in the urinary bladder representing bladder carcinoma.

FIGURE 7-59 An intravenous urogram of a patient after cystectomy. A portion of the cecum has been formed into a pouch to allow the collection of urine.

PATHOLOGY SUMMARY
The Urinary System

Pathology	Imaging Modalities of Choice	Additive or Subtractive Pathology
Congenital anomalies	Sonography in the fetus	
Lower urinary tract anomalies	Cystography and sonography	
Polycystic kidney disease	Sonography, CT with and without contrast, MRI with and without contrast	Subtractive
Medullary sponge kidney	Sonography	
Pyelonephritis	IVU, CT with and without contrast, sonography	
Cystitis	Abdominal and pelvic CT without contrast, cystography and sonography	Additive, if reflux is present
Nephrosclerosis	Angiography and sonography	
Nephrocalcinosis	Sonography, CT, and KUB	Additive
Renal failure	Sonography, CT, and angiography	
Calcifications	CT, sonography, KUB	Additive
Hydronephrosis	Sonography, CT, and IVU	Additive
Renal cyst	Sonography, CT with and without contrast, MRI with and without contrast	Subtractive
Renal cell carcinoma	CT, MRI, and chest radiography	
Nephroblastoma	Sonography	
	Sonography	
Bladder carcinoma	Sonography, MRI, CT, FDG-PET, and cystography	

CT, Computed tomography; *FDG-PET,* 18F-fluorodeoxyglucose positron emission tomography; *IVU,* intravenous urography; *KUB,* kidney, ureter, bladder radiography; *MRI,* magnetic resonance imaging.

REVIEW QUESTIONS

1. A malignant tumor of the kidney generally occurring in children under 5 years of age is:
   a. Adenocarcinoma
   b. Hypernephroma
   c. Fibroadenoma
   d. Nephroblastoma

2. Which of the following statements are true regarding the anatomy and function of the urinary system?
   1. The amount of urine formed in a typical day is about 1 to 1.5 L.
   2. Urine is formed and excreted in the nephron, the microscopic unit of the kidney.
   3. The left kidney lies lower than the right because of the spleen's presence above it.
   a. 1 and 2
   b. 1 and 3
   c. 2 and 3
   d. 1, 2, and 3

3. Urinary system disorders may be suggested by an abnormal:
   1. Blood urea nitrogen level
   2. Creatinine blood level
   3. Coloration of urine
   a. 1 and 2
   b. 1 and 3
   c. 2 and 3
   d. 1, 2, and 3

4. Horseshoe kidney is an anomaly of:
   a. Fusion
   b. Number
   c. Position
   d. Size

5. Which of the following statements are true of urinary system anomalies?
   1. Crossed ectopy exists when one kidney lies across the midline, fused to the other.
   2. Nephroptosis and a pelvic kidney are identical conditions.
   3. Ureteroceles are ureteral dilatations near the ureter's termination.
   a. 1 and 2
   b. 1 and 3
   c. 2 and 3
   d. 1, 2, and 3

6. *Vesicoureteral reflux* refers to the backward flow of urine into the:
   a. Bladder
   b. Major calyx
   c. Ureters
   d. Urethra
   e. Any of the above

7. Arterial and venous renal blood flow in a patient who has received a kidney transplant is best assessed by using:
   a. Computed tomography
   b. Conventional urography
   c. Doppler sonography
   d. Magnetic resonance imaging

8. Which of the following conditions can make the kidneys appear smaller than normal?
   1. Atrophy following obstruction
   2. Chronic pyelonephritis
   3. Hypoplasia
   a. 1 and 2
   b. 1 and 3
   c. 2 and 3
   d. 1, 2, and 3

9. Which of the following procedures may be performed to image a nonfunctioning kidney?
   1. Computed tomography (CT)
   2. Intravenous urography (IVU)
   3. Renal sonography
   a. 1 and 2
   b. 1 and 3
   c. 2 and 3
   d. 1, 2, and 3

10. Gradual and chronic deterioration of the renal parenchyma eventually results in:
    a. Glomerulonephritis
    b. Polycystic kidney disease
    c. Renal calculi
    d. Renal failure

11. Renal failure is characterized by the abnormal retention one of the following substances in blood. Which is it?
    a. Bilirubin
    b. Calcium
    c. Pus
    d. Urea

12. Which of the following statements are true of renal calculi?
    1. Precipitation of solutes out of urine is the pathogenesis of renal calculi.
    2. Renal colic causes referred pain into the subscapular area or epigastrium.
    3. Stones tend to be asymptomatic until they move or cause an obstruction.
    a. 1 and 2
    b. 1 and 3
    c. 2 and 3
    d. 1, 2, and 3
13. Significant dilatation of the renal pelvis and calyces as a result of an obstruction from a stone is characteristic of:
    a. Hydronephrosis
    b. Renal failure
    c. Nephroblastoma
    d. Vesicoureteral reflux
14. Which of the following statements are true of neoplastic diseases of the urinary system?
    1. Chronic inflammation from obstruction may result in adenocarcinoma.
    2. Wilms tumor is generally associated with older patients in renal failure.
    3. Early excision of nephroblastoma has shown a very high cure rate.
    a. 1 and 2
    b. 1 and 3
    c. 2 and 3
    d. 1, 2, and 3
15. A patient arrives in the CT department for a contrast-enhanced abdominal examination. What blood laboratory values must be checked before the patient is injected, and what are the maximum values allowed for contrast administration?
16. A delayed image of the abdomen in an IVU routine demonstrates only a portion of the ureters. Is this cause for concern? Why, or why not?
17. How can nephroptosis and a pelvic kidney be differentiated?
18. Identify at least three mechanisms through which bacteria can enter the urinary tract.
19. A 30-year-old pregnant woman presents with fever, flank pain, and general malaise. Although the IVU image looks normal, urinalysis demonstrates pyuria. What might you suspect?
20. In renal failure, what causes the kidney to lose its normal regulatory and excretory functions?

8

Central Nervous System

LEARNING OBJECTIVES

On completion of Chapter 8, the reader should be able to:

- Describe the anatomic components of the central nervous system and their general function.
- Discuss the roles of the various imaging modalities in evaluation of the central nervous system, particularly magnetic resonance imaging and computed tomography.
- Discuss common congenital anomalies of the central nervous system.

- Characterize a given condition as inflammatory, degenerative, vascular, or neoplastic.
- Identify the pathogenesis of the pathologies cited and typical treatments for them.
- Discuss the imaging modalities most commonly used for each type of central nervous system pathology discussed in this chapter.
- Describe, in general, the radiographic appearance of each of the given pathologies.

OUTLINE

KEY TERMS

Acoustic neuroma

Annulus fibrosus

Astrocytomas

Atherothrombotic brain infarction

Blood–brain barrier

Brain abscess

Cervical spondylosis

Craniopharyngioma

Encephalitis

Ependymoma

Glioblastoma multiforme

Gliomas

Herniated nucleus pulposus

Hydrocephalus

Lacunar infarction

Medulloblastomas

Meningioma

Meningitis

Meningocele

Meningomyelocele

Multiple sclerosis

Myelocele

Neurofibromas

Nucleus pulposus

Oligodendroglioma

Pituitary adenoma

Schwannoma

Subdural empyema

Sylvian triangle

Transient ischemic attacks

ANATOMY AND PHYSIOLOGY

The central nervous system (CNS) includes the brain and the spinal cord. The CNS is composed of neurons (nerve cells) and neuroglia (the interstitial tissue) and extends peripherally through nerves that carry motor messages through efferent nerves to muscles and sensory messages from skin and elsewhere back to the spinal cord and brain through afferent nerves. This chapter concentrates on conditions involving the brain and the spinal cord.

The brain consists of the cerebrum (right and left hemispheres), cerebellum, diencephalon (including the hypothalamus), and brainstem. The brainstem, composed of the midbrain, pons, and medulla oblongata, connects the cerebrum with the spinal cord. The innumerable motor and sensory nerves pass through the brainstem into the spinal cord. The spinal cord originates as an extension of the medulla oblongata at the foramen magnum in the base of the skull. It extends to approximately the level of the first or second lumbar vertebra and terminates with a cone-shaped area called the *conus medullaris*

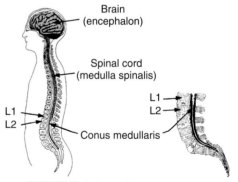

FIGURE 8-1 Central nervous system.

(Fig. 8-1). Spinal nerves beyond this point are referred to as the *cauda equina*.

Both the brain and the spinal cord are covered by the meninges, which consist of three distinct layers (Fig. 8-2). The dura mater is the outermost and is tough and fibrous. It has three major extensions: (1) the falx cerebri, which divides the cerebral hemispheres; (2) the falx cerebelli, which similarly divides the cerebellar hemispheres; and (3) the tentorium cerebelli, which separates the occipital lobe of the cerebrum from the cerebellum. The arachnoid is the middle layer of the meninges and has the appearance of cobwebs. The pia mater is innermost and adheres directly to the cortex of the brain and the spinal cord. The subarachnoid space, at its deepest at the base of the brain, is located between the arachnoid and the pia mater. It is filled with cerebrospinal fluid (CSF) to continuously bathe the brain and

the spinal cord with nutrients and to cushion them against shocks and blows. CSF is secreted by the choroid plexus, a network of capillaries located in the brain's ventricles.

The ventricles are four interconnected cavities within the brain. As noted earlier, they house the choroid plexus, which secretes CSF. The right and left lateral ventricles are located in their respective cerebral hemispheres (Fig. 8-3, A and B). They may be further divided into anterior, posterior, and inferior horns, as well as a body and a trigone. CSF flows from the lateral ventricles into the third ventricle via the interventricular foramina (of Monro). The third and fourth ventricles are midline structures connected to each other by the cerebral aqueduct (see Fig. 8-3, C). From there, CSF flows through a median and two lateral foramina (Magendie and Luschka, respectively) into the subarachnoid space surrounding the brain and the spinal cord.

Most of the brain's blood is supplied anteriorly via the bilateral internal carotid arteries and

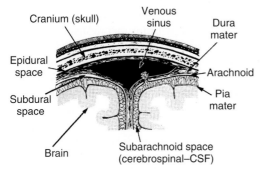

FIGURE 8-2 Coronal perspective of meninges and meningeal spaces.

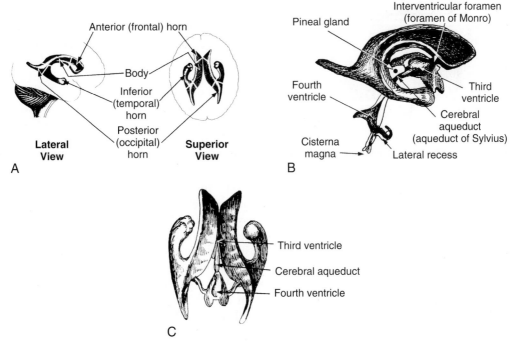

FIGURE 8-3 A, Lateral and superior views of the lateral ventricles. **B,** A lateral view of the ventricular system. **C,** A superior view of the ventricular system.

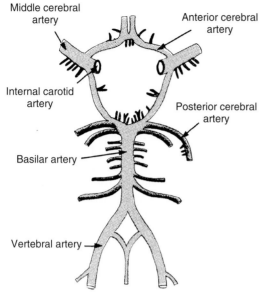

FIGURE 8-4 The circle of Willis.

Middle cerebral artery

Anterior cerebral artery

Internal carotid artery

Posterior cerebral artery

Basilar artery

Vertebral artery

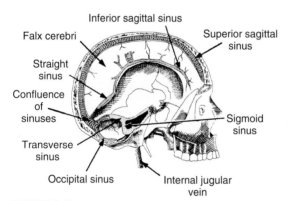

FIGURE 8-5 Dura mater sinuses and venous drainage of the brain.

Inferior sagittal sinus

Falx cerebri

Superior sagittal sinus

Straight sinus

Confluence of sinuses

Sigmoid sinus

Transverse sinus

Occipital sinus

Internal jugular vein

The capillaries that connect the arteries and veins function somewhat differently in the brain than in other organs. In the brain, they prevent passage of unwanted substances into the brain through a special function called the **blood–brain barrier**. This is accomplished in a number of ways, but especially as a result of these capillary cells having a very tight junction that prevents macromolecules and fluids from leaking out into the brain parenchyma. This protects the brain by keeping toxins out, yet it allows removal of the waste products of brain metabolism. These specialized capillaries are found everywhere in the brain except in the pineal and pituitary glands and the choroid plexus. The significance of the blood–brain barrier in terms of imaging is that enhancement of contrast media occurs in the brain where the barrier breaks down from inflammation, ischemia, or neoplastic growth (with its new vascularity). Also, glucose readily passes over this barrier and is the primary agent used in positron emission tomography (PET).

Neurons are the primary tissue comprising the nervous system, and they may vary greatly in size. At birth, the human body has an excess of neurons, which begin to die if they are not used. The three basic components of a neuron are the cell body, or soma, which is located within the CNS; dendrites, which carry nerve impulses toward the soma; and axons, responsible for carrying impulses away from the cell body. Most neurons have only one axon, which is covered by a delicate web of connective tissue of Schwann cells covered by a myelin sheath. Myelin is a lipid substance that acts as an insulator and assists in nerve impulse transmission. Neuroglia or supporting cells also play a major role in the nervous system and are much more numerous than neurons. In addition to Schwann cells, neuroglias include astrocytes, oligodendrocytes, ependymal cells, and microglia (Table 8-1).

Although the intervertebral disks are not part of the CNS, they may come into contact with it when they herniate and impinge on adjacent spinal nerves. Disks cushion the movement of the vertebral column. They are composed of a tough outer covering, known as the **annulus fibrosus**,

posteriorly via the bilateral vertebral arteries. After entering the cranial vault through the foramen magnum, the vertebral arteries converge to form the basilar artery. The basilar artery and the internal carotid arteries form the circle of Willis (Fig. 8-4) to distribute oxygenated, arterial blood through various branches to all parts of the brain. Venous blood is returned to large venous sinuses in the dura mater, which ultimately drain into the internal jugular veins (Fig. 8-5).

TABLE 8-1	Support Cells of the Nervous System
Cell Type	**Primary Functions**
Astrocytes	Form specialized contacts Provide rapid transport for nutrients and metabolites Believed to form an essential component of the blood–brain barrier Appear to be the scar-forming cells of the CNS, which may be the foci for seizures Appear to work with neurons in processing information and memory storage
Oligodendroglia (oligodendrocytes)	Formation of myelin sheath and neurilemma in the CNS
Schwann cells (neurolemmocytes)	Formation of myelin sheath and neurilemma in the PNS
Microglia	Responsible for clearing cellular debris (phagocytic properties)
Ependymal cells	Serve as a lining for ventricles and choroid plexuses involved in production of cerebrospinal fluid

CNS, Central nervous system; *PNS*, peripheral nervous system.
From: McCance, K. L., Huether, S. E.: *Pathophysiology: The biologic basis for disease in adults and children*, ed 5, St. Louis, MO, 2006, Mosby.

and a pulpy center called the **nucleus pulposus** (Fig. 8-6).

IMAGING CONSIDERATIONS

Radiography

Conventional radiographic demonstration of the various cranial structures provides information that is important in evaluation of the CNS. Its role, however, has largely been reduced to evaluation of cranial trauma because of the increased use of magnetic resonance imaging (MRI) and computed tomography (CT). In addition to visualization of fractures caused by trauma, plain skull films may also reveal normal variants. Blood vessels such as the middle meningeal artery commonly cause radiolucent impressions on the inner table of the cranial vault (Fig. 8-7). Their linear progression and bilateral appearance help distinguish them from fractures. Visualization of an enlarged or deformed pituitary fossa provides information about the presence of a pituitary tumor or increased intracranial pressure (ICP) (Fig. 8-8). A calcified pineal gland situated in the midline can be seen on about 60% of all plain skull radiographs (Fig. 8-9). Its displacement

FIGURE 8-6 An intervertebral disk.

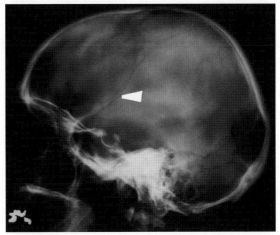

FIGURE 8-7 Normal appearance of the middle meningeal artery as indicated on this lateral skull radiograph.

FIGURE 8-8 An enlarged sella turcica on this lateral skull radiograph evidences a pituitary macroadenoma.

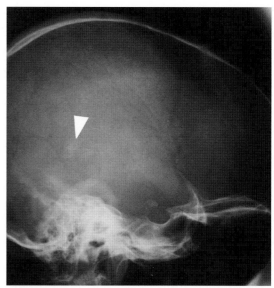

FIGURE 8-10 Normal calcification of the choroid plexus in the posterior horn of the lateral ventricle as seen in this lateral skull radiograph of a 60-year-old woman.

FIGURE 8-9 Normal calcification of the pineal gland as seen in this lateral skull radiograph of a 44-year-old man.

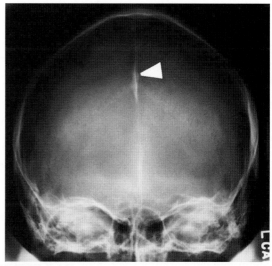

FIGURE 8-11 Normal calcification of the falx cerebri as seen in this posteroanterior skull projection of a 59-year-old man.

may indicate the presence of a pathologic lesion if it is greater than 2 to 3 millimeters (mm). The choroid plexus (Fig. 8-10), falx cerebri (Fig. 8-11), and falx cerebelli may also be calcified.

The role of radiography in the evaluation of the spine was described in Chapter 2. A number of conditions that affect the spinal cord can readily be demonstrated (Fig. 8-12). The fluoroscopic procedure of myelography has been a staple of radiology for years, allowing

visualization of conditions (such as herniated disks) that impinge on the spinal cord. Its role, however, is diminishing because of the significant specificity of MRI. When myelography is still performed, it is often followed by a CT myelographic examination of the spine.

FIGURE 8-12 An anteroposterior lumbar spine radiograph showing L1 through L4 fusion with stable hardware in place.

Magnetic Resonance Imaging

For a wide variety of conditions related to the CNS, MRI is the modality of choice (Fig. 8-13). Its sensitivity is excellent in evaluation of all types of spinal diseases, including tumors, abscesses, and disk disease. The ability of MRI to evaluate brain tumors and conditions such as stroke, cranial tumors, and infection surpasses that of CT. Because MRI does not image the dense petrous bone, it is excellent in evaluating the brainstem and anomalies of the posterior fossa (Fig. 8-14). Evaluation of demyelinating disease such as **multiple sclerosis** (MS) is substantively enhanced by MRI. It is, however, important to note that the high sensitivity associated with MRI

in the diagnosis of myelopathy may also prove to be a limitation at times. The ease with which MRI studies depict expansion and compression of the spinal cord may potentially lead to false-positive examinations and inappropriately aggressive therapies. These issues can be minimized by experienced observers meticulously correlating clinical and radiologic findings. Despite rapid evolution in technology, MRI currently has a small role in the evaluation of trauma, mainly limited to evaluation of spinal cord compression and, in some instances, vertebral fractures.

Magnetic resonance angiography (MRA) is used to evaluate the vascular anatomy of the head and neck (Fig. 8-15). It has been proven to accurately locate vascular occlusions within the large arteries of the brain that may lead to a stroke. MRA also demonstrates the major veins and dural sinuses within the brain and plays a large role in the diagnosis and treatment of cerebral venous thrombosis. To date, it has not replaced conventional cerebral angiography but is often used as an adjunct modality.

Functional MRI (fMRI) may be used to correlate and map motor functions to specific locations in the brain. This procedure identifies neural activation on the basis of hemodynamic changes within the brain. It provides useful information in demonstrating alterations in normal CNS function caused by structural changes in individuals with MS. fMRI is also helpful in identifying the regions of the cortex affected by neoplastic lesions within the brain and in assessing patients with a history of seizures and epilepsy. Currently, researchers are also using this modality to achieve a better understanding of the physiologic basis of autism by seeking information about neuroanatomic as well as physiologic changes resulting from this disorder.

Diffusion-weighted imaging (DWI) involves monitoring the extent to which water can freely move in any volume element (voxel). When the motion of water molecules within a voxel is restricted, greater magnetization will result, and the associated voxels will appear brighter. Reduced water diffusivity has been correlated with more aggressive tumor behavior and is

FIGURE 8-13 A, A normal magnetic resonance image of a young woman with a history of seizures as seen in a sagittal, T1-weighted view without gadolinium contrast. **B,** A normal T1-weighted axial view with gadolinium contrast of the same patient. **C,** A normal T1-weighted coronal view with gadolinium contrast of the same patient.

sometimes seen with high cellular density and tumor recurrence as well as ischemic stroke (Fig. 8-16). Diffusion-tensor imaging (DTI) capitalizes on the expected relative increase in restricted water molecules among neurologic fiber tracts by acquiring a three-dimensional map of the fiber tracts with a postprocessing technique referred to as *tractography*. The higher information content of the voxels makes DTI extremely sensitive to subtle pathology in the brain, which may be preventing the natural movement of water in the brain.

Perfusion-weighted imaging (PWI) involves the use of paramagnetic contrast agents to assess the cerebral hemodynamic status of a patient. By utilizing acquisition times that are short enough to capture the changes in signal intensity as a bolus of contrast material passes through the brain, PWI provides useful information on the vascular supply of various tumors, which is only implied from conventional MRI. The relative cerebral blood volume (rCBV) within a tumor can also be measured and compared with the contralateral normal white matter, typically displayed on color maps. The perfusion curves that are generated provide additional prognostic information by distinguishing between the characteristics of benign and malignant tumors.

FIGURE 8-14 A, A computed tomography scan of the posterior fossa region demonstrating the dense petrous portion of the temporal bone and associated artifacts. **B,** A magnetic resonance imaging scan of the posterior fossa region; note how the brain structures are visualized because the bone is not visible.

FIGURE 8-15 A, A magnetic resonance angiogram (MRA) without contrast enhancement readily showing vasculature within the head and neck. **B,** An MRA without contrast enhancement demonstrating the circle of Willis within the brain.

FIGURE 8-16 A magnetic resonance imaging diffusion-weighted apparent diffusion coefficient map image of the brain.

FIGURE 8-17 A magnetic resonance imaging perfusion scan of the brain.

Investigative studies that are now under way indicate that intraarterial MRI perfusion methods could be useful in better understanding the perfusion characteristics of some tumors and may also be useful in monitoring the delivery of therapeutics (Fig. 8-17).

Computed Tomography

CT continues to play a significant role in the evaluation of the CNS. It is rapid, noninvasive, and reasonably accurate. Because CT has excellent contrast resolution, it readily differentiates among the sulci, ventricles, and the gray and white matter within the brain (Fig. 8-18). It is particularly useful in evaluating cerebral bleeding after trauma because it readily reveals the extent of hematomas, if present. In many institutions, it is common practice to routinely perform CT examinations of the head and neck after significant trauma. CT of the brain is also performed to evaluate the ventricles, as in the case of hydrocephalus; to demonstrate cortical atrophy, as in the case of dementia; and to identify neoplasms within the brain, which may or may not

FIGURE 8-18 An axial computed tomography scan of a normal brain distinguishing between white and gray matter and demonstrating ventricular anatomy.

create a mass effect or shifting of the midline of the brain. In cases of infarction, edema, abscess, or cyst formation, tissue density is decreased (Fig. 8-19). Tissue density is increased by fresh blood or recent hemorrhage and calcifications

FIGURE 8-19 A computed tomography scan of the brain showing a decreased density in brain tissue as a result of infarction.

FIGURE 8-20 A sonogram of a normal premature neonate head with no evidence of periventricular hemorrhage.

within the brain. Other related roles include routine anatomic evaluation such as assessment of shunt (an artificial passageway) functioning and assessment of the bony cerebral and visceral skull. Contrast-enhanced CT of the brain is used to demonstrate anomalies in the cerebral vasculature and to delineate neoplastic growth within the cranial vault. It should be noted, however, that CT-related artifacts that may occur in association with bone at the margins of the posterior fossa often require the use of MRI to optimally evaluate pathology in this region of the brain. As discussed earlier, postmyelographic CT of the spine is also fairly prevalent. CT myelograms demonstrate encroachments of the spinal cord and nerve roots, as does MRI, but bone detail is best visualized with CT. CT is also used to evaluate vertebral fractures, as discussed in Chapter 2.

Sonography

Sonography is useful in evaluating the brains of neonates before closure of the fontanels because the fibrous tissue covering the fontanels provides a ready window into the brain (Fig. 8-20). Sonography readily detects cerebral hemorrhage and hydrocephalus. In premature infants, brain tissue around the ventricles (periventricular germinal matrix) is prone to hemorrhage, often resulting in intraventricular hemorrhage. In addition, premature infants are at an increased risk for periventricular white matter infarction. Portable sonography is a noninvasive method of evaluating cerebral anatomy and can be performed in the neonatal intensive care unit (NICU) to evaluate the status of affected infants.

Duplex Doppler sonography is a noninvasive modality useful in evaluating carotid blood flow. It demonstrates vascular occlusion and ulceration within the carotid arteries, most commonly at the point of bifurcation. Although it cannot provide the same level of detail compared with traditional angiography, it is a cost-effective and radiation-free alternative that is useful for evaluating patients experiencing carotid artery transient ischemic attacks (TIAs).

Nuclear Medicine

In nuclear medicine, radionuclide brain scans are primarily used to confirm brain death in patients with the appropriate clinical signs, generally after trauma or an intracranial bleed (Fig. 8-21). Technetium-labeled flow agents in combination with single photon emission computed tomography (SPECT) may be used experimentally to

FIGURE 8-21 A, A portable radionuclide brain scan confirming brain death by the absence of intracranial blood flow. The brain death occurred after an intracranial hemorrhage from preeclampsia in a postpartum woman. **B,** A portable brain scan also confirming brain death in a patient after a subarachnoid hemorrhage.

assess tumors, areas of stroke and ischemia, and Alzheimer disease. To complement the more traditional anatomic evaluation of other modalities, PET scanning allows imaging of the body's normal chemical processes and provides physiologic evaluation (Fig. 8-22). In high-risk patients with identified intracranial pathology, PET and SPECT both assist in differentiating tumors from infections.

Vascular and Interventional Radiology

Cerebral angiography is used to demonstrate vessel anatomy within the neck and brain (Fig. 8-23). Because of the increased use of MRA and CT angiography (CTA) vascular studies, conventional angiography is most frequently utilized when an interventional therapeutic procedure is warranted. It is used to diagnose and treat neoplastic lesions, stenosis, aneurysms, arteriovenous malformations (AVMs), and congenital anomalies of the CNS. Cerebral blood flow may be visualized by placing the catheter in the aortic arch or in selected vessels such as the carotid or vertebral arteries. Therapeutic devices such as stents and shunts and therapeutic medications are also placed by the interventionalist via catheters, often eliminating the need for surgical intervention.

FIGURE 8-22 An axial image from a positron emission tomography scan demonstrating an infarct in the posterior left parietotemporal region, with shunting of blood to hypermetabolic basal ganglia.

Interventional techniques include angioplasty, stent or shunt placement, thrombolysis, or embolization. Percutaneous transluminal angioplasty (PTA) and intraarterial thrombolysis are used to open stenotic vessels and improve blood flow within the vessel treated. Laser-tipped angioplasty and percutaneous atherectomy may also be performed to open stenotic vessels, especially

FIGURE 8-23 Carotid arteriogram showing vasculature of the head and neck.

in the neck. Spheres, coils, or beads are used to embolize or occlude cerebral vasculature, as in the case of aneurysms or AVMs. If an AVM is suspected, contrast-enhanced MRI, MRA, and CTA, as well as traditional myelography images can be utilized to initially identify abnormal spinal vasculature and guide spinal arteriography and intervention, potentially limiting the number of direct vascular injections required.

CONGENITAL AND HEREDITARY DISEASES

Meningomyelocele (Spina Bifida)

As mentioned in Chapter 2, spina bifida is a condition in which the bony neural arch that encloses and protects the spinal cord is not completely closed (Fig. 8-24). It most commonly occurs in

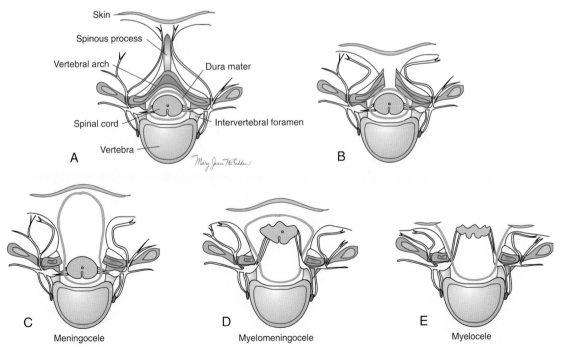

FIGURE 8-24 A normal neural arch in comparison with congenital defects. **A,** Normal. **B,** Spina bifida occulta. The median segment of the vertebral arch is missing and covered by skin. **C,** Meningocele. The arch is mostly absent with a bulging dura; however, the spinal cord remains in the vertebral canal. **D,** Myelomeningocele with a deformed spinal cord within the protruding dural sac. **E,** Myelocele: the area is totally exposed.

the lumbar region, and the spinal cord and its meninges may or may not herniate through the resultant opening. Elevated α-fetoprotein (AFP) levels in the mother's blood and on amniocentesis may allow spina bifida to be diagnosed prenatally. The defect and soft tissue sac are confirmed with fetal sonography. Complications depend on the extent of protrusion and range from treatable to life threatening. Any opening of the sac to the exterior of the body risks meningeal infection, so surgical closure is critical. If only the meninges protrude, the condition is termed a **meningocele** (Fig. 8-25). These are treated surgically without difficulty and usually have an excellent prognosis. A **myelocele** is a protrusion of the spinal cord, minus its meningeal coverings, which may also be treatable surgically. A **meningomyelocele** is the most common and most serious of possible conditions, affecting approximately one in every 800 infants and consisting of a protrusion of both the meninges and the spinal cord into the skin of the back (Figs. 8-26 and 8-27). Affected patients

FIGURE 8-25 A, The circular defect seen in the middle of the occipital bone of this newborn is the site of a meningocele. **B,** A lateral skull radiograph demonstrates the soft tissue density associated with the meningocele superimposed over the occipital bone.

FIGURE 8-26 A, A T1-weighted sagittal magnetic resonance imaging (MRI) view without gadolinium in this newborn readily demonstrates a meningomyelocele, with the arrow indicating the herniated spinal cord. **B,** A T1-weighted axial MRI view without gadolinium in the same patient similarly demonstrates the meningomyelocele, with the arrow indicating the herniated spinal cord.

FIGURE 8-27 A, A T1-weighted sagittal magnetic resonance imaging (MRI) view without gadolinium in this infant demonstrates a surgically repaired meningomyelocele. **B,** A T1-weighted axial MRI view without gadolinium similarly demonstrates the surgically repaired meningomyelocele, with the arrow pointing to the surgical site.

often have severe neurologic deficits, the extent of which depends on the level of herniation. Associated neurologic difficulties include paraplegia and diminished control of the lower limbs, bladder, and bowel. Hydrocephalus may affect as many as 90% of children diagnosed with meningomyelocele.

Some structural anomalies of the brain have been associated with the presence of meningomyelocele, in which MRI techniques have proven useful in further evaluation. One such example is the use of DTI to demonstrate the compromised integrity of some specific white matter pathways. Other structural anomalies that may be identified with MRI include cerebellar hyperplasia as well as altered development of the corpus callosum and posterior fossa.

Hydrocephalus

Normally, CSF flows around the spinal cord and over the convexity of the brain before reabsorption into the venous sinuses. This normal circulation may be interrupted by causes such as an obstruction to flow (noncommunicating hydrocephalus) and impaired absorption (communicating hydrocephalus); increased CSF production may also disturb normal circulation. The ventricles then distend proximal to the site of obstruction, which results in compression atrophy of the brain tissue around the dilated ventricles. In such cases, the sulci are obliterated, and the gyri are flattened. **Hydrocephalus** refers to an excessive accumulation of CSF within the ventricles and can be either congenital or acquired.

In noncommunicating hydrocephalus, an obstruction may occur congenitally or result from tumor growth, trauma (hemorrhage), or inflammation. It interferes with or blocks normal CSF circulation from the ventricles to the subarachnoid space. It is also commonly associated with malformations of the posterior fossa such as Arnold-Chiari malformation, which is a congenital defect in which the cerebellar tonsils are displaced downward below the level of the foramen magnum and are clearly visible on a sagittal T1 MRI examination of the brain.

Poor reabsorption of CSF by arachnoid villi results in communicating hydrocephalus. It may arise from a number of factors, including increased ICP caused by tumor compression, raised intrathoracic pressure impairing venous drainage, inflammation from meningitis, or subarachnoid hemorrhage. Hydrocephalus may also occur from overproduction of CSF, although this is the least common cause.

CT and MRI provide excellent visualization of hydrocephalus (Fig. 8-28). In neonates, sonography is used to demonstrate the ventricular system through the infant's fontanels, which permit passage of the beam until their eventual closure. Treatment may consist of surgery. In some cases, a shunt is surgically inserted to divert excess fluids. Placed between the ventricles and the internal jugular vein, the heart, or the peritoneum, it drains excess CSF. The shunt contains a one-way valve to prevent the backflow of blood into the ventricles. Radiographs are taken to demonstrate shunt placement after insertion (Fig. 8-29), and CT is used for periodic follow-up to

FIGURE 8-28 Comparison of normal and hydrocephalic brains.

FIGURE 8-29 A lateral projection of the skull showing ventriculojugular shunt placement.

evaluate ventricular size, which indirectly allows assessment of shunt function.

INFLAMMATORY AND INFECTIOUS DISEASES

Meningitis

An inflammation of the meningeal coverings of the brain and spinal cord is termed **meningitis**. It may be caused by bacteria, viruses, or other organisms that reach the meninges from elsewhere in the body via blood or lymph or may occur as a result of trauma and penetrating wounds or from adjacent structures (e.g., the mastoids) that become infected. Bacterial infection is the most common cause of meningitis (Fig. 8-30). Pathogens responsible for acute bacterial meningitis include meningococci, streptococci, and pneumococci. These are pus-forming (pyogenic) types of bacteria, and they may be carried to the meninges via the middle ear or the frontal sinus. Meningococcal meningitis is most common in infants, streptococcal meningitis in children, and pneumococcal meningitis in the adult population. In addition, a few cases result from infection by the tubercle bacillus *Mycobacterium tuberculosis*, which is not a pus-forming pathogen. This type of bacterial meningitis is more

difficult to diagnose because it does not have the same acute symptoms as those of the other types of bacterial meningitis. Tuberculous meningitis is usually spread from the lung in association with miliary tuberculosis.

In cases of bacterial meningitis, CSF is under increased pressure and may contribute to hydrocephalus. Acute bacterial meningitis may follow an upper respiratory infection or sore throat. Symptoms include fever, headache, stiff neck, vomiting, and changes in consciousness, with the patient becoming severely ill within 24 hours. Because bacterial meningitis can become lethal within a short period, accurate and immediate diagnosis and treatment are imperative. The primary means of diagnosing meningitis is the increased ICP detectable via the results of a lumbar puncture (spinal tap) procedure. On laboratory examination, CSF contains both bacteria responsible for the infection and a large number of polymorphonuclear leukocytes (pus cells).

A brain CT or MRI may be performed before the lumbar puncture to rule out the presence of abnormalities such as a midline shift of the central brain structures secondary to a brain mass. If a mass is present, it should be assumed that an increase in ICP exists; therefore, a lumbar puncture is contraindicated because of the risk of subsequent further CNS pressure changes and potential herniation of brain tissue. Antibiotics, in particular, have been very successful against many forms of meningitis, and antibiotic therapy may begin before a definite diagnosis has been established. If antibiotic therapy is started early, the mortality rate from bacterial meningitis is less than 10%. Contrast-enhanced MRI scans help identify subarachnoid inflammation and inflammation of the mastoids or sinuses. CT scans may also be helpful in assessing the presence of pathologic skull fractures or a brain abscess.

Chronic meningitis is most commonly caused by fungi and is often seen in patients with acquired immunodeficiency syndrome (AIDS) or in individuals undergoing immunosuppressant drug therapy. The symptoms are similar to those associated with acute meningitis; however, unlike in acute meningitis, the symptoms of chronic

FIGURE 8-30 A, A T1-weighted coronal magnetic resonance imaging (MRI) view with gadolinium demonstrates a ring lesion that communicates with the left lateral ventricle in this 17-year-old boy, creating meningitis as a result of transplantation into the brain of a bacterial (*Staphylococcus*) infection. **B,** A T1-weighted axial MRI view with gadolinium of the same patient demonstrates the presence of multiple infectious lesions. **C,** An axial computed tomography view of the same patient demonstrates the presence of an infectious lesion as well as slightly widened ventricles, as characteristic of meningitis.

meningitis occur over weeks rather than days. Treatment depends on the infecting agent, with amphotericin B being the preferred drug for all fungal infections. Although the disease may progress at a slower rate, the outcome may still be fatal.

Encephalitis

An infection of the brain tissue is termed **encephalitis**. In contrast to meningitis, which is most frequently a bacterial infection, encephalitis is usually viral in nature (Fig. 8-31) and may also occur subsequent to conditions such as chickenpox, smallpox, influenza, and measles. Primary viral encephalitis may be caused by the arbovirus transmitted by mosquitoes during warm weather or by herpes simplex virus. The symptoms and signs most commonly associated with encephalitis are headache, malaise, and coma. This condition is more serious than meningitis because individuals who acquire encephalitis more frequently develop permanent neurologic disabilities. The viral infection results in cerebral edema

FIGURE 8-31 A, A T2-weighted coronal magnetic resonance imaging (MRI) view demonstrates the infectious response in the brain of this boy with herpes encephalitis. **B,** A T2-weighted axial MRI view demonstrates the extent of the infectious process in the same patient with herpes encephalitis.

with numerous hemorrhagic spots scattered throughout the cerebral hemispheres, brainstem, and cerebellum.

MRI is especially valuable because it can detect brain inflammation earlier compared with CT, nuclear medicine studies, or electroencephalography (EEG). MRI can also rule out other anomalies such as a brain abscess or a subdural empyema or hematoma, which may mimic the clinical signs associated with viral encephalitis.

Herpes simplex encephalitis is treated with the antiviral medication acyclovir. Survival rates depend on the cause of the disease. In some instances, it may be fatal.

Brain Abscess

A **brain abscess** is an encapsulated accumulation of pus within the cranium resulting from a cranial infection, a penetrating head wound, or an infection spread through the bloodstream. A brain abscess may also result from the direct spread of organisms associated with a complicated case of sinusitis, chronic otitis, or mastoiditis. The symptoms are similar to those of encephalitis and include fever, headache, nausea and vomiting, seizures, and personality changes. An early diagnosis of a brain abscess or of cerebritis, which is its earlier stage, guides appropriate treatment, including careful selection of antibiotics, drainage of the abscess cavity, and correction of the original source of the infection, particularly if the abscess is secondary to a sinus or middle ear infection. Brain abscesses are fatal unless they are treated with antibiotic therapy. The specific antibiotic agent depends on the infecting organism, and treatment lasts approximately 4 to 8 weeks (Fig. 8-32).

FIGURE 8-32 A magnetic resonance imaging scan demonstrating a brain abscess.

The diagnosis of a brain abscess is usually made by CT or MRI evaluation of the brain. Since the introduction of CT, the overall mortality rate from abscesses has decreased from more than 40% to less than 5%. Serial CT examinations are often performed during antibiotic therapy to assess the progression of treatment. Although it is less sensitive than CT for detecting small calcifications related to brain abscesses, MRI provides greater sensitivity in the assessment of intracranial abscesses and may be more specific. The demonstration of a mature abscess on MRI includes shortening of the T1 and T2 relaxation times in the abscess wall, which results in hyperintensity on T1-weighted and hypointensity on T2-weighted images. However, the CT or MRI appearance of such a lesion is not specific enough to preclude histologic confirmation before initiation of treatment.

If pus associated with the abscess accumulates within the meningeal layers between the dura mater and the arachnoid, it is termed a **subdural empyema**. Like brain abscesses, subdural empyemas are diagnosed with CT or MRI of the brain. Symptoms are the same as those of a brain abscess; however, subdural empyemas require

immediate drainage. After drainage, the patient is treated with antibiotic therapy similar to that used for brain abscesses.

DEGENERATIVE DISEASES

Degenerative Disk Disease and Herniated Nucleus Pulposus

A **herniated nucleus pulposus**, or herniated disk, may result from either degenerative disease (Fig. 8-33) or trauma. A weakened or torn annulus fibrosus is subject to rupture, which allows the nucleus pulposus to protrude and compress spinal nerve roots. The disk may prolapse in any direction and, in some instances, may not produce pain. However, pressure may be placed on the spinal cord as the nucleus pulposus spreads beyond its normal confines posteriorly (Fig. 8-34), resulting in pain along the course of adjacent nerve roots and a weakening of the muscles supplied by these nerves. The most common locations for disk herniation are in the lower cervical and lower lumbar regions. In the lumbar region, over 80% occur at the L5–S1 nerve roots, and in the cervical region, C6–C7 herniations are most common.

Symptoms may include a sudden and severe onset of pain in the distribution of the compressed nerve root, in combination with weakened muscles, although at times symptoms may be more insidious. Compression of the nerve roots in the cervical area causes pain in the neck and upper extremities, whereas compression in the lumbar area results in pain of the hip, posterior thigh, calf, and foot. The extent of nerve root compression may be demonstrated through myelography, CT, and MRI, with MRI remaining the imaging modality of choice (Fig. 8-35). Patients with complicated low back pain can be evaluated for edema associated with facet arthropathy through the use of short-tau inversion recovery (STIR) and fat-saturated T2 spin-echo pulse sequences. In postoperative patients, contrast-enhanced MRI studies allow for a distinction between vertebral disks and scar tissue that extends beyond the vertebral interspace. It should

FIGURE 8-33 A, An anteroposterior projection of the lumbar spine demonstrating degenerative joint disease of the lower lumbar spine. **B,** A lateral lumbar projection of the same patient as in *A*.

FIGURE 8-34 A T1-weighted sagittal magnetic resonance imaging view of the spine in this 75-year-old man readily demonstrates severe degenerative disk disease as well as fusion of L1 and L2.

FIGURE 8-35 A sagittal magnetic resonance image demonstrating degenerative disk disease in the lumbar vertebral column.

also be noted that with normal aging, the nucleus pulposus tends to dehydrate, and the change in water content is well demonstrated on the basis of subsequent alteration in MRI relaxation times.

CT scans provide superior bone detail but are not as useful in depicting extradural soft tissue pathologies such as disk disease compared with multiplanar MRI. Myelography examinations are usually combined with postmyelography CT. The combined study serves as a complement to standard CT or MRI and occasionally leads to a more accurate diagnosis of disk herniation. Myelography may also be useful in surgical planning, with weight-bearing and flexion-extension views aiding in a comprehensive image-guided assessment.

Diskography is a radiographic technique that evaluates the vertebral column after injection of radiopaque material into an intervertebral disk of interest. This examination may have a role in localizing the source of back pain that cannot be defined with other less invasive studies as well as in patients with multifocal abnormalities on MRI. Although radiography, MRI, and postinjection CT may depict nonspecific aging or degenerative changes, the diskography injection itself may reproduce or provoke the patient's pain, which can be of diagnostic value. Used alone, diskography has limited specificity in disease diagnosis; however, recent research indicates that certain signal intensity changes on MRI may have a high positive predictive value in identifying pain generation during the diskography examination.

Physical therapy and analgesics are used as treatment, with 95% of patients recovering within 3 months without surgical intervention. If these fail to relieve pain, microscopic diskectomy, surgical decompression, or laminectomy with spinal fusion may be performed.

Cervical Spondylosis

Osteoarthritic conditions may also affect the vertebral column, leading to nerve disorders caused by chronic nerve root compression. These osteoarthritic changes of the neck are referred to as cervical spondylosis and are well demonstrated radiographically, most notably on an oblique projection of the cervical spine. Osteophytes (bone spurs) form in the articular facets of the cervical vertebrae and compress the nerves located in the intervertebral foramina. They may also compress the spinal cord (Fig. 8-36).

The ability of MRI to depict the spinal cord directly and assess its contour and internal signal characteristics reliably and noninvasively has resulted in general acceptance of MRI as the study of choice in evaluating cervical myelopathy, especially in cases of suspected spondylosis. Current research indicates that bone scintigraphy SPECT imaging, followed by a limited CT if scintigraphy is positive, has been found to be more sensitive than MRI; however, this imaging protocol has yet to be adopted in routine clinical practice. When MRI is contraindicated or is unavailable or to answer specific questions prior to surgical intervention, cervical myelography and CT myelography may be useful. Standard CT imaging, with multiplanar reformatted sagittal and coronal planes, is also useful in depicting bone structural problems related to spondylosis and in the postsurgical evaluation process.

As with degenerative disk disease, treatment is conservative at first but may include laminectomy and decompression procedures.

Multiple Sclerosis

MS, a chronic, progressive disease of the nervous system, most commonly affects individuals between the ages of 20 and 40 years. It affects women more often than men. The etiology of this disease is unknown, but research indicates that it may result from a latent herpesvirus or retrovirus infection. It also appears more often in individuals living in a temperate climate than in those living in a tropical environment. Although the disorder does not exhibit a defined inheritance pattern, 15% of individuals diagnosed with MS have an affected relative. Furthermore, a single gene, *DR2*, is implicated in this potential genetic susceptibility. MS involves degeneration of the myelin sheath covering the nervous tissue

FIGURE 8-36 A, A T1-weighted sagittal magnetic resonance imaging (MRI) view demonstrates compression of the spinal cord in this older man with cervical spondylosis. Cerebrospinal fluid (CSF) is dark adjacent to the gray spinal cord. **B,** A T2-weighted sagittal MRI image indicates the constriction of CSF flow (white) at C2 through C5.

of the spinal cord and the white matter within the brain. This demyelination impairs nerve conduction, beginning with muscle impairment and loss of balance and coordination. As MS progresses, tremors, vision impairment, and urinary bladder dysfunction develop, along with continued weakening of muscles. Numerous patchy areas of demyelinated nerves develop, forming scar tissue or sclerotic lesions throughout the nervous system. These scars are called *MS plaques* and present as multiple oval periventricular regions of increased T2 signal intensity, making MRI the modality of choice for evaluating individuals with suspected MS (Fig. 8-37). In cases of established MS diagnoses, contrast-enhanced MRI aids in differentiating new onset of active inflammation from older brain plaques by demonstrating ring enhancement of the newer lesions. Other MRI features of MS include generalized

cerebral volume loss and lesions involving the corpus callosum and the optic nerve. On occasion, the use of advanced MRI techniques such as diffusion imaging, spectroscopy, perfusion imaging, and magnetization transfer imaging may be useful in supporting, though not establishing, a diagnosis of MS. fMRI may also be used to assess alterations in normal CNS function resulting from structural changes within the brain.

MS runs a long and unpredictable course, eventually leading to permanent neurologic disabilities. Except in severe cases, however, the patient's life span is not shortened by MS. Patients may be placed on corticosteroids to shorten the symptomatic periods, but long-term use of corticosteroids is contraindicated. Interferon-β is a more promising drug that has also been used to reduce the frequency of symptomatic periods,

FIGURE 8-37 An axial fluid-attenuated inversion recovery (FLAIR) magnetic resonance imaging (MRI) scan from a patient with known multiple sclerosis (MS). The examination demonstrates MS plaques on the white matter of the brain.

FIGURE 8-38 An axial fluid-attenuated inversion recovery magnetic resonance imaging scan of the brain demonstrating an infarct in the left parietal lobe.

and it may actually delay the progression of the disease. Most patients benefit from regular exercise, alterations in diet, and physical therapy in conjunction with medications to reduce muscle spasticity and improve range of motion.

VASCULAR DISEASES

Cerebrovascular Accident

Atherosclerotic disease affecting the blood supply to the brain may eventually result in a cerebrovascular accident (CVA), commonly referred to as a *stroke*. About 795,000 strokes per a year occur in the United States, resulting in an average of 1 per 40 seconds, with 185,000 cases being recurrent attacks. Strokes are the third leading cause of death in the United States, behind heart disease and cancer. Strokes occur in essentially two ways, and they are classified as *ischemic* and *hemorrhagic*. Ischemic strokes make up 87% of

all strokes and are caused when a blood clot blocks a blood vessel in the brain. In contrast, hemorrhagic strokes, 10% being intracerebral in nature and 3% classified as subarachnoid, occur when a blood vessel in the brain ruptures and bleeds into the adjacent brain tissues and structures. Hemorrhagic strokes generally have a more sudden onset compared with ischemic strokes. Both CT and MRI (Fig. 8-38) examinations of the brain distinguish between ischemic and hemorrhagic causes.

Carotid duplex sonography and contrast-enhanced magnetic resonance angiography (CE-MRA) are also useful in the diagnosis of a stroke when carotid stenosis is believed to be the cause of the reduced cerebral blood flow. Although CTA, CE-MRA, and duplex sonography exhibit an accuracy ranging from 70% to 99% in diagnosing internal carotid artery (ICA) stenosis, only sonography offers a cost-effective method of initial screening in a large patient population. However, dependency on sonographer performance, presence of calcified plaque artifact, and difficulty distinguishing subtotal occlusion from total occlusion preclude endorsement of its routine use as the sole examination prior to treatment. For this reason, combined use of sonography and CE-MRA is becoming an increasingly common practice.

Ischemic Strokes

Under normal circumstances, the natural blood clotting cascade slows and eventually stops the bleeding and is beneficial. In an ischemic stroke, however, blood clots are dangerous because they may block blood flow and cause vessel occlusion. An ischemic stroke may occur in two ways: (1) infarction caused by thrombosis of a cerebral artery or (2) embolism to the brain from a thrombus elsewhere in the body. A *thrombus* is a blood clot that obstructs a blood vessel, and an *embolus* is a mass of undissolved matter (solid, liquid, or gas) present in a blood vessel brought there by blood current. Vessel occlusion or ischemia lasting over 1 hour usually results in the development of an infarct and permanent neurologic damage. Infarcts are often diagnosed with CT or MRI. However, angiography may be performed if the diagnosis with these imaging modalities is questionable. Two types of thromboses may cause stroke: (1) large vessel thrombosis and

(2) small vessel disease, also known as **lacunar infarction**. Large vessel thrombosis most often occurs in the large arteries as a result of long-term atherosclerosis followed by rapid blood clot formation. Typical sites are the bifurcation of the common carotid artery, within the carotid sinus, or the termination of the internal carotid artery, giving rise to the cerebral arteries (Figs. 8-39 and 8-40). An infarct caused by thrombosis of a cerebral artery is termed an **atherothrombotic brain infarction** (ABI). Symptoms associated with ABI develop slowly over a period of hours or days and include confusion, hemiplegia, and aphasia. This type of CVA may be preceded by a temporary episode of neurologic dysfunction, which is termed **transient ischemic attack** (TIA), and includes hemiparesis, hemiparesthesia, or monocular blindness. In 70% of the cases, these symptoms should clear within 2 hours or less. Furthermore, patients with TIA will exhibit positive signs for ischemic injury on MRI-based DWI in 30% to 50% of cases. This calls for an evaluation of stroke risk arising from a 10% to 15% increase in the likelihood that these patients will eventually suffer a debilitating stroke. Patients with a thrombotic stroke are also likely to have coronary artery disease, and heart attack is a

FIGURE 8-39 A, An unenhanced computed tomography (CT) scan of the brain of an 83-year-old woman reveals a large infarct along the distribution of the middle cerebral artery on the right side. **B,** A similar unenhanced CT scan taken 4 days later reveals worsening of the edema with early shift of the right lateral and third ventricles to the left.

FIGURE 8-40 A, A magnetic resonance imaging scan of the head of a 54-year-old woman who experienced sudden left facial paralysis and slumped forward while shopping reveals a large infarct along the distribution of the middle cerebral artery. **B,** A magnetic resonance angiogram of the same patient demonstrates occlusion of the middle cerebral artery, thought to be secondary to an embolus from carotid artery disease.

frequent cause of death in those who have a thrombotic stroke.

Small vessel disease, or lacunar infarction, occurs when blood flow to a very small arterial vessel is blocked. *Lacune* is the French term for "hole" and describes the small cavity that remains after products of a deep infarct have been removed by other cells. Although little is known about small vessel disease, it is closely linked to hypertension. About 20% of all strokes are caused by small vessel disease.

An embolism may also cause infarction in the brain from a thrombus elsewhere in the body, most commonly from the left side of the heart. CVAs resulting from cerebral embolism have a sudden onset of symptoms without warning. The mortality rate associated with ischemic strokes is approximately 20%. The prognosis depends on the location and extent of the stroke in addition to the patient's age and general health. Complete recovery is very rare, and deficits that are present 6 months following the stroke incident most likely are permanent neurologic changes. Between 50% and 70% of stroke survivors eventually regain functional independence, but 15% to 30%

become permanently disabled, and 20% require institutional care at 3 months after onset. One of the most common treatments involves the administration of recombinant tissue plasminogen activator (rtPA) within 3 hours of the onset of symptoms.

Noncontrast brain CT is most commonly used to diagnose patients with strokelike symptoms, especially before treatment with thrombolytic agents. This is primarily because of its wide availability and high sensitivity to acute hemorrhage, although it is relatively insensitive to acute ischemia and infarction with only one third to two thirds of such lesions being detected. According to the latest stroke management guidelines from the American Heart Association (AHA), ischemic stroke victims treated with thrombolytic agents (rtPA) have the best success if the CT examination is completed and results interpreted within 45 minutes from the onset of the stroke. Advanced MRI and CT techniques may be used to diagnose the stroke subtype and to guide other management decisions. However, garnering this additional diagnostic information should never result in a delay of rtPA after exclusion of an acute hemorrhage within the first 3 hours following ictus. Follow-up brain CT or transcranial Doppler sonography is used after the administration of rtPA to monitor the success of thrombolysis. Although traditional T1- or T2-weighted MRI is of limited value, DWI-MRI is a highly sensitive tool for imaging the onset of an acute ischemic stroke, and in many cases, it is more accurate than CT in identifying early infarct signs. DWI can be used in combination with PWI to identify potentially salvageable ischemic tissue, especially 3 hours after symptom onset.

CTA, MRA, and sonography may offer information about vessel patency in the brain and carotid arteries. In the future, PET may also prove to be a valuable asset in managing patients who have suffered an ischemic stroke, as the use of oxygen-15 PET shows promise in its ability to identify regions of decreased blood flow and to demonstrate oxygen consumption within the brain.

Hemorrhagic Strokes

In a hemorrhagic stroke, brain hemorrhage results from a weakening in the diseased vessel wall. Typically, the ruptured vessel has been weakened by arteriosclerosis from hypertension; however, hemorrhage may also result from congenital aneurysms or vascular anomalies. The onset of this type of CVA is sudden and often lethal because it expands rapidly. Brain hemorrhages account for approximately 10% to 15% of all CVAs and are of two types: (1) subarachnoid and (2) intracerebral. Most bleeds occur in the cerebrum and bleed into the lateral ventricle. Most commonly, they are preceded by an intense headache that is often accompanied by vomiting. Loss of consciousness follows within minutes and leads to total contralateral hemiplegia or death. Brain CT is often used in the case of a hemorrhagic stroke because fresh blood appears denser than surrounding brain tissue, which makes this imaging modality highly specific for this particular condition. However, if CT is negative but a hemorrhage is still suspected, a lumbar puncture may be performed to confirm

the negative result. MRI identification of acute intracranial hemorrhage may be variable and nonspecific. For this reason, although MRI is potentially more sensitive than CT, it is not generally used as a substitute for CT to detect acute intracranial hemorrhage.

Surgical intervention is necessary when the bleed causes brain displacement (midline shift) or when an aneurysm must be clipped to prevent fatal bleeding. The prognosis of this type of CVA is very poor, with approximately 35% of patients dying after the stroke and another 15% dying within a few weeks, usually from a subsequent vessel rupture.

NEOPLASTIC DISEASES

In the United States, the annual incidence rate of primary brain tumors is 46 per 100,000, and deaths from these tumors comprise about 10% of deaths from cancer. Primary brain tumors are often difficult to classify as purely benign or malignant. In many cases, the location of the brain neoplasm is of equal or greater importance than its malignancy or benignancy because of the complications produced by mass effect (Fig. 8-41). Edema accompanying a tumor causes an increase in ICP, which, in turn, causes headaches, vomiting, blurred vision, and seizures. Hemorrhage and brainstem herniation may occur, resulting in death as brainstem function (e.g., control of respiration) fails.

Other characteristics of primary brain tumors include a greater incidence in young to middle-aged adults and a relative infrequency of metastasis. Brain tumors often tend to occur in the posterior fossa in children, whereas the anterior portion of the cerebrum is a more prevalent site in adults. In addition, primary brain tumors are among the most common brain neoplasms in children, and metastases to the brain from other areas are more common in adults.

Primary brain tumors may be classified according to the site such as the specific lobe of the brain or according to histologic composition. The two categories of brain tumors based on histologic type are *glial* and *nonglial*

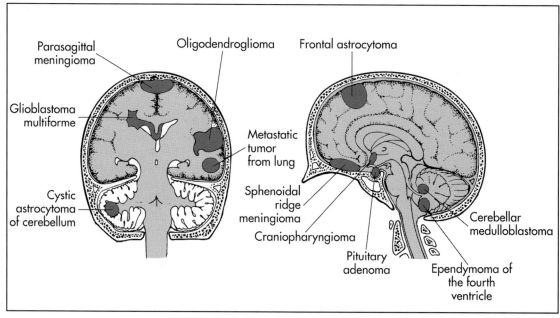

FIGURE 8-41 Common sites of intracranial tumors.

neoplasms. Glial tumors generate from the supporting tissues of the brain and spinal cord. **Gliomas** account for about half of all primary brain tumors. Their growth occurs through infiltration, making them difficult to treat surgically through resection. Nonglial tumors grow through expansion and are more treatable surgically. Meningiomas are the most frequently occurring nonglial tumors.

The modalities of choice in imaging brain tumors of all types are MRI and CT. As mentioned earlier, since optimal details of the posterior fossa structures may be obscured by beam-hardening artifact associated with CT, MRI is usually the initial modality of choice for evaluating patients of all ages unless an apparent contraindication exists. CT imaging, PET imaging, or both are indicated when an underlying primary is not evident with MRI examination. In addition to surgical intervention, radiation therapy and chemotherapy also play an important role in the treatment of brain tumors. Functional MRI and DTI may be used for mapping of the neural pathways to delineate motor and speech areas and assess any tumor-induced deflection of nerve

fibers, subsequently contributing to surgical and radiation treatment planning.

When patients previously treated for brain neoplasms present with new neurologic complaints, distinguishing between radiation necrosis and tumor recurrence may be a diagnostic challenge. These lesions, which may have a similar appearance on contrast-enhanced MRI, call for significantly different clinical management. Nuclear medicine SPECT imaging, PET, MR spectroscopy, and dynamic PWI-MRI studies may provide some improved specificity in making the differential diagnosis. Catheter angiography may also play a role in the treatment planning process by providing information related to tumor vascularity.

Gliomas

The most common type of primary brain tumor is the glioma (Fig. 8-42), accounting for approximately 45% of all intracranial tumors. Although derived from glial (supporting) cells, their precise classification is still being debated. However, several growth factors and their receptors have

FIGURE 8-42 A, A "butterfly" glioma seen in this T1-weighted coronal magnetic resonance imaging (MRI) view with gadolinium in a 54-year-old woman. **B,** A T1-weighted axial MRI view with gadolinium of the same "butterfly" glioma.

FIGURE 8-43 A, A T1-weighted axial magnetic resonance imaging view with gadolinium demonstrates a glioblastoma multiforme in a 70-year-old man. **B,** Computed tomography study of the brain without contrast demonstrates an intra-parenchymal hemorrhage after biopsy in the same patient with the glioblastoma multiforme.

been identified and are associated with the development of gliomas. These tumors may contain different types of cells in the same tumor, but one commonality is loss of genetic information from chromosome 17p. Gliomas commonly occur in the cerebral hemispheres and the posterior fossa, with nearly half of all gliomas classified as the malignant glioblastoma variety (Fig. 8-43).

Other types of gliomas include benign astrocytomas, oligodendrogliomas, and ependymomas. In terms of MRI results, gliomas are evaluated on the basis of associated edema (Fig. 8-44), mass effect, and amount of contrast enhancement. An association exists between the aggressiveness of the tumor and these three factors. Malignant gliomas may be extremely

FIGURE 8-44 A, A T1-weighted sagittal magnetic resonance imaging (MRI) view with gadolinium of a large glioma with surrounding edema in a 25-year-old man. **B,** A T2-weighted axial MRI view without gadolinium of the same glioma in the right parietal region, again with edema (white on T2) surrounding the tumor.

vascular, demonstrating pathologic vessels on angiographic examination. Low-grade malignant gliomas, however, are relatively avascular. CT images generally demonstrate an ill-defined area of decreased density (attenuation) with displacement of the midline structures and ventricular compression. Without contrast enhancement, it is difficult to differentiate the surrounding edema from the actual tumor, so the use of an iodinated intravenous (IV) contrast agent is necessary to enhance the lesion. Surgical biopsy generally provides the final diagnosis of the exact type of glioma. As described earlier, signs and symptoms include severe headaches, vision impairment, personality changes, and seizures as a result of increased ICP.

Astrocytomas account for about a third of all gliomas (Fig. 8-45) and are composed of astrocytes, which are star-shaped neuroglial cells with many branching processes. Astrocytomas are white, usually slow-growing, infiltrative tumors with a low grade of malignancy. Although their etiology remains unconfirmed, multiple genetic deletions, additions, duplications, mutations, and amplifications of specific genes have been linked with these tumors in different stages of malignant progression. Early detection leads to a good prognosis. A **glioblastoma multiforme** (an advanced astrocytoma) is highly malignant. An **oligodendroglioma** is a slow-growing astrocytic tumor, and histologically, it is often relatively benign (Fig. 8-46). It typically calcifies so that its appearance in a punctate or stippled pattern on a skull radiograph is virtually diagnostic. **Ependymoma** is a firm, whitish tumor that arises from the ependyma, the lining of the ventricles (Fig. 8-47). Typically, it derives from the roof of the fourth ventricle, but it may also appear from the central canal of the spinal cord.

Stereotactic biopsy of the brain lesion is generally used to confirm the diagnosis of a glioma. Treatment begins with surgical resection of the tumor followed by radiation therapy and chemotherapy. However, the prognosis is very poor, with only 25% of patients surviving after 2 years.

Medulloblastoma

Like astrocytic tumors, **medulloblastomas** are soft, infiltrating tumors of neuroepithelial tissue. These rapidly growing tumors are highly malignant and most often occur in the cerebellum of children and young adults (Fig. 8-48) and usually extend from the roof of the fourth ventricle. They

FIGURE 8-45 A, A T1-weighted sagittal magnetic resonance imaging (MRI) view with gadolinium demonstrates a pineal gland astrocytoma in this 32-year-old man. **B,** A T2-weighted axial MRI view demonstrates the same pineal gland astrocytoma.

FIGURE 8-46 An axial computed tomography view without contrast demonstrates the presence of an oligodendroglioma and surrounding edema.

are more common in boys and rarely seen in adults. Because MRI does not image bone or demonstrate artifacts associated with the dense bone within the base of the skull, it is an excellent modality for the demonstration of a medulloblastoma on both enhanced and nonenhanced examination. These tumors may also be demonstrated on CT, with the medulloblastoma visible as a midline lesion that is denser than normal brain tissue and surrounded by edema. In addition, tumor dissemination throughout the subarachnoid space often blocks the flow of CSF, causing hydrocephalus. Shunting is used to relieve the hydrocephalus. Surgical excision of the tumor as much as possible and radiation to the entire CNS (brain and spinal cord) have improved the 5-year survival rate to over 50% and the 10-year survival rate to about 40%. Unfortunately, recurrence is common with this tumor, and chemotherapy regimens have not been found to be consistently effective in controlling the recurrence.

Meningioma

A **meningioma** is a slow-growing, generally benign tumor that originates in the arachnoid tissue. It is the most common nonglial tumor,

FIGURE 8-47 A, A T1-weighted sagittal magnetic resonance imaging (MRI) view of the lumbosacral spine demonstrates an ependymoma at the L3–L4 interspace in this young man. **B,** A T1-weighted axial MRI view with gadolinium demonstrates the same ependymoma.

FIGURE 8-48 A, A T1-weighted sagittal magnetic resonance imaging (MRI) view without gadolinium demonstrates a medulloblastoma in the cerebellum of this 25-year-old man. **B,** A T1-weighted sagittal MRI view with gadolinium demonstrates the medulloblastoma, illustrating more of its actual size.

accounting for about 15% of all intracranial tumors. Meningiomas are more frequent in women than in men, and although meningiomas may affect individuals at any age, they usually arise in adults between the ages of 40 and 60 years. Furthermore, a loss of chromosome 22 has been isolated as a possible genetic etiology of this tumor type. Meningiomas are most often found adhering to the dura in relation to the intracranial venous sinuses. These tumors do not invade the brain but compress it with their growth. Resultant neurologic deficits are generally less in proportion to the tumor size compared with gliomas.

In some instances, the skull may thicken over the site of the meningioma, with the increased calcification visible on conventional skull radiographs. This area of hyperostosis may be palpable on physical examination. Because these tumors are fed by the meningeal arteries, plain skull radiography may also demonstrate an enlarged foramen spinosum and increased meningeal vascular markings on the inner table of the skull. Catheter angiography, when performed during preoperative embolization of the meningioma, is useful in identifying the feeding arteries of the tumor. Reports of the use of nuclear medicine imaging with radiolabeled agents such as ^{111}In-octreotide, which have an affinity for somatostatin receptors, can be useful in detecting and localizing meningiomas. This benefit is diminished, however, by the lack of specificity in differentiating meningiomas from other lesions such as high-grade gliomas or pituitary adenomas. PET is attractive for investigating the metabolic activity of tumors, but its role in the evaluation of meningiomas is complicated by variable metabolic presentations in different meningioma types. In general, nuclear medicine techniques provide capabilities that are sensitive for meningiomas but have relatively low specificity.

On MRI and CT, meningiomas show a typical yet variable appearance. For this reason, these modern imaging tools usually suggest the histologic diagnosis, but usually not the grade of tumor. CT studies of patients with a diagnosis of meningioma demonstrate a well-defined mass of increased attenuation, with calcifications visible in approximately 20% of the lesions. The extent of the meningioma is clearly visible on enhancement with an IV contrast agent. In comparison, nonenhanced MRI is not as sensitive as CT in detecting meningiomas because a significant inherent contrast difference does not exist between these tumors and normal brain tissue. However, an IV gadolinium contrast agent clearly demonstrates meningiomas on MRI examination (Fig. 8-49). Perfusion and diffusion imaging have also been useful tools for diagnosis, especially in suggesting alternative histologies and predicting aggressive histologic features.

Surgical removal is the method of treatment for a symptomatic meningioma. However, if the meningioma is surgically inaccessible, stereotactic radiosurgery using a gamma knife may be required.

Pituitary Adenoma

A **pituitary adenoma** is usually a benign tumor of the pituitary gland, and these tumors comprise about 15% of all intracranial tumors. Anatomically, these tumors are classified according to size, based on radiologic findings, as either microadenomas (less than <10 mm) or macroadenomas (≥10 mm). Hormones produced by the pituitary are affected, with one type of adenoma of the anterior pituitary resulting in gigantism if it develops before puberty and acromegaly if it occurs in adults because of excessive production of growth hormone (GH). Prolactin-secreting adenomas cause amenorrhea–galactorrhea syndrome, in which the breasts spontaneously secrete milk and menstrual periods cease. Pituitary adenomas may grow out of the sella turcica. As they grow, they compress structures such as the optic chiasm, resulting in vision problems.

A common radiographic demonstration of this growth is an enlargement and erosion of the sella turcica on a lateral skull radiograph. Angiography might demonstrate a displacement of the Sylvian triangle but generally only after the adenoma has assumed a considerable size. The **Sylvian triangle** is an anatomic landmark created by the middle cerebral artery and its branches. A

FIGURE 8-49 A, A T1-weighted sagittal magnetic resonance imaging (MRI) view with gadolinium of a large meningioma in the posterior occipital area with marked hydrocephalus in this 31-year-old woman. **B,** A T1-weighted axial MRI view with gadolinium of the same meningioma. Displacement of the fourth ventricle is seen, as well as a distortion of the vascular structures within the meningioma.

brain CT is useful to confirm the diagnosis of pituitary adenomas and to detect the extent of these lesions, especially when the tumor extends above the sella turcica. Enlargement of the sella turcica and suprasellar extension into the optic chiasm are generally demonstrated. These neoplasms are generally slightly denser than surrounding brain tissue and show obvious enhancement on IV injection of contrast medium. Small microadenomas are best demonstrated on thin slice, contrast-enhanced MRI images (Figs. 8-50 and 8-51) or high-resolution CT.

Generally, pituitary adenomas are treatable through surgical extraction, possibly followed by radiation therapy. Small adenomas may also be treated medically by drugs such as bromocriptine, which increase prolactin inhibitory factor (PIF) and suppress tumor growth.

Craniopharyngioma

A **craniopharyngioma** is a cystic, benign tumor growing from remnants of the development of the pituitary gland. It is thought to be developmental in origin and most commonly manifests

in childhood. Craniopharyngiomas usually arise above the sella and extend upward into the third ventricle (Fig. 8-52). Occasionally, they are seen within the sella, causing erosion of the sella turcica. Although traditional radiography of the skull has been superseded by newer imaging techniques, it still may be useful in cases of tumor wall calcification. Furthermore, it has been reported that in 46% to 87% of cases, skull radiography may show an abnormal sella with widening of its outlet, uniform expansion, and shortening or erosion of the dorsum sellae.

The CT appearance of craniopharyngiomas depends on the proportion of the solid and cystic components of the tumor. They are usually of mixed attenuation, with the cyst fluid having a low density and the contrast medium enhancing any solid portion as well as the cyst capsule. For this reason, pre- and postcontrast enhanced images in the axial plane followed by postcontrast coronal images are typically recommended.

MRI, especially after contrast administration, is valuable for topographic and structural analyses of craniopharyngiomas. Similar to CT, the appearance of the craniopharyngioma on MRI

FIGURE 8-50 A, A T1-weighted coronal magnetic resonance imaging (MRI) view demonstrates a suprasellar macroadenoma of the pituitary in this 37-year-old man. **B,** A T1-weighted sagittal MRI high-resolution scan with gadolinium demonstrates the same suprasellar macroadenoma of the pituitary.

FIGURE 8-51 A, Large pituitary adenoma extending downward into the right cavernous sinus in a 79-year-old woman as seen on this magnetic resonance imaging (MRI) T2-weighted coronal scan. **B,** A high-resolution T1-weighted sagittal MRI view of the same pituitary adenoma with gadolinium.

FIGURE 8-52 A, A T1-weighted axial magnetic resonance imaging (MRI) view with gadolinium demonstrates a mass, later confirmed by biopsy to be a craniopharyngioma, in this 53-year-old woman. **B,** A T1-weighted coronal MRI view with gadolinium demonstrates the relative size of the craniopharyngioma in the same patient.

will depend on the proportion of the solid and cystic components, the content of the cyst (cholesterol, keratin, hemorrhage), and the amount of calcification present. The signal of a solid tumor is isointense or hypointense relative to surrounding brain tissue on precontrast T1-weighted sequences, showing enhancement after gadolinium, whereas it is usually of mixed hypointensity or hyperintensity on T2-weighted sequences. The cystic component is usually hypointense on T1-weighted sequences and hyperintense on T2-weighted sequences. Postcontrast T1-weighted images demonstrate the thin peripheral contrast-enhancing rim of the cyst. Additionally, edema in the adjacent brain parenchyma, either due to a reaction to the craniopharyngioma itself or an associated disturbance in CSF flow caused by the tumor, may be present and provide useful information for distinguishing craniopharyngiomas from other common parasellar tumors.

Cerebral angiography may be useful for clarifying the anatomic relationship between the tumor and blood vessels. Occasionally, images revealing displacement of the Sylvian triangle as caused by a pituitary adenoma can be visualized if the tumor is large. Furthermore, in cases of craniopharyngioma in which angiography was

performed, displacement or encasement of the carotid artery was identified in 54% of the cases, with an additional 22% involving the basilar artery. Although craniopharyngiomas are treated surgically, excision is often difficult because of their location and proximity to structures such as the third ventricle and the optic nerves. Radiation therapy is used to enhance the effects of surgery.

Tumors of Central Nerve Sheath Cells

Two tumors of the peripheral nerve sheath are the **acoustic neuroma** (Fig. 8-53), and **schwannoma** (Fig. 8-54). They account for up to 10% of all intracranial tumors and are most common in middle-aged and older adults. The most common site is the eighth cranial (vestibulocochlear or acoustic) nerve. At this location, the tumor compresses the adjacent brain tissue and erodes the temporal bone. Symptoms of acoustic neuromas include facial paralysis, tinnitus, and partial hearing loss on the affected side. Nerve sheath tumors may also be found on other cranial nerves, especially the fifth cranial nerve (trigeminal), and on spinal nerve roots and peripheral nerves. The imaging method of choice for

FIGURE 8-53 A, A T2-weighted axial magnetic resonance imaging (MRI) view of a right acoustic neuroma that is not readily visible without gadolinium in this 24-year-old man. **B,** A high-resolution T1-weighted coronal MRI view with gadolinium readily reveals the acoustic neuroma. Compare the appearance of the tumor with the appearance of the normal vasculature and anatomy on the left side.

acoustic neuromas is MRI. In general, high-field strength magnets (1.5T to 3.0T) are preferred to low-field strength units because of the optimal signal-to-noise ratios, gradient strength, and spatial resolution that are achievable. In extreme cases, erosion and expansion of the internal auditory canal may be visible on an anteroposterior (AP) axial projection of the skull. The use of CT is primarily indicated in relation to tumors involving the skull base foramina and for evaluating calcific matrices within lesions and tumor-related osseous erosions. Stereotactic radiosurgery or conventional surgical excision of the tumor is the method of treatment.

Metastases from Other Sites

Secondary metastases from another site can involve any intracranial structure and account for about 10% of all brain tumors (Fig. 8-55). The metastatic lesions may be solitary or multiple. Brain metastasis usually arises from lung carcinoma. Other significant causes include adenocarcinoma of the breast, bronchogenic carcinoma, and malignant melanoma. Signs and symptoms of brain metastasis are similar to those of other brain tumors. Patients with metastases from other sites usually have signs of increased ICP, especially headache and ataxia; those with primary brain tumors are more likely to have seizures. Diagnosis and follow-up are done with MRI and CT. Treatment includes resection using either conventional surgical techniques or radiosurgery followed by radiation therapy. Prognosis depends on the number of metastatic lesions and the primary type of malignant disease.

Spinal Tumors

Primary tumors of the spinal cord are even less common than those of the brain. They are commonly divided into extradural and intradural groups, with the latter further divided into extramedullary (outside the spinal cord) and intramedullary (within the spinal cord) (Fig. 8-56). The most common types (>60%) of primary spinal neoplasms are **meningiomas** (Fig. 8-57) and **neurofibromas** (Fig. 8-58), both of which are extramedullary tumors. Neurofibromatosis is an inherited autosomal dominant disorder, and the gene for type 1 is located on chromosome 17, while the gene for type 2 is on chromosome 22. The most common intramedullary tumors are **astrocytoma** and **ependymoma**.

FIGURE 8-54 A, A T1-weighted sagittal magnetic resonance imaging (MRI) view of the lumbar spine with gadolinium shows a schwannoma at L3–L4 before surgery in this 27-year-old woman. **B,** A T1-weighted sagittal MRI view of the same lumbar spine without gadolinium after surgery demonstrates that apparent total excision of the tumor has been accomplished. Note also the excision of the spinous processes from the surgical site. **C,** A T1-weighted axial MRI view with gadolinium of the L3–L4 interspace demonstrates that some residual tumor is present in the left neural foramina.

Symptoms of extramedullary tumors may be similar to those of a herniated nucleus pulposus in that spinal tumors also compress the nerve roots, leading to pain and muscular weakness. In contrast, intramedullary tumors cause progressive paraparesis and sensory loss. In terms of imaging, CT myelography may be necessary to identify extradural tumors. Enlargement of the spinal cord by intramedullary masses may also be well depicted with myelography, but this is possible only in cases when large masses are present. For this reason, when evaluating spinal cord tumors, contrast-enhanced MRI is the examination of choice and has essentially replaced myelography. Differentiating syrinx from tumor, location of tumor nodules, and extent of cystic pathology, and differentiating nodules and cysts from edema are all factors that

FIGURE 8-55 Brain metastases from renal cell carcinoma as seen in this T1-weighted axial magnetic resonance imaging view with gadolinium after craniotomy in this 59-year-old woman.

FIGURE 8-57 A T1-weighted sagittal magnetic resonance imaging view of the spine with gadolinium demonstrates the presence of a meningioma in this 45-year-old woman with ataxia.

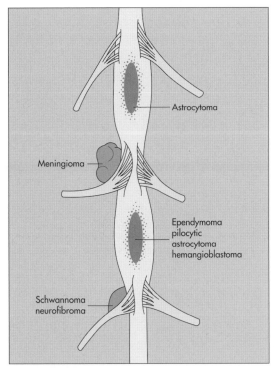

FIGURE 8-56 Distribution of some spinal tumors.

are crucial to the treatment planning process for intramedullary disease, so MRI imaging becomes a practical necessity. Conventional spine radiography is primarily reserved for demonstrating bone destruction and widening of the vertebral pedicles related to tumor growth.

Both intramedullary and extramedullary tumors may be surgically resected, depending on the location and degree of damage. Approximately 50% of patients undergoing surgery experience a reversal of clinical anomalies resulting from the neoplasm. In cases in which surgery is not a viable alternative, radiation therapy is the primary means of treating the tumor.

FIGURE 8-58 A, A T1-weighted coronal magnetic resonance imaging (MRI) view demonstrates the presence of a "dumbbell" neurofibroma showing clear compression of the spinal cord of this young female patient with back pain and leg weakness. **B,** An axial T1-weighted MRI image similarly demonstrates the lesion and compression of the spinal cord (*arrow*) into a narrow space.

PATHOLOGY SUMMARY
Central Nervous System

Pathology	Imaging Modalities of Choice	Additive or Subtractive Pathology
Hydrocephalus	CT, MRI, sonography in the neonate	
Meningitis	MRI, CT without contrast	
Encephalitis	MRI, CT without contrast	
Brain abscess	CT, MRI	
Herniated nucleus pulposus	MRI, CT without contrast, myelography, and postmyelography CT	
Cervical spondylosis	Radiography	Subtractive
Multiple sclerosis	MRI	
CVA	MRI, CT, sonography with Doppler, CTA, MRA	
Glioma	MRI, CT	
Medulloblastoma	MRI, CT	
Meningioma	CT, MRI	
Pituitary adenoma	CT, MRI	
Craniopharyngioma	CT	
Acoustic neuroma	MRI	
Spinal tumor	MRI, radiography, CT, myelography	Both
Metastases from other sites	MRI, radiography, CT	Subtractive

CT, Computed tomography; *CTA,* computed tomographic angiography; *CVA,* cerebrovascular accident; *MRA,* magnetic resonance angiography; *MRI,* magnetic resonance imaging.

REVIEW QUESTIONS

1. Under normal conditions, the central nervous system (CNS) within the cranial vault is well protected from damage by all of the following except:
   a. The cauda equina
   b. Cerebrospinal fluid (CSF)
   c. The diploë
   d. The dura mater

2. The correct order of meninges from outermost to innermost is:
   a. Arachnoid, pia, dura
   b. Dura, arachnoid, pia
   c. Dura, pia, arachnoid
   d. Pia, arachnoid, dura

3. The blood–brain barrier prevents passage of unwanted substances into the CNS through the cerebral:
   a. Arteries
   b. Capillaries
   c. Dura mater
   d. Veins

4. Erosion of the sella turcica is most commonly associated with neoplasms of the:
   a. Meninges
   b. Pineal gland
   c. Pituitary
   d. Pons

5. "Protrusion of both the spinal cord and the meninges into the skin of the back" describes a:
   a. Meningocele
   b. Meningomyelocele
   c. Myelocele
   d. Spinal hydrocephalus

6. The most typical cause of meningitis is:
   a. Bacterial infection
   b. Trauma
   c. Tumor compression
   d. Viral infection

7. The imaging modality of choice for demonstration of herniated nucleus pulposus is:
   a. Computed tomography (CT)
   b. Magnetic resonance imaging (MRI)
   c. Conventional myelography
   d. Sonography

8. The term *atherothrombotic brain infarction* denotes:
   a. Brain hemorrhage caused by atherosclerosis
   b. Infarction caused by thrombosis of a cerebral artery
   c. An embolism to the brain from a left heart thrombus
   d. None of the above

9. Which of the following neoplastic conditions is highly malignant and often occurs in the cerebellum of children?
   a. Astrocytoma
   b. Medulloblastoma
   c. Meningioma
   d. Pituitary adenoma

10. Which cranial nerve is the most common site for tumors of the peripheral nerve sheath (e.g., schwannoma)?
    a. 4
    b. 6
    c. 7
    d. 8

11. Where is CSF manufactured and absorbed? Explain the physiologic basis for the development of hydrocephalus.

12. Why is MRI the modality of choice for demonstrating diseases in the posterior fossa?

13. What is the most common cause for a cerebrovascular accident, and what is its most common site?

14. What are the major differences between meningitis and encephalitis?

15. Explain the differences between glial and nonglial tumors, and give an example of each type.

9

Hemopoietic System

LEARNING OBJECTIVES

On completion of Chapter 9, the reader should be able to:
- Identify the major constituents of blood and describe the function of each constituent.
- Specify the various blood types.
- Explain the role of the lymphatic system in terms of immunity.

- Describe the pathogenesis, prognosis, and signs and symptoms of the disease processes discussed in this chapter.
- Identify the various imaging modalities used in diagnosing hemopoietic disorders.

OUTLINE

KEY TERMS

Acquired immunodeficiency syndrome
Acute lymphocytic leukemia
Acute monoblastic leukemia
Acute myelocytic leukemia
Agglutination
Anemia
Chronic lymphocytic leukemia
Chronic myelocytic leukemia
Erythrocytes
Hematocrit
Hemocytoblasts
Hemophilia A
Hemophilia B

Hemophilia C
HIV protease
Hodgkin lymphoma
Human immunodeficiency retrovirus
Kaposi sarcoma
Leukemia
Leukocytes
Lymph
Lymph nodes
Lymphocytes
Multiple myeloma
Myeloid tissue
Non-Hodgkin lymphoma

Pneumocystis carinii pneumonia
Reed-Sternberg cells
Reticuloendothelial system
Reverse transcriptase
Rh factor
Rh-negative

Rh-positive
Sickle cell anemia
Spleen
Thalassemia
Thrombocytes
von Willebrand disease

ANATOMY AND PHYSIOLOGY

The hemopoietic system consists of blood, lymphatic tissue, bone marrow, and the spleen. Circulating blood contains both plasma and blood cells, with the plasma constituting approximately 55% of the total blood volume. The plasma is about 90% water and 10% solutes such as proteins, glucose, amino acids, and lipids. Plasma proteins are classified as globulins, albumins, and clotting factors. With the exception of immunoglobulins (Igs), all of these proteins are synthesized by the liver. Immunoglobulins are synthesized by the lymphatic system, specifically by mature lymphocytes termed *plasma cells*. Immunoglobulins are responsible for fighting infectious organisms and include IgA, IgB, IgM, IgD, and IgE. Albumins regulate the passage of water and solutes through the capillaries. Clotting factors found within the plasma are primarily fibrinogen, the precursor of the fibrin clot.

Three basic types of blood cells—erythrocytes, leukocytes, and thrombocytes (Table 9-1)—make up the remaining 45% of the total blood volume.

Erythrocytes, or red blood cells (RBCs), are very small in relation to the other blood cells. They do not possess a nucleus and are shaped like biconcave disks. Erythrocytes are responsible for transporting oxygen and carbon dioxide to and from the various organs of the body. This is accomplished via the hemoglobin in erythrocytes, which allows oxygen or carbon dioxide molecules to attach to the cell for transport. Individuals with a hemoglobin level of less than 12 grams (g) per 100 milliliters (mL) of blood have **anemia** and are considered "anemic" because

TABLE 9-1	Blood Cell Types		
Type	**Formed By**	**Function**	**Life Span**
Erythrocyte	Myeloid tissue within red bone marrow	Transporting oxygen and carbon dioxide	120 days
Leukocyte			
Granular	Red bone marrow	Body defense	2 weeks
Nongranular	Lymphatic tissue	Immunity	Years
Thrombocyte	Myeloid tissue within red bone marrow	Blood clotting	10 days

less than normal oxygen or carbon dioxide transportation occurs in them. The total percentage of RBCs in blood volume is determined by a laboratory test termed **hematocrit.**

Erythrocytes are formed by specialized cells called **hemocytoblasts,** which are located in the myeloid tissue found within red bone marrow. These cells live approximately 120 days and are phagocytosed by the **reticuloendothelial system,** which consists of specialized cells in the liver, spleen, and bone marrow. During phagocytosis, the iron within the hemoglobin is released, and bilirubin is formed. The released iron is used again in the development of new erythrocytes, and bilirubin is excreted in bile.

Erythrocytes may contain various antigens that determine blood type. This is especially critical for blood transfusions because blood type incompatibility could have fatal results. Erythrocytes may contain no antigens, either the A or the B antigen, or both the A and the B antigens. The resulting blood types are O (no antigen), A, B, and AB. If incompatible blood types are mixed (e.g., a type O patient receives type AB blood), erythrocytes from the donor clump together in the serum of the recipient. Because the type O recipient does not possess the A or B antigen, antibodies are formed to fight against the foreign RBCs. This is termed **agglutination.** Eventually, donor erythrocytes are destroyed, and the rejection possibly results in immediate shock. In some cases, the reaction may be delayed and may result in fever, pain, and ultimate renal failure as the kidneys try to excrete the byproducts from the destruction of the donor erythrocytes. Cross-matching of blood types to eliminate the risk of transfusion of incompatible blood is essential.

The person with type O blood is considered the universal donor because this type does not contain any antigens and can be given to anyone regardless of the recipient's blood type. The person with type AB blood is considered the universal recipient because this type of blood possesses both antigens, which enables the person to receive any type of blood (Table 9-2). In addition, the Rh blood factor should be considered. The **Rh factor** is termed such because it was first discovered in the blood of the rhesus monkey. Approximately 85% of the human population has this factor; these people are classified as **Rh-positive.** Individuals not possessing the Rh factor are **Rh-negative.** The Rh factor becomes a problem if an Rh-positive father transmits the Rh factor to a fetus carried by an Rh-negative mother. The first pregnancy generally progresses normally, but in subsequent pregnancies, the mother's anti-Rh antibodies, made during the first pregnancy, attack the Rh-positive fetal blood. This scenario can be avoided by Rh-immunization of the mother before pregnancy.

Leukocytes, or white blood cells (WBCs), may be classified as *granular* or *nongranular.* Granular leukocytes contain cytoplasmic granules and

TABLE 9-2	Cross-Matching of Blood Types			
	Acceptable Donor Type			
Recipient Blood Type	**A**	**B**	**AB***	**OE†**
A	Yes	No	No	Yes
B	No	Yes	No	Yes
AB*	Yes	Yes	Yes	Yes
O†	No	No	No	Yes

*AB, Universal recipient.
†O, Universal donor.

irregular nuclei. They are formed within the red bone marrow and include basophils, neutrophils, and eosinophils. The names of these cells correspond to the manner in which they respond to certain dyes for microscopic inspection. Nongranular leukocytes do not contain cytoplasmic granules, and they possess regular nuclei. They are mainly formed in the lymphatic tissue of the spleen and include lymphocytes and monocytes. Leukocytes play an important role in the body's defense system. They are able to move out of capillaries into tissue to "attack" and phagocytose foreign substances. The life span of leukocytes varies, depending on the type of cell. Granular leukocytes live for only about 2 weeks, whereas lymphocytes may live for years. Normal blood contains between 5000 and 9000 leukocytes per milliliter. Changes in the number of leukocytes often indicate the presence of disease.

The third major type of blood cells is the **thrombocytes,** or platelets. These cells are necessary for blood to clot properly and respond within seconds to initiate the coagulation process. Thrombocytes are also formed in the myeloid tissue within the red bone marrow and have a life span of approximately 10 days. The normal platelet count is 140,000 to 340,000 per cubic millimeter (mm^3). Platelet activation is increased by an inflammatory response. Vascular damage results in a physiologic response to maintain homeostasis, including vasoconstriction, the development of a platelet plug, the activation of

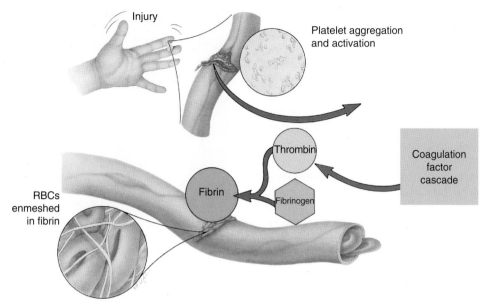

FIGURE 9-1 The blood clotting mechanism involves the release of platelet factors at the injury site, formation of thrombin, and trapping of red blood cells in fibrin to form a clot.

blood coagulation (thrombin), and the formation of a blood clot. This process is critical in preventing hemorrhage and is dependent on the availability of the proper number of platelets (Fig. 9-1).

The lymphatic system is a subsystem of the circulatory system. Its major function is ensuring immunity through production of lymphocytes and antibodies, but it is also responsible for absorbing fat from the intestinal tract and for manufacturing blood under certain circumstances. The lymphatic system is composed of both lymphatic vessels and nodes. Lymphatic vessels contain a milky liquid substance termed **lymph**. **Lymph nodes** are small ovoid bodies attached in a chainlike pattern along the vessels. They filter out particles and foreign materials from blood. Major areas of lymph node chains include the neck, the mediastinum, and the axillary, retroperitoneal, pelvic, and inguinal regions. These lymph nodes often become enlarged when the body is invaded by an infectious agent and in cases of neoplastic disease.

Mature **lymphocytes** are the most important cells in the development of immunity. T lymphocytes are derived from lymphatic tissue of the thymus gland, and B lymphocytes are derived from bone marrow. These two types of lymphocytes work together with macrophages to ingest foreign substances and process specific foreign antigens. Through a complex process, an antibody that is capable of attacking the foreign antigen is formed. An *antibody* is an immunoglobulin produced by plasma cells and is categorized into one of five classifications: IgG, IgM, IgA, IgD, and IgE. The formation of antibodies is the systemic response that could have a negative effect on tissue grafts and organ transplants. The human body sees the transplant as foreign, so the lymphocytes and macrophages try to destroy the foreign antigens, which results in rejection of the graft or transplant.

Although the risk of whole-body radiation exposure is of little concern in diagnostic radiology, it is important for the radiographer to remember that exposure to x-rays or gamma-rays can have a harmful effect on blood marrow and lymphoid tissue. It takes a whole-body dose of approximately 0.5 to 0.75 Gray (Gy) (50 to 75 rad) to cause a detectable change in blood cells. The most radiosensitive blood cells are lymphocytes, followed by leukocytes and thrombocytes.

The **spleen** is the largest lymphoid organ and is located in the upper left quadrant of the abdomen. Its chief function is production of lymphocytes and plasma cells. It serves as a reservoir for blood and contains mononuclear phagocytes that cleanse the blood and lymphocytes to fight infectious bloodborne microorganisms. The splenic artery arises from the trifurcation of the celiac trunk off the abdominal aorta and supplies fresh blood to the spleen. This blood is cleansed by macrophages, which remove old or defective blood cells and microorganisms. The splenic vein empties into the portal vein. The spleen is occasionally ruptured in abdominal trauma and can be removed without detrimental effects.

Myeloid tissue, or bone marrow, is located within the spongy bone cavities formed by the outer layer of compact bone and may be classified as red or yellow marrow. This tissue contains blood vessels, nerves, stem cells, blood cells, mononuclear phagocytes, and fatty tissue. Red marrow is myeloid tissue that is still active in the production of blood cells, whereas yellow marrow is inactive tissue that is primarily composed of fatty tissue. Red bone marrow is predominantly found in flat bones (cranium, ribs, pelvis, and vertebrae) and in the proximal end of long bones such as the humerus and femur.

IMAGING CONSIDERATIONS

Radiography plays a limited role in the diagnosis and treatment of hemopoietic disorders. Skeletal survey radiography may be used in cases of multiple myeloma, a neoplastic disease of plasma cells, and for some types of leukemia. Chest radiography is helpful in identifying lymphatic changes within the mediastinum often associated with lymphomas. Chest radiography is also warranted in diagnosing various opportunistic infections resulting in acute respiratory infections in immunocompromised patients such as those with **acquired immunodeficiency syndrome** (AIDS).

FIGURE 9-2 Computed tomography of the lower chest and upper abdomen demonstrates enlargement of lymph nodes on a 27-year-old man with lymphoma.

Although abdominal computed tomography (CT) is useful in the assessment of lymph node enlargement (Fig. 9-2) and to further determine the location and extent of neoplastic diseases of the lymphatic system, positron emission tomography (PET) is now considered the modality of choice in the follow-up treatment for patients with Hodgkin lymphoma. Compared with CT, PET has been shown to have a higher specificity in demonstrating relapses of the disease. CT of the brain, without contrast enhancement, and magnetic resonance imaging (MRI) of the brain, with or without contrast enhancement, are highly recommended by the American College of Radiology (ACR) in assessing focal neurologic deficits associated with human immunodeficiency virus (HIV) infection. CT of the chest without contrast enhancement is also appropriate in evaluating acute respiratory infections associated with HIV.

MRI is quite useful in imaging bone marrow and the diseases that affect the marrow. Although MRI produces a signal void in areas of compact bone, changes in the marrow pattern are quite visible and useful in the diagnosis of many disorders (Fig. 9-3).

Nuclear medicine technetium-99m (^{99m}Tc) bone scans are indicated for metastatic bone disease such as multiple myeloma, and follow-up radiography after a positive bone scan may be

FIGURE 9-3 A, A T2-weighted sagittal magnetic resonance imaging (MRI) view without gadolinium demonstrates an obvious L4 lesion. **B,** A T2-weighted sagittal MRI view with gadolinium demonstrates L4 destruction consistent with multiple myeloma in this 55-year-old man.

appropriate. As mentioned above, PET is increasingly used in the initial staging and follow-up of patients with Hodgkin lymphoma and has been deemed highly predictive of patient outcomes by the ACR. In addition, PET or CT is used in the radiation treatment planning process and posttreatment follow-up of patients undergoing radiation therapy for Hodgkin lymphoma.

Many bloodborne pathogens may be transmitted from patients to health care workers. Therefore, it is of utmost importance that radiographers always practice standard precautions in terms of blood and bodily fluids. Gloves should be worn when performing venipuncture or whenever the possibility of contamination with blood or other bodily fluids exists. Additional protective apparel may be necessary if large amounts of bodily fluids may be encountered. Needles should not be recapped; they should be placed in puncture-proof containers for hazardous waste disposal. The importance of hand washing cannot be overemphasized because it is a vital part of infection control practices. It is the single most significant factor in infection control.

ACQUIRED IMMUNODEFICIENCY SYNDROME

AIDS was first recognized in 1981. It is caused by one of two related **human immunodeficiency retroviruses,** HIV-1 and HIV-2, and results in a wide range of clinical manifestations. HIV-1, identified in 1984, paralyzes the normal immune mechanisms within the human body, which results in severe immunosuppression, or AIDS. It is responsible for most cases of AIDS in the Western hemisphere. In late 2008, the Centers for Disease Control and Prevention (CDC) estimated that almost 683,000 individuals in the United States had a diagnosis of HIV infection. Less virulent than HIV-1, HIV-2 is the principal agent of AIDS in West Africa. In 2007, HIV infection affected nearly 33 million individuals worldwide and is considered a pandemic.

Retroviruses contain **reverse transcriptase,** an enzyme that converts viral ribonucleic acid (RNA) into a deoxyribonucleic acid (DNA) copy that becomes integrated into the host cell DNA. Each time the cell divides, the retroviral DNA is duplicated. Both types of HIV also contain **HIV protease,** an enzyme that converts immature, noninfectious HIV to its infectious state within the cell. HIV infects a part of the T lymphocyte, termed *T4* or *CD4*, responsible for immune response to infection, as well as non-lymphoid cells such as macrophages. Infected individuals experience a brief antibody-negative period immediately after infection, during which time the virus rapidly reproduces until the immune system begins to react to the infectious agent.

Because HIV inhibits the body's defensive response to the presence of a variety of diseases, one major sign of AIDS is the presence of unusual opportunistic infections (Box 9-1) such as *Pneumocystis carinii, Toxoplasma gondii,* cryptococci, *Mycobacterium avium,* and herpes. AIDS is also directly linked to an increased incidence of malignancies such as Kaposi sarcoma, non-Hodgkin lymphoma (NHL), Hodgkin lymphoma, and primary central nervous system (CNS) lymphoma. It is the most common disease associated with lymphocytopenia, or the depletion of lymphocytes. This occurs through the destruction of CD4+ T cells infected by the virus. Anemia, thrombocytopenia, and leukopenia also commonly occur in HIV-infected patients (Fig. 9-4).

Signs and symptoms associated with HIV and AIDS are broad and may mimic those of other diseases. Symptoms of HIV infection include generalized lymphadenopathy, malaise, fever, and joint pain within 1 to 4 weeks after infection. These early-stage HIV symptoms may last up to 10 years before progressing to AIDS. Left untreated, approximately 99% of HIV infections progress to AIDS. As this progression takes place, weight loss may occur as a result of nausea, vomiting, and diarrhea. As mentioned earlier, leukopenia, anemia, and thrombocytopenia also occur. AIDS may affect the CNS, which results in apathy, memory loss, inability to concentrate, and dementia. Headaches, fever, or photophobia associated with acute aseptic meningitis, encephalopathy with seizures, or motor, sensory, or gait deficits may be the first manifestations of the disease. Atrophy of the brain cortex is commonly

---

BOX 9-1	**AIDS-Defining Opportunistic Infections and Neoplasms Found in Individuals with Human Immunodeficiency Virus Infection**

Infections
Protozoal and Helminthic Infections
Cryptosporidiosis or isosporiasis (enteritis)
Pneumocystosis (pneumonia or disseminated infection)
Toxoplasmosis (pneumonia or CNS infection)
Fungal infections
Candidiasis (esophageal, tracheal, or pulmonary)
Cryptococcosis (CNS infection)
Coccidiomycosis (disseminated)
Histoplasmosis (disseminated)

Bacterial Infections
Mycobacteriosis (atypical, e.g., *Mycobacterium avium-intracellulare,* disseminated or extrapulmonary; *Mycobacterium tuberculosis,* pulmonary or extrapulmonary)

Nocardiosis (pneumonia, meningitis, disseminated)
Salmonella infections (disseminated)

Viral Infections
Cytomegalovirus (pulmonary, intestinal, retinitis, or CNS infections)
Herpes simplex virus (localized or disseminated)
Varicella-zoster virus (localized or disseminated)
Progressive multifocal leukoencephalopathy

Neoplasms
Kaposi sarcoma
B-cell non-Hodgkin lymphomas
Primary lymphoma of the brain
Invasive cancer of the uterine cervix

AIDS, Acquired immunodeficiency syndrome; *CNS,* central nervous system.
From: Kumar, V., Abbas, A., Fausto, N.: *Robbins and Cotran pathologic basis for disease,* ed 7, Philadelphia, PA, 2005, Saunders.

Brain
glial cells

Thymus gland

Bone marrow

Colon, duodenum,
and rectum
enterochromaffin cells

Lymphocytes
in blood, semen,
and vaginal fluid

Brain
macrophages
(microglial cells)

Lymph
nodes

Lung,
alveolar
macrophages

Skin,
Langerhans'
cells

Bone marrow

FIGURE 9-4 Distribution of tissue that can be infected by human immunodeficiency virus (HIV). Infection is closely linked to the presence of CD4 receptors or chemokine co-receptors on host tissue, particularly T cells and macrophages.

demonstrated on brain CT and MRI studies in patients with subacute encephalitis related to AIDS. In cases of toxoplasmic encephalitis, CT and MRI will demonstrate contrast-enhanced lesions within the basal ganglia.

With no known cure, AIDS remains a major health crisis and places a burden on the health care system in the United States and throughout the world. As a result of advances in the production and use of antiretroviral therapy (ART) in the United States, the number of individuals diagnosed with AIDS and the number of deaths associated with AIDS have continually declined

since 1996 with the median age at death increasing to 47 years in 2008. However, according to the CDC, AIDS still remains one of the leading causes of death in the United States in individuals aged 22 to 44 years of age.

ART has reduced the incidence of opportunistic infections and extended the lives of individuals infected with HIV. However, the use of antiviral drugs in the treatment of HIV infection is continually being reevaluated because the use of only one drug results in mutation of the virus as well as resistance to the drug and loss of efficacy of the therapy. HIV infection must be staged prior to placing an individual on an ART regimen. Staging includes HIV antibody testing, CD4 T-cell count, viral load, a complete blood cell (CBC) count and chemistry profile, as well as genotypic resistance testing. The CD4 T-cell count is the primary indicator of immune function, and the CDC recommends that CD4 T-cell counts should be monitored quarterly. Current ART regimens may reduce HIV-associated morbidity and improve the quality of life. Currently, the most common therapy calls for an individualized two- or three-drug regimen of a combination of 20 antiretroviral drugs that have been approved by the U.S. Food and Drug Administration (FDA) and categorized into six mechanistic drug classifications. Guidelines for preventing opportunistic infections in persons with HIV infection were updated in 2009 by the CDC, the National Institutes of Health, and the HIV Medicine Association of the Infectious Diseases Society of America. Additional information can be accessed at the CDC Web site. Bone marrow evaluation is common in HIV-positive individuals. This diagnostic tool is used to evaluate decreased blood cell counts, stage malignancies, and obtain cultures for determining associated infections.

Although it can affect anyone, regardless of age or sexual orientation, in the United States, HIV most frequently affects homosexual and bisexual men and intravenous (IV) drug users. The virus is transmitted through sexual contact and exposure to infected blood and bodily fluids.

One of the most common lung infections associated with HIV is tuberculosis (TB). TB may be the first indication of HIV infection in areas of the world where TB is prevalent. In developed countries such as the United States, HIV has caused an increase in the rates of TB. The lungs are also a common site for opportunistic infections associated with AIDS, such as *Pneumocystis carinii* pneumonia, often in combination with a cytomegalovirus. In the early stages of disease, the small multifocal infiltrates of the lungs associated with this pneumonia are often termed *ground glass lesions*. This fungal infection occurs in over half of all patients with AIDS; however,

in developed countries, the risk of these infections has been reduced through the use of effective prophylactic treatment. Bacterial pneumonias are also common in IV drug users infected with HIV. Chest radiography demonstrates localized consolidation, which usually indicates a bacterial infection (Fig. 9-5). *P. carinii* infections (Fig. 9-6) generally reveal bilateral perihilar reticular–interstitial infiltrates that rapidly progress within 3 to 5 days to diffuse consolidation.

Kaposi sarcoma is the most common malignancy in patients with AIDS, especially in homosexual or bisexual men who are often co-infected with herpes virus 8. It is present in approximately 25% to 30% of patients with AIDS and may affect connective tissue in various sites in the body. It most often affects skin, lymph nodes, and the gastrointestinal system. About 20% of patients with Kaposi sarcoma also demonstrate pulmonary involvement. Radiographically, hilar adenopathy, nodular pulmonary infiltrates, and pleural effusion are demonstrated (Fig. 9-7). Endobronchial Kaposi sarcoma is common among patients with AIDS and may result in atelectasis or postobstruction pneumonia.

CONGENITAL AND HEREDITARY DISEASES

Sickle Cell Disease

Sickle cell disease is a hereditary autosomal recessive disorder that affects RBCs, causing abnormal hemoglobin levels. It is caused by a mutation of the β-chain of the hemoglobin molecule and results in chronic hemolytic anemia leading to organ failure. It is present during infancy, most commonly in individuals of African, Near Eastern, Mediterranean, or Indian descent. Deoxygenation causes the erythrocyte to stiffen and elongate to a crescent or sickle shape, prohibiting the normal movement of the blood cell through the circulatory system. This results in acute pain from poorly oxygenated tissue due to vessel occlusion, atypical pneumonias caused by pulmonary vessel infarction, and the development of a variety of infectious diseases. Sickle cell

FIGURE 9-5 A, Posteroanterior and **B,** left lateral chest radiographs of a patient with known acquired immunodeficiency syndrome demonstrate a left lower lobe infiltrate.

FIGURE 9-6 Chest radiograph of a 53-year-old man diagnosed with acquired immunodeficiency syndrome. The radiograph demonstrates *Pneumocystis carinii* pneumonia with diffuse bilateral airspace parenchymal infiltrative densities.

FIGURE 9-7 Chest radiograph of a 27-year-old man with Kaposi sarcoma of skin and pulmonary involvement. The radiograph shows nodular diffuse patchy parenchymal infiltration with nodular densities in the upper lobes.

disease generally affects the abdomen, the chest, and the skeletal system. The clinical course of sickle cell disease is highly variable, and medical imaging plays a small role in the diagnosis and management of this disease. Treatment is limited to supportive care to prevent anemia and infection.

Thalassemias

Thalassemias are inherited disorders caused by a mutation on the α-chain or β-chain of the hemoglobin molecule. Like sickle cell disease, this disorder tends to occur most frequently in individuals of Mediterranean or African descent. Thalassemias are classified as α-major, α-minor, β-major, and β-minor. The effects of the disorder vary, depending on the number of defective genes and the mode of inheritance. As with sickle cell anemia, evaluation is based on family history and laboratory tests. Radiography does not play a role in the diagnosis and treatment of these disorders.

Hemophilias

Hemophilias are inherited hemorrhagic diseases that involve a congenital deficiency of three plasma clotting factors. **Hemophilia A** results from a deficiency in plasma clotting factor VIII and is the most common type of hemophilia. This disorder only affects males, but it is transmitted by females. **Hemophilia B** results from a deficiency in plasma clotting factor IX and is clinically indistinguishable from hemophilia A. These hemophiliac conditions may be mild, moderate, or severe. **Hemophilia C** results from a deficiency in plasma clotting factor XI and occurs equally in both males and females. The severity of this deficiency is less than that of either hemophilia A or B.

In individuals with hemophilia, clinical manifestations begin to appear before the age of 4 years, and these patients experience persistent bleeding from minor injuries. As with other hereditary hemopoietic diseases, radiography does not play a role in the diagnosis and treatment of hemophilia. Evaluation is based on family history and laboratory tests.

von Willebrand Disease

von Willebrand disease, the fourth type of hereditary bleeding disorder, is relatively common in both males and females. This disorder results from a defect in the plasma clotting factor termed *von Willebrand factor* (vWF) and is not diagnosed in adulthood. Many variants of this disorder exist, but the most common clinical signs include spontaneous bleeding from the nose, mouth, and gastrointestinal tract. The bleeding episodes are not as severe as those associated with hemophilia A, B, or C, and the only treatment is usually preventive, and includes avoidance of aspirin ingestion.

NEOPLASTIC DISEASES

Multiple Myeloma

Multiple myeloma, a neoplastic disease of B cells in plasma, results in cell proliferation. The cause of multiple myeloma is unknown, but it is thought to be the result of deletion of chromosome 13q and translocations of the IgG locus of chromosome 14. The disease is usually confined to bone marrow and forms discrete osteolytic tumors that weaken the affected bone. Multiple myeloma most frequently affects the pelvis, spine, ribs, and skull, which results in multiple osteolytic lesions, renal insufficiency, and hypercalcemia. It is typically seen in persons over the age of 60 years, and its signs and symptoms include progressive bone pain, especially in the back and thorax, anemia, fatigue, bleeding disorders, renal insufficiency or failure, hypercalcemia, and recurrent bacterial infections, especially pneumococcal pneumonia. The incidence is slightly more common in men than in women and in blacks than in whites.

The abnormal plasma cells produce large amounts of monoclonal paraprotein (*M protein*), specifically IgG, IgA, IgD, and IgE, which create a variety of problems in addition to skeletal involvement. This protein is excreted via urine and disrupts normal renal function. The protein can be detected in both blood and urine. Blood tests for hypercalcemia, elevated erythrocyte sediment rate (ESR), and renal failure, as well as bone marrow biopsies, are most commonly used in the diagnosis of multiple myeloma. Radiography plays a vital role in the diagnosis and treatment of multiple myeloma because about 90% of these patients have bone involvement. Skeletal survey radiography demonstrates diffuse osteoporosis with discrete punched-out, osteolytic regions (Figs. 9-8 and 9-9). These patients are at risk for pathologic fractures and vertebral compression fractures because multiple myeloma primarily affects the axial skeleton. A 30% bone loss should have occurred before the disease can be visualized with conventional radiography, but MRI is useful in the diagnosis and management of early-stage multiple myeloma. In addition, approximately 90% of patients exhibit proteinuria, and 50% of patients develop renal insufficiency. High levels of protein in blood increase the viscosity of blood, thus affecting circulation to the brain, kidneys, and extremities.

Treatment involves the use of thalidomide drugs in combination with a corticosteroid. However, treatment is currently advancing with the development and use of new pharmaceuticals. Chemotherapy and stem cell transplantation may be prescribed, especially in patients under the age of 70 years. Radiation therapy may also be used to treat bone lesions that do not respond to chemotherapy. The prognosis for multiple myeloma is poor, the median survival rate being approximately 2 to 3 years.

Leukemia

Leukemia is a term associated with neoplastic disease of leukocytes that results in an overproduction of WBCs. This increase in leukocytes interferes with normal blood cell production and may lead to anemia, bleeding, and infection. Leukemias may infiltrate lymphatic tissue and organs such as the liver and spleen. The causes of leukemia are unknown and most likely vary

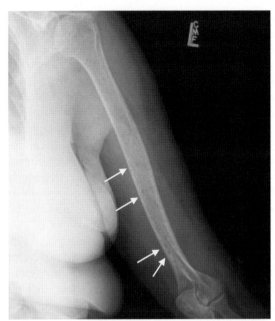

FIGURE 9-8 Humerus radiograph of a patient with multiple myeloma. The radiograph demonstrates the presence of discrete, lytic, well-circumscribed skeletal defects.

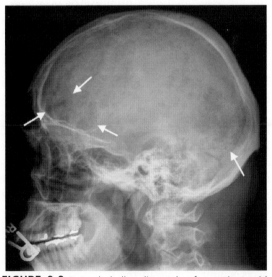

FIGURE 9-9 Lateral skull radiograph of a patient with multiple myeloma. The radiograph demonstrates the presence of discrete, lytic, well-circumscribed skeletal defects.

according to the type of leukemia. However, exposure to radiation and to certain chemicals (especially benzene) and genetic defects such as Down syndrome seem to predispose individuals to developing these disorders. Current research also indicates an association between leukemia and two viruses: (1) the Epstein-Barr virus and (2) the human T-cell leukemia and lymphoma virus. Structural molecular changes disrupting the genes that regulate normal blood cell development have been observed. Most frequently, these disruptions include the translocation of chromosomes, the inversion of chromosome 16, and the deletion of part of chromosome 6.

Leukemias are classified according to cell type and cell maturity. *Myelocytic leukemias* develop from primitive or stem cells. *Monocytic leukemias* develop from precursor cells (the cells from which leukocytes are derived) and are the least common type of leukemia. *Lymphocytic leukemias* arise from lymphoid cells. In addition, leukemias are classified as either acute or chronic. *Acute leukemias* have an abrupt onset and may manifest as a hemorrhagic episode. They generally are associated with primitive or poorly differentiated cells. *Chronic leukemias* progress at a relatively slow pace with nonspecific signs such as fatigue and weakness. They are associated with mature or well-differentiated cells. All of the above-mentioned terms are used in combination to describe the specific type of leukemia.

Acute lymphocytic leukemia (ALL) affects both children and adults. **Chronic lymphocytic leukemia** (CLL) predominantly affects individuals over age 60 years. **Chronic myelocytic leukemia** (CML) most often affects older adults. **Acute myelocytic leukemia** (AML) and **acute monoblastic leukemia** (AMOL) affect anyone at any age. Leukemias, in general, account for approximately 33% of all cancer-related deaths in children under the age of 15 years. Radiography plays a limited role in the diagnosis and treatment of most leukemias.

Common symptoms and signs associated with acute leukemia include fatigue, anemia, low-grade fever, night sweats, weight loss, bruising due to a decreased platelet count, and bone pain

caused by the expansion of the bone marrow. Patients with ALL may also present with an enlarged spleen and liver, whereas patients with AML often exhibit infiltration of the malignant cells to skin and other soft tissues within the body. In some instances, the leukemic cells may pass the blood–brain barrier, causing cranial nerve palsies, headaches, lethargy, confusion, and seizures. The definitive diagnoses of acute leukemias are primarily established through blood tests, bone marrow biopsies, and cytogenetic studies used to determine chromosomal abnormalities. CT of the chest, abdomen, and pelvis are frequently performed to identify sites of the disease. Additionally, lumbar puncture under fluoroscopic guidance is also common for analysis of the cerebrospinal fluid to assess involvement of the CNS. The primary treatment of acute leukemia is chemotherapy, although stem cell transplantation and bone marrow transfusions may also be used in patients under the age of 50 years. Most patients with acute leukemias die within 6 months without treatment. ALL therapies carry a 5-year survival rate of 80% or better in children and 40% in adults. In all cases, survival depends on complete remission.

Individuals with CLL are often asymptomatic, and the disease is often discovered during routine blood counts. With progression of the disease, lymph node involvement, which leads to an enlarged spleen and liver, becomes evident. Symptoms at this stage of the disease include fever, abdominal pain, and weight loss. These patients will also present with anemia and susceptibility to other infectious pathogens such as *Streptococcus pneumoniae*, *Staphylococcus aureus*, and *Haemophilus influenzae*. The treatment for individuals with CLL varies, as many patients may remain stable for years, whereas others may require chemotherapy or bone marrow irradiation and stem cell transplantation.

Patients with CML present with a slow chronic phase of variable length. During this phase, these individuals are asymptomatic, but as the disease progresses to the short accelerated stage, they present with weakness, weight loss, splenomegaly, low-grade fever, bone pain, dysfunctional platelets, and anemia. The final stage of CML is the blast crisis stage, in which the number of myeloid precursor blast cells increases dramatically (>100,000 cells per microliter [cells/µL]). CML is progressive, with an average survival of about 3 to 4 years after the onset of the disease and a 5-year survival rate of approximately 20%. Patients reaching the blast crisis stage only survive an average of 3 months. Treatment for CML is constantly evolving; however, the only curative treatment currently available is bone marrow or stem cell transplantation.

Non-Hodgkin Lymphoma

NHL is a malignancy of the lymphoid cells found in the lymph nodes, bone marrow, spleen, liver, and gastrointestinal system. It is the most common type of lymphoma, and its incidence increases with age, most commonly occurring in individuals aged 50 years or older. Some patients tolerate NHL very well, and others die very quickly from the disease. Although its etiology is unknown, it is believed to result from translocation chromosomal alterations. Research indicates that the chances of developing NHL increase with exposure to certain chemicals; an impaired immune system, as occurs with HIV or in immunosuppressant patients following organ transplantation; or chronic *Helicobacter pylori* infection. Most cases arise from B cells (80% to 85%), and approximately 15% arise from T cells. Currently, multiple methods of classifying NHLs exist, with approximately 40 types of lymphomas identified. The most common classification system has been established by the World Health Organization (WHO), and in this system, lymphomas are designated by cell type, cell maturation, and anatomic site. B-cell lymphomas include both precursor B-cell lymphoma and a multitude of mature B-cell lymphomas, whereas T-cell lymphomas include one precursor T-cell lymphoma and two mature T-cell lymphomas.

The signs and symptoms of NHL are varied. In a few cases, the patient manifests general lymphadenopathy before developing lymphoma.

FIGURE 9-10 Chest computed tomography of a patient with non-Hodgkin lymphoma. The scan demonstrates a necrotic lymph node in the cardiophrenic angle.

Many patients also have anemia. Diagnosis is made from histologic examination of the diseased tissue via lymph node biopsy to differentiate NHL from Hodgkin lymphoma, leukemia, and metastatic disease. CT scans of the neck, chest, abdomen, and pelvis are commonly used to stage the disease and to demonstrate the extent of disease in the lymphatic system around the aorta and mesentery (Figs. 9-10 and 9-11). PET or CT is gaining popularity, and MRI of the chest and abdomen may also be indicated. A bone marrow biopsy may be performed as well, as bone marrow involvement and organ infiltration are more common with NHL than with Hodgkin lymphoma. Treatment of NHL depends on the stage of the disease. It consists of chemotherapy and radiation therapy, either independently or in combination. In some advanced cases, radiolabeled antibody therapy may also be used.

Hodgkin Lymphoma

Hodgkin lymphoma is another neoplastic disease that affects lymphoid tissue. Its cause is unknown, and it commonly affects individuals between the ages of 20 and 40 years and those over 60 years of age. It tends to affect men slightly more often than women and whites more than blacks. The presence of **Reed-Sternberg cells** differentiates Hodgkin lymphoma from other types of lymphatic diseases. Reed-Sternberg cells are believed to be mutant B cells that secrete and release cytokines, which leads to inflammatory cellular response. However, the genetic etiology of Hodgkin lymphoma is unknown.

Common signs and symptoms associated with Hodgkin lymphoma are general malaise, fever, night sweats, weight loss, splenomegaly, and enlarged lymph nodes (Fig. 9-12). Mediastinal and hilar lymph nodes are often visible on a chest radiograph, although a definitive diagnosis is made via biopsy of lymphatic tissue. As with other neoplastic disorders, Hodgkin lymphoma is staged according to the extent of the disease.

Hodgkin lymphoma and NHL generally have different nodal distributions as seen on CT, as Hodgkin disease is generally retroperitoneal with less mesenteric involvement compared with NHL. CT examinations of the chest, abdomen, and pelvis, which are used to stage the disease, commonly demonstrate enlarged retroperitoneal nodes. However, PET is gaining popularity in the initial staging of Hodgkin lymphoma. Nuclear medicine gallium scans and MRI of the abdomen may also be useful in staging Hodgkin lymphoma. In some cases, a laparotomy, including splenectomy, may also be indicated. Stage I denotes one anatomic node location, and stage IV denotes extranodal spread to bone marrow, the lungs, or the liver. Chest radiography, PET, and CT are frequently used for follow-up studies.

Hodgkin disease is most commonly treated and cured with a combination of radiotherapy, bone marrow and stem cell transplantation, and chemotherapy. Stage I and stage IIA Hodgkin lymphoma may be treated with radiation therapy alone and is associated with a 5-year survival rate of 85% to 90%. Stage IV Hodgkin lymphoma has approximately a 70% to 80% complete remission rate, with more than 50% of patients remaining disease-free for up to 15 years.

FIGURE 9-11 Pelvic computed tomography of a patient with non-Hodgkin lymphoma. The scan demonstrates enlarged inguinal lymph nodes.

PATHOLOGY SUMMARY
Hemopoietic System

Pathology	Imaging Modalities of Choice
AIDS	CT and MRI
Multiple myeloma	MRI, skeletal radiography, and nuclear medicine bone scan
Non-Hodgkin lymphoma	CT, PET, and MRI
Hodgkin lymphoma	Chest radiography, PET, CT, and MRI

AIDS, Acquired immunodeficiency syndrome; *CT,* computed tomography; *MRI,* magnetic resonance imaging; *PET,* positron emission tomography.

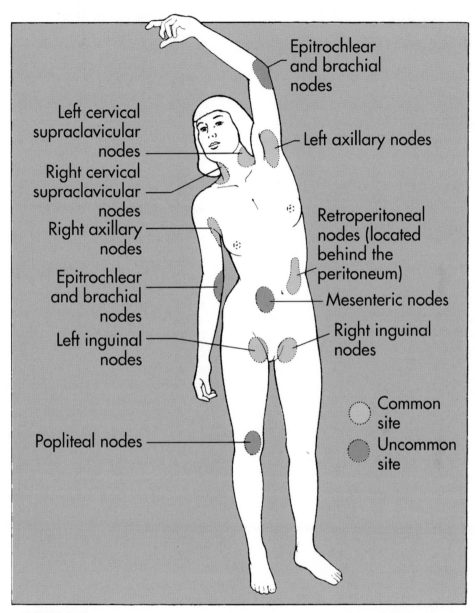

FIGURE 9-12 Common and uncommon involved lymph node sites for Hodgkin lymphoma.

REVIEW QUESTIONS

1. The majority of blood volume is composed of:
   a. Erythrocytes
   b. Leukocytes
   c. Plasma
   d. Thrombocytes
2. Bilirubin is formed during the destruction of:
   a. Erythrocytes
   b. Leukocytes
   c. Plastocytes
   d. Thrombocytes
3. Which of the following is considered the universal donor type of blood?
   a. A
   b. B
   c. AB
   d. O
4. Which cells are most important in the development of immunity?
   a. Erythrocytes
   b. Lymphocytes
   c. Platelets
   d. Thrombocytes
5. The most common pulmonary complication resulting from acquired immunodeficiency syndrome (AIDS) is:
   a. *Pneumocystis carinii* pneumonia
   b. Pneumococcal pneumonia
   c. Legionnaire pneumonia
   d. Tuberculosis
6. Kaposi sarcoma is frequently associated with AIDS, and it may affect:
   a. The gastrointestinal system
   b. Lymph nodes
   c. Skin
   d. All of the above

7. A neoplastic disease of the plasma is:
   a. Hodgkin lymphoma
   b. Leukemia
   c. Non-Hodgkin lymphoma
   d. Multiple myeloma
8. Which type of leukemia predominantly affects children?
   a. Acute lymphocytic
   b. Chronic lymphocytic
   c. Chronic myelocytic
   d. Acute myelocytic
9. With what type of neoplastic disease are Reed-Sternberg cells associated?
   a. Leukemia
   b. Hodgkin lymphoma
   c. Multiple myeloma
   d. Non-Hodgkin lymphoma
10. What blood cells are affected by non-Hodgkin lymphoma?
    a. Erythrocytes
    b. Lymphocytes
    c. Plastocytes
    d. Thrombocytes
11. Explain why researchers currently believe that an association exists between viral agents and the development of lymphomas.
12. Identify two means of transmission of human immunodeficiency virus (HIV) infection.
13. What is the difference in cellular origin between multiple myeloma and leukemia?
14. What is the risk of using radiation or antileukemic drug therapy in treating leukemias?
15. Identify at least three signs and symptoms of Hodgkin lymphoma.

Reproductive System

KEY TERMS

Adenocarcinoma of the prostate
Bicornuate uterus
Breast carcinoma
Cervical carcinoma
Cervical dysplasia
Corpus luteum ovarian cysts
Cryptorchidism
Cystadenocarcinoma
Cystic teratomas
Dermoid cysts
Ectopic pregnancy
Endometrial carcinoma
Endometriosis
Epididymo-orchitis
Fibroadenoma
Fibrocystic breasts
Follicular ovarian cysts
Hydatidiform mole
Hydrocele
Hysterosalpingography
Leiomyomas
Mastalgia
Mastitis

Nongravid
Oligohydramnios
Peau d'orange
Pelvic inflammatory disease
Pessary
Placenta previa
Placental abruption
Placental percreta
Polycystic ovaries
Polyhydramnios
Prostatic calculi
Prostatic hyperplasia
Sonohysterography
Spermatoceles
Testicular choriocarcinomas
Testicular embryonal carcinomas
Testicular seminomas
Testicular teratomas
Transurethral resection of the prostate
Unicornuate uterus
Uterine fibroids
Uterus didelphys

Female Reproductive System

ANATOMY AND PHYSIOLOGY

The female reproductive system consists of one pair of ovaries, which are the primary sex organs, and the secondary sex organs, which include one pair of fallopian tubes, the uterus, the vagina, and two breasts (Fig. 10-1). The primary function of the system is to provide a female reproductive cell (the ovum), hormones, and a site for the development of the zygote.

The external genitalia (the vulva) include the mons pubis, the labia majora and minora, the clitoris, the openings of the urethra and vagina, and the perineum. The vagina connects the external genitalia with the uterus and is the mode of exit for menstrual fluids and conception products.

FIGURE 10-1 Female pelvic organs.

The uterus is a pear-shaped organ, and its primary purpose is to provide an environment for fetal growth and development. Located within the pelvic cavity, it can be divided into the upper portion, termed the *fundus;* the midportion, termed the *body;* and the lower portion, termed the *cervix.* The cervix connects the uterine cavity with the upper vagina. Anatomically, the uterus is flexed so that the cervix and lower portion of the body lie anterior to the rectum. The body of the uterus follows the contour of the posterior urinary bladder wall. The upper portion, or fundus, normally lies superior to the bladder. The walls of the uterus include an inner, endometrial layer; a middle, muscular, myometrial layer; and an outer layer, termed the *parietal peritoneum*. In actuality, the parietal peritoneum drapes over the fundus and the upper three fourths of the body but does not enclose the lower fourth of the body or the cervix. The actual cavity within the uterus is fairly small and can be well visualized with ultrasonography. It is divided into the *internal os,* leading to the cervical canal, and the *external os,* which opens into the vagina. The uterus is held in place within the pelvic cavity via eight ligaments.

Occasionally, lack of proper uterine support is present, and a device known as the **pessary** (Fig. 10-2) is inserted into the vagina to provide proper support. Current research has demonstrated that the majority of women who use the pessary are very satisfied, as the device relieves the majority of urinary symptoms. Some women report that although the use of a pessary helps improve urinary symptoms, stress incontinence remains an ongoing problem. However, the use of the pessary continues to be the treatment for pelvic organ prolapse and may assist with the quality of life for many of these patients.

The fallopian tubes extend from the upper, outer edges of the uterus and expand distally into the infundibulum located close to, but not attached to, the ovaries. Suspended in place by the broad ligament, they are 8 to 12 cm long and tend to fall behind the uterus. These tubes serve as a passageway for the mature ova and are the normal site of fertilization. In a normal pregnancy, the fertilized ovum continues to travel through the fallopian tube and implants itself into the endometrium of the uterus.

The ovaries are the primary reproductive glands and are responsible for ovulation and for secretion of estrogen and progesterone. Attached to the broad ligament and the posterior uterine

FIGURE 10-2 A pessary, inserted into the vagina for uterine support, is readily visible on this abdominal radiograph of an 88-year-old woman.

wall, each ovary contains numerous graafian follicles enclosing ova. After puberty, several graafian follicles and ova grow and develop each month. Normally only one follicle matures, migrates to the surface of the ovary, and degenerates, thus expelling a mature ovum, which is the hallmark of the *ovulation* process.

Breasts—like the fallopian tubes, uterus, and vagina—are considered secondary sex organs. Breast parenchyma differs according to age and parity. Women in their 20s and 30s, especially nulliparous women, have dense, fibroglandular parenchyma that may conceal breast masses during a clinical breast examination and imaging. However with advancing age, decline in estrogen and progesterone causes breast tissue to undergo what is known as *involutional change.* Involution is the conversion of glandular breast tissue into adipose as well as loss of the supportive

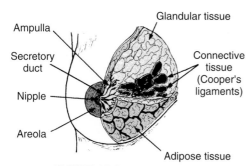

FIGURE 10-3 Breast, anterior.

tissue. As a result of this slow process, the breast changes its architecture, and fibroglandular tissue is replaced by fat. This process is variable, but it typically begins at the back of the breast and progresses forward to the nipple. The term **mastalgia** applies to conditions that result in pain in one or both breasts. Many patients fear that mastalgia is indicative of breast cancer; however, it is more closely related to architectural changes in breast tissue. Involution aids the imaging professional and the interpreting physician because fatty tissue is radiolucent and enhances the radiographic visibility of many breast masses.

Anatomically, breasts are attached via Cooper ligaments to the pectoral muscles, and this gives the breast its contour and shape. The breast consists of about 12 lobes separated by connective tissue, much like the spokes of a wheel. The lobes are further divided into lobules clustered around small ducts. These small ducts join to form larger ducts, which terminate at the nipple (Fig. 10-3). Breasts function as accessory reproductive glands to secrete milk for the newborn. During pregnancy, changes in estrogen and progesterone levels prepare breasts for lactation. Approximately 3 days after delivery, a lactogenic hormone stimulates the secretion of milk.

IMAGING CONSIDERATIONS

Hysterosalpingography

One of the most common radiographic studies of the female reproductive system is the **hysterosalpingography** (HSG). It is an examination

FIGURE 10-4 Free spillage of contrast medium bilaterally, as seen in this hysterosalpingogram, in a 38-year-old woman indicates that the uterine tubes are open.

performed for screening of the **nongravid** (nonpregnant) woman, especially in cases of suspected infertility. A common finding in cases of infertility is nonpatent fallopian tubes. In addition, although HSG does not define the extent of certain conditions such as endometriosis, it is useful in revealing the shape of the uterus and certain characteristics of the fallopian tubes other than their patency. The practice guideline of the American College of Radiology (ACR) for the performance of HSG is to inject approximately 10 to 30 mL of contrast medium into the uterine cavity and the injection should be done slowly to avoid causing spasms and discomfort. Spillage of the contrast medium from the fallopian tubes indicates the patency of the tubes (Fig. 10-4). Typically, HSG is used for diagnostic purposes, but it can also be used therapeutically for restoring tubal patency or to dilate or stretch the fallopian tubes.

An adjunct procedure that has the potential to replace the conventional HSG is known as **sonohysterography** (SHG). This examination is similar to hysterosalpingography in procedural approach; however, with SHG, normal saline, instead of an iodinated contrast agent, is injected into the uterus. Because saline is devoid of the complications associated with iodinated contrast agents, the procedure may be better tolerated by the patient. In the current application of SHG, saline is used to pry apart the layers of the endometrium to reveal abnormalities within the uterus. The saline fluid is expelled via the fallopian tubes, and this may also indicate their patency. This procedure is viewed via a transvaginal sonographic probe as the physician injects the saline. With real-time images, the dynamics of the reproductive system can be assessed without radiation to the patient.

In a study of a group of 100 patients with infertility, HSG was compared with SHG. These patients' HSG results were matched to their laparoscopic results. In this small group of women, HSG and SHG were equally effective in the evaluation of tubal disease.

Mammography

The use of mammography as a diagnostic procedure for symptomatic patients is well documented. Mammography provides important information about specific clinical problems such as a breast mass, pain, nipple discharge, and abnormalities of the skin and lymph nodes. With modern mammographic equipment and techniques, radiation exposure is minimal, and evidence does not suggest significant risk to women over 35 years of age. If a risk does exist, it is thought to be so minimal that it has never been observed, but only inferred scientifically.

The use of mammography in asymptomatic patients for screening purposes is based on its ability to detect nonpalpable breast lesions at an early stage when they are too small to be identified by physical examination. Current literature suggests that mammography can detect some cancers 2 years before they are palpable; survival depends on tumor size and lymph node involvement. It is generally agreed that women 50 years of age and older should undergo regular mammographic screening because in this age group, breast tissue is less sensitive to radiation and the incidence of breast cancer increases with age.

This also takes advantage of the involutional process, making occult lesions easier to identify on a radiograph. The benefits far outweigh the associated risks from radiation exposure.

Mammography is also a valuable examination tool in the detection and evaluation of breast disease in individuals with augmentation prostheses. Although experience with patients who have undergone augmentation mammoplasty is limited, current research indicates that mammography can demonstrate both palpable and nonpalpable breast lesions. For mammographic screening of these patients, it is important to displace the implant so that the native breast tissue can be imaged and assessed for disease. To demonstrate the underlying breast parenchyma in these individuals, implant-displaced views are required. Technologists are encouraged to use the Eckland maneuver to displace the implant from the native breast tissue to radiograph as much of the native breast tissue as possible. The Eckland maneuver is accomplished by the technologist applying pressure at the area of the nipple and then carefully rolling the native breast tissue away from the implant. The implant-displaced view is performed for both craniocaudal and mediolateral projections of the breast. Once the implant is pushed upward and away from the native breast tissue, the compression paddle is used to continue to hold the implant so that the native breast tissue can be more fully imaged. Because of the variations in patients' breast tissue and their implants, manual exposure techniques are commonly used.

Needle guidewire localization is a specialized procedure to identify nonpalpable, mammographically detected abnormalities of the breast. It helps direct the surgeon to the lesion in question and allows excision of the suspect tissue for biopsy. Needle guidewire localizations cause minimal morbidity, with complications including hematoma formation, intraoperative wire dislodgement, and wire breakage. The development and refinement of localization techniques have greatly increased the percentage of positive findings on surgical biopsy and allow more accurate diagnosis and treatment of early-stage carcinoma of the breast. Fine-needle and large-core biopsy techniques offer an alternative to surgical biopsy as an initial step in the investigation of breast masses. These procedures are performed on an outpatient basis by the mammographer and the radiologist or by the surgeon in the mammography area using a specially designed stereotactic localization unit. Ductal lavage of the breast may also be performed in cases of suspected intraductal disease to obtain a specimen for laboratory analysis. Use of sonography-guided aspiration and biopsy is also common because sonography provides the ability to visualize the area in question and note whether the area has been completely removed while the needle or biopsy gun is still in situ. This may prevent additional punctures into the patient's skin during the biopsy procedure.

In patients who have a positive finding on screening mammography, according to the ACR Appropriateness Criteria, diagnostic mammography is rated as highly appropriate as the next step in a patient's diagnostic workup. The only finding on screening mammography that would not result in the use of diagnostic mammography is a mass that has circumscribed margins, no additional malignant qualities, and has not enlarged compared with the last mammogram. In this case, the use of breast sonography would be highly appropriate.

Sonography

Sonography is the primary modality for examining the gravid or nongravid female reproductive system because of its excellent accuracy and because it presents no radiation hazards to the fetus or the mother. Not only is sonography applicable in pregnancy, but it is also useful in normal gynecologic examinations to visualize the reproductive organs or to monitor the progress of a regimen of fertility medication.

Transabdominal pelvic sonography requires a distended urinary bladder to serve as an "acoustic window" for good visualization of the pelvic organs. In addition, the fluid within the urinary bladder displaces bowel gas away from the area of interest. Sonography of the uterus and ovaries

has been greatly enhanced by the use of the transvaginal transducer, which provides more accurate clinical information with magnification of the images of internal pelvic structures. The most common indications for sonography in the nongravid female include evaluation of pelvic, uterine, and ovarian masses because sonography can provide information about mass size, location, internal characteristics, and effect on surrounding organs. Obstetrically, sonography is the method of choice for visualizing the position of the placenta, multiple gestations, or ectopic pregnancies and for determining gestational age. It is used to assist and guide the physician during amniocentesis and is invaluable in assessing fetal abnormalities such as anencephaly, hydrocephaly, congenital heart defects, polycystic kidney disease, urinary tract obstructions, and gastrointestinal (GI) tract obstructions and in determining fetal death.

The use of sonography to assess the pregnant uterus for determining fetal growth, any disturbances, or risk of growth restriction is recommended by the ACR. Sonography is the best imaging modality to assess the fetus, growth, and amniotic fluid and for an overall survey of fetal well-being.

Sonography is an excellent modality for differentiating cystic masses from solid masses within the breast. However, sonography has limitations in the diagnosis of malignant breast disease because of the solid nature of most breast cancers. Recently, researchers and clinicians have made great strides in the use of sonography to evaluate the dense breast for disease. To reduce the radiation dose to young patients, research continues to strive to perfect an accurate and safe screening modality. However, currently, breast sonography is not advocated as a screening modality for breast cancer because of the difficulty in consistently differentiating between a solid benign mass and malignant disease.

Magnetic Resonance Imaging

Magnetic resonance imaging (MRI) is now often used in conjunction with sonography in the evaluation of the female pelvis (Figs. 10-5 and 10-6). MRI, like sonography, uses no ionizing radiation and is noninvasive. MRI gives detailed information on pelvic, uterine, and ovarian masses (Fig. 10-7). In cases of ovarian cancer, MRI accurately demonstrates proliferation into other pelvic structures. In addition, multiple leiomyomas can be detected and localized in a short period.

MRI is increasingly being used to assist in differentiating between malignant and benign solid lesions within the breast. Fat suppression imaging is used before and after contrast enhancement. This technique suppresses the normal, fatty tissue of the breast, allowing easier identification of malignant masses through contrast enhancement (Fig. 10-8). MRI is also used to detect faulty or

FIGURE 10-6 An example of a sagittal T2-weighted magnetic resonance imaging scan of a normal female pelvis demonstrating the bladder and the uterus.

FIGURE 10-5 A sagittal sonographic image of the normal uterus.

FIGURE 10-7 A, A sagittal T2-weighted fat-suppressed magnetic resonance imaging (MRI) scan demonstrating a large mass, most likely a subserosal fibroid, posterior to the endocervical junction. **B,** An axial T2-weighted fat-suppressed MRI image depicting the large subserosal fibroid shown in A.

Sc1/12

P.

W 651
L 292

FIGURE 10-8 A sagittal T2-weighted fat-suppressed magnetic resonance imaging scan of the left breast.

leaking breast implants. Again, fat suppression imaging is used to suppress the normal breast tissue and detect the presence of silicone in surrounding tissue.

A review of published studies on the value of adding MRI as a screening tool for breast cancer found that it was better for screening patients compared with mammography alone or a combination of mammography, sonography, and clinical breast examination. One concern about using MRI as a screening tool for breast cancer was that it raised the return rate for additional imaging; therefore, it has been suggested that MRI be used as an adjunct to mammography. MRI has also proven to be a safe, more effective screening tool in women who have a family history of breast cancer and are positive for the *BRCA* oncogene, for whom early screening is recommended.

Computed Tomography

Computed tomography (CT) of the pelvis and abdomen is often performed to diagnose diseases of the female and male reproductive systems. It is quite helpful in assessing neoplastic growth and abscess formation resulting from inflammatory processes. It is often used in conjunction with transvaginal sonography to evaluate ovarian lesions, especially cystic teratomas in females, and is used extensively in staging cancers of the female reproductive system. In the male patient, CT is also used in conjunction with sonography to demonstrate anomalies of the seminal vesicles and prostate gland. CT and positron emission tomography (PET) fusion studies (CT-PET) are also of value in the diagnosis and staging of neoplastic disease of the reproductive system, as well as the assessment of disease progression.

Sonography is highly recommended by the ACR for suspected gynecologic adnexal masses. CT of the pelvis, with or without contrast, is also equally indicated for nongravid women in the reproductive age group who have a complex or solid mass that is growing in the short term.

CONGENITAL ANOMALIES

Congenital anomalies of the female reproductive system occur in approximately 1% to 2% of women in the United States. The most common anomaly is the **bicornuate uterus,** in which paired uterine horns extend into the fallopian tubes (Figs. 10-9 and 10-10). A **unicornuate uterus** occurs when the uterine cavity is elongated and has a single fallopian tube emerging from it. Often, the kidney on the side of the missing fallopian tube is also absent. **Uterus didelphys** is a rare congenital anomaly with complete duplication of the uterus, cervix, and vagina. The most serious complication of these anomalies is problems with reproduction, although various surgical corrections can be performed.

In the normal female reproductive system, the fundus of the uterus lies anterior to the cervix and away from the rectum and is said to be *anteverted.* Occasionally, the normal uterus may lie in an abnormal position. If the uterus is more vertical than normal and points backward toward the bowel, it is said to be *retroverted.* If the uterus is completely bent back and lies against the rectosigmoid region of the bowel, it is said to be *retroflexed.* A uterus that is tilted vertically forward is *anteflexed,* and it lies on top of the urinary bladder.

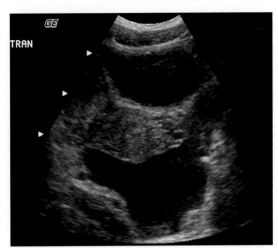

FIGURE 10-11 A transverse sonographic image of bacterial fluid in the posterior cul-de-sac.

FIGURE 10-9 A hysterosalpingogram demonstrating bicornuate uterus.

FIGURE 10-10 A transverse sonographic image of a bicornuate uterus.

Although neither position is normal, this is generally of little clinical significance.

INFLAMMATORY DISEASES

Pelvic Inflammatory Disease

Pelvic inflammatory disease (PID) is a bacterial infection of the female reproductive system, specifically the fallopian tubes. One third of cases is caused by *Gonococcus*, one third is caused by a mixture of infections, and the last third of cases is caused by *Staphylococcus* or *Streptococcus*. The disease may result from an unsterile abortion or introduction of a pathogen from other sources. This inflammation is generally bilateral, and without treatment, the infection spreads to the peritoneum, resulting in bacteremia. Tubo-ovarian abscess formation may also occur with PID, often resulting in sterility. The clinical presentation of this entity involves pelvic pain and tenderness, guarding, rebound tenderness, or both. Patients often have fever and chills, elevated white blood cell (WBC) count, nausea and vomiting, and purulent cervical discharge.

The most common treatment for PID is aggressive antibiotic therapy, but healing often results in scarring and obstruction of the fallopian tubes, which predisposes the individual to ectopic pregnancy because of tubal narrowing. Rupture of the fallopian tubes because of infection results in septic shock and can be a life-threatening situation. Sonography is commonly indicated as an imaging method for determining the presence of infection and the extent of the disease (Fig. 10-11). Severe cases with abscess formation may also require surgical intervention.

Mastitis

Inflammation of the breast, or **mastitis,** is most often caused by *Staphylococcus aureus.* Acute mastitis begins when bacteria gain access to breast tissue via the ducts. This bacterial route of infection occurs because of cracks or fissures in the nipple that may develop during the first weeks of lactation and the subsequent nursing of an infant. Common signs and symptoms of mastitis include pain, redness, and swelling of the affected breast, elevated temperature, and, in severe cases, abscess formation. Mastitis is treated medically with antibiotic therapy and heat application to the affected breast. Risk factors for lactational mastitis are diabetes, steroid use, cigarette smoking, and inverted nipples. Mammography is difficult to perform on these patients because of the substantial engorgement of breast tissue. Mammographic imaging to document mastitis may result in higher doses owing to the thickness of the tissue and is of little value in the diagnosis and treatment of mastitis.

NEOPLASTIC DISEASES

Ovarian Cystic Masses

Simple ovarian cysts are fairly common in women in the reproductive age group. They are frequently asymptomatic but may cause abdominal aching and pressure. Acute, sharp abdominal pain may indicate rupture or hemorrhage of the cyst. They include follicular ovarian cysts and corpus luteum ovarian cysts. Follicular and corpus luteum cysts form as part of the normal menstrual cycle. **Follicular ovarian cysts** result from faulty reabsorption of the fluid from incompletely developed follicles (Fig. 10-12). **Corpus luteum ovarian cysts** occur when reabsorption of any blood leaked into the cavity after ovulation leaves a small cyst behind. Changes in the sizes of follicular and corpus luteum cysts occur quickly and vary with the menstrual cycle. These cysts may occasionally increase in size and cause pelvic discomfort or abnormal pressure on the

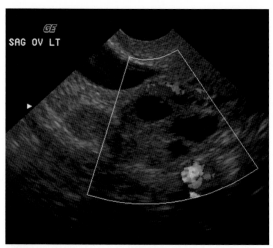

FIGURE 10-12 A transvaginal sonographic image of a follicular cyst on an ovary.

FIGURE 10-13 A coronal T2-weighted fat-suppressed magnetic resonance imaging scan of the female pelvis demonstrating a cyst of the right ovary (*arrow*).

urinary bladder. These cysts are readily visible with sonography, MRI (Fig. 10-13), and CT (Fig. 10-14) of the pelvis. Treatment is generally not necessary because these cysts often disappear completely without medical intervention.

Multiple cystic masses may indicate **endometriosis,** a disease caused by the presence of

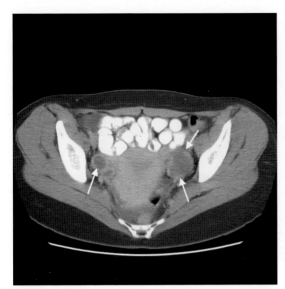

FIGURE 10-14 A computed tomography scan of a female pelvis demonstrating bilateral cysts. The patient is currently taking fertility drugs.

FIGURE 10-15 A transvaginal sonographic image of a dermoid mass.

endometrial tissue or glands outside the uterus in abnormal locations within the pelvis. External endometriosis commonly involves the ovaries, the uterine ligaments, the rectovaginal septum, and the pelvic peritoneum; however, it may also attach to the rectal wall, the ureters, or the urinary bladder. Endometriosis is believed to arise from lymphatic spread, seeding from retrograde menstruation, or from direct surgical spread. The endometrial implants appear to respond to normal hormonal stimuli and are clinically significant in women between the ages of 20 and 40 years. The external endometrial tissue implants contain normal functioning endometrium. Responsive to hormonal changes, it continues to bleed cyclically. These blood-filled cysts (also referred to as *chocolate cysts*) are often visible on ultrasonographic examination. Longstanding endometriosis results in the development of fibrosis, adhesions, scarring, and eventually sterility. Common signs and symptoms include pelvic and low back pain, dysmenorrhea, intermittent constipation and diarrhea, and infertility. Although sonography is useful in the diagnosis of endometriosis, a positive

diagnosis is generally made via laparoscopy. Mild cases of endometriosis may be treated with hormone therapy; severe cases generally require surgical therapy.

Polycystic ovaries consist of enlarged ovaries containing multiple small cysts. The ovaries are bilaterally enlarged and have a smooth exterior surface, with multiple cysts lying just below the outer surface. Polycystic ovaries are often associated with Stein-Leventhal syndrome, a fairly rare disease. Women with Stein-Leventhal syndrome rarely ovulate because of an endocrine abnormality that inhibits maturation and release of the ovarian follicle. In addition, these individuals may experience amenorrhea and sterility. The primary treatment is drugs to induce ovulation.

Benign **cystic teratomas** of the ovary, often referred to as **dermoid cysts,** account for approximately 15% to 25% of ovarian tumors and are the most common type of germ cell tumor containing mature tissue. These masses arise from an unfertilized ovum that undergoes neoplastic change. Cystic teratomas are composed of tissue derived from the ectoderm, endoderm, and mesoderm, and they often contain hair, thyroid tissue, keratin, sebaceous secretions, and occasionally teeth (Fig. 10-15). Cystic teratomas have only a 1% to 2% chance of containing malignant cells. Some of the complications associated with a cystic teratoma are torsion of the mass and, in some cases, bleeding that may result in rupture and severe peritonitis. The treatment for cystic teratomas is surgical removal of the mass.

FIGURE 10-16 A sagittal and transverse sonographic image of an ovarian mass.

Cystadenocarcinoma

Cystadenocarcinoma is a malignant tumor of the ovary, accounting for more than 60% of all ovarian cancers (Figs. 10-16 and 10-17). It primarily occurs in perimenopausal and postmenopausal women over age 40 years. Cystadenocarcinoma is the second most commonly diagnosed female genital carcinoma, occurring in 1 out of 70 women in the United States. It is the most lethal gynecologic malignancy, and the prognosis depends on the stage at which the tumor is discovered. Late stage tumors that have broken through the capsule of the ovary carry a very poor prognosis.

The cause of this neoplasm is unknown. However, known risk factors include a diet high in fat, a history of late childbearing or nulliparity, delayed menopause, a family history of cancers of the endometrium, breast, or colon, and the presence of an inherited autosomal dominant gene known as the *BRCA* gene. Sonographic evaluation demonstrates a rough, irregular ovarian surface, with the tumor often containing both cystic and solid areas. Serous tumors are frequently bilateral, whereas mucinous tumors are more likely to be unilateral.

The signs and symptoms of cystadenocarcinoma are very vague and include urinary bladder

FIGURE 10-17 Computed tomography scan of an ovarian mass in the female pelvis that confirms the mass seen on the sonogram.

or rectal pressure, back pain, and bloating. In many cases, the disease is completely asymptomatic and discovered only on routine pelvic examination. This tends to delay diagnosis and treatment, thus reducing the chance for cure. As a woman's age increases, the probability of an enlarged ovary testing positive for ovarian cancer increases proportionately. These tumors often spread to other pelvic organs, the small intestines, the omentum, and the stomach and less frequently to the liver and lungs, resulting in associated ascites and pleural effusions. Common treatment of cystadenocarcinoma includes surgery in combination with chemotherapy or radiation therapy.

According to the most recent literature, the laboratory test, CA 125, is the best noninvasive technique to detect ovarian cancers, as it provides the most specific diagnosis. Additionally, PET-CT is also highly sensitive in the detection of ovarian cancer, and the literature indicates that the use of PET-CT is an important imaging technique for the surveillance of patients with elevated levels in CA 125 or questionable results from sonographic studies.

Carcinoma of the Cervix

Cervical carcinoma or dysplasia is a common malignancy of the female reproductive system caused by an abnormal growth pattern of epithelial cells around the neck of the uterus. It is the third most common carcinoma of the female genital organs and the eighth most common malignancy in American women. Cervical intraepithelial neoplasias (CINs) are classified or staged as mild (I), moderate (II), or severe (III) and are generally diagnosed with a Papanicolaou test and confirmed with surgical biopsy. Cervical cancer is essentially a sexually transmitted disease, as a history of multiple sexual partners or prior sexually transmitted infections predisposes women to this disease. The development of cervical cancer is strongly associated with infection with human papillomavirus type 16, 18, 31, 33, 35, or 39. Associated risk factors include cigarette smoking and immunodeficiency. Multiple clinical trials are ongoing to investigate vaccines against the different strains of the virus. To date, Gardasil (Quadrivalent Human Papillomavirus Recombinant Vaccine) is the only vaccine approved by the U.S. Food and Drug Administration (FDA), and it is effective in preventing HPV types 6, 11, 16, and 18. This is a major breakthrough, as HPV 16 accounts for almost half of all cervical cancers. Gardasil is currently available to young females aged 9 to 26 years for vaccination against HPV and cervical cancer. The National Cancer Institute is also supportive of programs that are attempting to develop a therapeutic vaccine for those already infected with HPV.

Symptoms commonly associated with **cervical dysplasia** include abnormal bleeding, especially postcoital bleeding. In addition, impaired renal function resulting from ureteral obstruction is often seen. If the cancer is invasive, radiography of the chest, urinary system, and skeletal system, in combination with CT or MRI of the abdomen and pelvis, is performed to assist in staging the disease. The treatment of cervical dysplasia varies according to the classification. The Pap test allows early detection of this disease, thus improving the chance of cure and survival. The 5-year survival rate ranges from 90% for stage I dysplasia to less than 15% for advanced disease. The primary treatments are radiation therapy and surgical intervention. Chemotherapy may also be administered in combination with radiation therapy to act as a radiosensitizer.

Postoperative radiation therapy planning is essential to minimize the adverse effects of the treatment and also to prevent extension of extracervical disease. The ACR recommends the use of several techniques to spare radiation exposure to the small bowel, including displacement of the small bowel from the radiation treatment field.

UTERINE MASSES

Leiomyomas (Uterine Fibroids)

Leiomyomas are benign, solid masses of the uterus, which develop from an overgrowth of the uterine smooth muscle tissue. They are present in approximately 30% of all women and in 40% to 50% of women over age 50 years. Uterine fibroids are the most common benign tumors of the female reproductive system. Symptoms include uterine enlargement and distortion, low back pain, pressure on the bowel and the bladder, intermenstrual bleeding, and acute pain. The cause of this neoplasm is unknown; however, leiomyomas tend to grow under the influence of estrogen, may enlarge during pregnancy, and stop growing at menopause. After menopause, leiomyomas are replaced largely by fibrous scar

RT BR 6:00 A-RAD 2.5 CM FTN

FIGURE 10-18 A sagittal sonographic image of a uterus with fibroids that are located in the fundus of the uterus.

tissue, which has led to the misnomer **uterine fibroids**. In addition, they often contain radiographically visible calcifications (Fig. 10-18). The tumors vary in size and number (usually occurring in multiples). About 70% to 80% of uterine fibroids are located in the wall of the uterus. They may remain asymptomatic until they grow large enough to place pressure on surrounding structures, and they are usually detected on pelvic examination. Sonography, CT, and MRI are all useful in confirming the presence of leiomyomas. Sonographically, fibroids appear as sharply circumscribed, encapsulated lesions and may contain cystic areas. Malignant transformation is rare, and treatment depends on patient symptoms, ranging from no treatment to surgical removal of the uterus. Uterine artery embolization is the most successful radiologic treatment for most uterine leiomyomas. The only exception is a fibroid that is found by MRI in an older patient suffering from constipation. This type of fibroid likely compresses the rectum, and the best treatment for this older patient is myomectomy or hysterectomy to relieve the pressure.

Adenocarcinoma of the Endometrium

Adenocarcinoma of the endometrium is, by far, the most common malignancy of the uterus,

accounting for more than 80% of all endometrial cancers. It is often termed **endometrial carcinoma** of the uterus, and it is histopathologically different from cervical carcinoma. Endometrial cancer is one of the most common cancers of the female reproductive system, second only to breast cancer. The incidence of adenocarcinoma of the endometrium has remained fairly static; the disease ranks as the fourth most common malignancy in women in the United States, occurring mainly in postmenopausal women and increasing in incidence with age. The development of this neoplasm has strong ties to hormonal changes in woman and is more common in nulliparous women. Obesity is a major risk factor, as are tamoxifen use, late menopause, a family history of breast or ovarian cancer, or a history of previous pelvic radiation therapy.

Adenocarcinoma of the endometrium is usually preceded by endometrial hyperplasia. It then passes through an in situ stage before reaching its final invasive stage, often completely filling the uterine cavity. The cancer is graded according to cellular differentiation and staged according to the extent of the disease. The most frequent symptom is irregular or postmenopausal bleeding. Treatment varies with the stage of the disease. Stage 0 is curable via hysterectomy, and stages I and II are usually treated with a combination of surgery and radiation therapy, with the 5-year survival rate ranging from 70% to 95%. Stage III and IV endometrial adenocarcinomas are best treated with chemotherapy, but they have a lower 5-year survival rate of 10% to 60%.

BREAST MASSES

Fibroadenoma

A **fibroadenoma** is a common benign breast tumor. It is usually unilateral and consists of a solid, well-defined mass that does not invade surrounding tissue. The neoplasm is formed by an overgrowth of fibrous and glandular tissues and is commonly located in the upper, outer quadrant of the breast. Fibroadenomas almost always occur in women under 30 years of age and most

FIGURE 10-19 Needle localization of fibroadenoma of the breast pinpoints the location of the mass for surgical biopsy.

FIGURE 10-20 A sonographic image of a juvenile fibroadenoma.

frequently in those 21 to 25 years of age. Fibroadenomas appear to be estrogen dependent and may grow rapidly during pregnancy. These lesions are often painless and can usually be moved about within the breast. Mammography, in conjunction with physical breast examination and sonography, plays a vital role in the detection of fibroadenomas (Figs. 10-19 and 10-20) and is useful in distinguishing them from mammary dysplasia (fibrocystic breast disease) and breast carcinoma. Surgical removal of the lesion is curative.

Fibrocystic Breasts

An overgrowth of fibrous tissue or cystic hyperplasia results in **fibrocystic breasts**. This is the most common disorder of the female breast and occurs to some degree in 60% to 75% of all women. This condition may be unilateral; however, it is most frequently bilateral, with variably sized cysts located throughout the breasts (Figs. 10-21 and 10-22). The severity of this disorder varies greatly, and it is believed to result from fluctuations in hormone levels during the menstrual cycle. The most common sign or symptom associated with fibrocystic breasts is a mass or masses that increase in size and tenderness immediately before the onset of the menstrual period. The texture of the breast tissue is ropy and thick, especially in the upper outer quadrant of the breast. Sonography is extremely useful as a follow-up to mammography in differentiating solid masses from cystic masses in women with fibrocystic breasts (Fig. 10-23). Large cysts are commonly aspirated for cytologic evaluation of the fluid. If this evaluation does not yield definitive results, surgical biopsy is often performed. Although controversy exists about the correlation between fibrocystic breasts and an increased incidence of breast cancer, it is well known that a fibrocystic condition may mask a coexistent cancer. Treatment of the condition is largely symptomatic, including a monthly breast self-examination and proper support.

Carcinoma of the Breast

Breast carcinoma is a very common malignancy among women in the United States and the

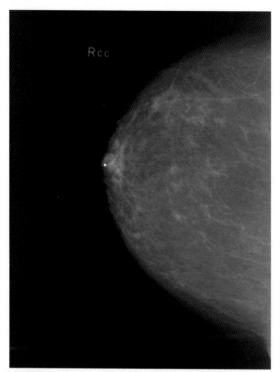

FIGURE 10-21 Craniocaudad mammographic projection of a moderately fibroglandular breast.

FIGURE 10-22 A sonographic image of a typical breast cyst.

second leading cause of cancer deaths in women, behind only lung cancer. Current literature suggests that 1 of every 8 women in the United States will develop breast cancer during her lifetime, with an increased incidence between ages 30 and 50 years. The incidence continues to rise throughout the postmenopausal years because of changes in estrogen levels, with the mean age for breast cancer being age 60 years. Approximately 60% of all palpable lesions occur in the upper outer quadrant of the breast.

Although the exact cause of breast cancer is unknown, it is believed to be a multifactorial disorder. Heredity, endocrine influence, oncogenic factors (such as viruses), and environmental factors (such as chemical carcinogens) appear to play a role in the development of this disease. The amount of biologically available estrogen and progesterone is a key endocrine factor in the development of breast cancer. Those individuals with an early onset of menstruation (menarche) or late menopause and women with a first pregnancy after age 30 years are at a higher risk for developing breast cancer. Women using oral contraceptives or estrogen replacement therapy over a 10-year period also have a very small increase in the risk of developing breast cancer. In terms of heredity, a family history including a parent, sibling, or child with breast cancer increases a woman's risk to two to three times that of the normal population. In addition, women who carry *BRCA1* or *BRCA2*, two known breast cancer genes, and men who carry *BRCA2* are at an increased risk for developing breast cancer. Current data also indicate that hereditary ovarian cancers are caused by *BRCA1* or *BRCA2* gene mutations. This syndrome is termed *hereditary breast ovarian cancer syndrome.*

Breast cancers may be classified as in situ carcinoma, ductal carcinoma in situ, lobular carcinoma in situ, invasive ductal or lobular carcinoma, or inflammatory carcinoma. Breast cancers generally are discovered as a lump in the breast by the patient. With the exception of inflammatory breast cancer, which is very virulent and associated with diffuse inflammation and breast

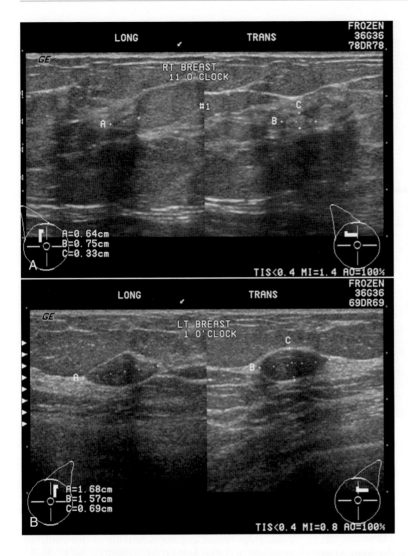

FIGURE 10-23 A, A sonogram of the breast demonstrating an enlarged lymph node and cyst in the eleven o'clock axis of the right breast, right upper quadrant. **B,** A sonogram of a hypoechogenic solid breast mass in the left upper quadrant in the one o'clock axis.

enlargement, most begin as slow-growing, relatively painless masses, but as they grow, they may infiltrate the suspensory ligaments, causing them to shorten and retract the overlying skin. Physical signs of advanced breast cancer include nipple retraction and distorted breast contour. The neoplasm may infiltrate and block the lymphatic vessels, the major route of metastases, especially to the axilla. This infiltration causes edema in the overlying skin and enlargement of the axillary or supraclavicular lymph nodes. As the infiltrating breast carcinoma blocks the lymphatic exchange, the skin pores open to allow the fluid to escape, thus causing a rough skin texture from chafing and pore enlargement. The edematous skin is described as having a **peau d'orange** (orange peel) appearance. As the tumor progresses, it may attach to surrounding fascia and ulcerate surrounding skin.

Mammography plays a very important role in the diagnosis and management of breast cancer. Routine screening mammography in asymptomatic women may lead to early detection and thus reduce breast cancer mortality by up to 30%. It has also been reported that breast cancer mortality could be reduced by as much as 50%

FIGURE 10-24 A mammogram of the left breast of a 63-year-old woman demonstrating a stellate mass commonly associated with carcinoma of the breast. Note the irregular borders of the mass.

FIGURE 10-25 A mammogram of the right breast in an older woman demonstrating a stellate mass containing microcalcifications commonly associated with carcinoma of the breast.

if all women older than age 40 years received annual screening mammography. However, annual screening of women between the ages of 40 and 50 years remains controversial.

Many breast tumors commonly appear radiographically as dense, irregular, stellate masses that infiltrate surrounding tissue (Fig. 10-24). Many contain numerous microcalcifications that are radiographically visible (Fig. 10-25). In some instances, fine-needle aspiration with cytologic evaluation may be sufficient to make a definitive diagnosis. Core needle biopsy or incisional biopsy is often performed to obtain a specimen of suspect tissue for further evaluation. For patients requiring an incisional biopsy, needle localization of mammographically detected, nonpalpable

cancerous breast lesions is reliable in directing the surgeon to the lesion in question and allows excision of suspect tissue. The tissue specimen is radiographed and forwarded to a pathologist for histologic evaluation. Statistics demonstrate that this method of localization causes minimal morbidity, and the development and refinement of mammographic localization have greatly increased the percentage of positive findings on surgical biopsy. This invasive technique allows more accurate diagnosis and treatment of early-stage carcinoma of the breast. If the tumor can be removed before the lesion is palpable, the survival rate is greatly increased. Specimens are routinely analyzed for estrogen and progesterone receptors because receptor status information is useful in determining a course of therapy. Patients with estrogen-receptor–positive (ER+) tumors have a better prognosis and tend to benefit from endocrine therapy.

As discussed earlier in this chapter, MRI may be used to detect breast cancer. PET is often used as a valuable adjunct imaging method for predicting the clinical outcome in patients who have been previously treated for breast cancer. Use of 18-fluorodeoxyglucose (FDG) PET provides both qualitative and quantitative information that helps detect the primary tumor and identify tumor spread via the lymphatic system, and it also has the potential to reduce the need for lymph node dissection. It is useful in assessing breast tumor metabolism and biologic behavior.

Treatment of breast carcinoma depends on the extent of the disease. Once the carcinoma is confirmed through biopsy, an axillary lymph node resection is performed to assist in the management of the disease. The 10-year survival rate for patients without node involvement is over 80% but drops to about 40% in patients with one to three positive nodes and to about 25% in patients with four or more positive nodes. Much controversy exists in terms of determining the best approach to the management and treatment of breast cancers. In the past 40 years, the 5-year survival rate for breast cancer has remained virtually unchanged. Currently, two surgical options are recommended for invasive breast cancers: (1) modified radical mastectomy and (2) breast-conserving surgery followed by radiation therapy. Both methods require axillary lymph node resection, and the difference between the survival rates of these two surgical options is insignificant. Inflammatory cancers are usually treated with a combination of chemotherapy and radiation therapy.

Treatment with an established combination of chemotherapeutic drugs is considered standard care for premenopausal women who have lymph node involvement. The chemotherapy may be continued for months or years after the primary therapy, but the adjuvant therapy may decrease the chance of death by 35% in this patient population. Breast carcinomas are also classified by a hormone receptor test. Many tumors require hormones for continued growth, and these carcinomas may undergo temporary regression if hormonal balances are altered.

DISORDERS DURING PREGNANCY

Diagnostic medical sonography is often used as positive proof of pregnancy, in addition to aiding in the diagnosis of multiple and ectopic pregnancies. With the use of transvaginal sonography, the sac and early fetal pole can been seen and a fetal heart detected at as early as 3 weeks of gestation. Sonographic examination may be indicated if the pregnant uterus is too small or too large for the calculated delivery date. Depending on the obstetrician's policy, many pregnant women may also have sonography performed at 6 to 8 weeks of gestation to screen for fetal anomalies. Additional laboratory tests such as amniocentesis, chorionic villus sampling, and deoxyribonucleic acid (DNA) analysis are performed in cases of suspected congenital anomalies of the fetus. Infant deaths are usually attributed to congenital anomalies or prematurity. Premature delivery may be associated with many anomalies of pregnancy. Examples include multiple pregnancies, placental anomalies, preeclampsia, and eclampsia, as well as congenital anomalies of the uterus such as bicornuate uterus or cervical incompetence. Preeclampsia is the development of hypertension in combination with proteinuria or edema and usually occurs after the twentieth week of gestation. The condition in which convulsions occur in a female patient with preeclampsia is termed *eclampsia*. Cervical incompetence can be demonstrated via sonography of the cervix during the first trimester of pregnancy.

Amniotic Fluid

Amniotic fluid is produced by various physiologic functions within the mother and the fetus. The amount of amniotic fluid present varies with the stage of pregnancy. **Oligohydramnios** refers to too little amniotic fluid, and **polyhydramnios** refers to an excess of amniotic fluid. The normal fetus swallows several hundred milliliters of fluid per day. This fluid is absorbed by the fetal intestines, with a portion excreted via the fetal urinary system and a portion transferred across the placenta into the mother's circulatory system. The major source of amniotic fluid arises from the fetus urinating fluid once the kidneys are developed. Therefore, oligohydramnios often results from poor fetal kidney function or blockage of the ureters associated with congenital anomalies of the fetal urinary system. If a fetus is unable to swallow because of anencephaly or a high GI obstruction, polyhydramnios may occur. It is also an indication of severe growth retardation and fetal death.

Ectopic Pregnancy

Ectopic pregnancy refers to the development of an embryo outside the uterine cavity. It occurs in approximately 10% to 15% of 1000 pregnancies. The most common site for an ectopic pregnancy is the fallopian tube (Fig. 10-26), but it may also occur in the ovary, cervix, or abdominal cavity. With tubal pregnancy, the fallopian tube distends to accommodate the growing embryo, causing blood vessels to rupture. This may produce serious internal hemorrhage and

can be life-threatening. If a tubal pregnancy goes untreated, the embryo will develop and survive for only 2 to 6 weeks.

Common signs and symptoms associated with ectopic pregnancy are the same as those of early pregnancy, but distension of the tube causes acute abdominal pain and tenderness. If internal hemorrhage occurs, loss of blood may cause fainting and shock. Ectopic pregnancies are more common in women who have had PID or have a partial obstruction of the uterine tube. The cause of tubal pregnancies is obstruction of the normal passageway for the ovum. Although sonography is useful in assessing ectopic pregnancies, diagnosis is confirmed via laparoscopy. Increasing evidence indicates that MRI may provide additional information on the location of an ectopic pregnancy that is located in the cervix or the interstitial area of the tube. The treatment is surgical removal of the embryo and the affected uterine tube.

Disorders of the Placenta

The placenta is a temporary organ associated with pregnancy. Its purpose is to exchange nutrients and oxygen from mother to fetus and waste products from fetus to mother for excretion. If a woman begins to bleed during the third trimester of pregnancy, ultrasonography should be

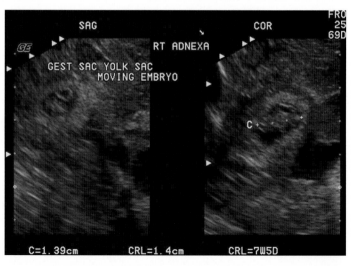

FIGURE 10-26 A transvaginal sonographic image reveals a live fetus in an ectopic location.

FIGURE 10-27 Placenta previa seen on this sagittal sonographic view reveals the placenta covering the internal os of the cervix.

performed to evaluate the placenta because the bleeding places both mother and fetus at high risk. The most common causes of third-trimester bleeding are placenta previa and abruption of the placenta. **Placenta previa** is a condition in which the implantation of the placenta leaves part or all of the cervical os covered. Several degrees are recognized: total, partial, marginal, and low-lying previa. These degrees of previa are related to the position of the placenta in relation to the internal cervical os. In placenta previa (Fig. 10-27), the mother experiences painless vaginal bleeding during the later stages of pregnancy because of the partial separation of the placenta from the uterine wall. Hemorrhage may occur, and this condition can be life-threatening to both mother and fetus. Sonography is an effective method for determining the location of the placenta in cases of suspected previa and is useful in the management of the pregnancy. Normal delivery cannot occur in patients with placenta previa, so a cesarean section is routinely performed.

Occasionally, a normally implanted placenta may prematurely separate from the uterus. This condition is termed **placental abruption** and may be life-threatening to the fetus. Predisposing factors for abruption include a history of a prior abruption, pregnancy-induced hypertension, smoking, alcohol abuse, cocaine abuse, external abuse, and multiple gestation. **Placental percreta** is a condition in which the placenta extends into the myometrium, causing an unduly firm attachment that bleeds at delivery because it will not separate normally. In rare cases, failure of the placenta to separate after birth results in the need for an immediate hysterectomy. The use of sonography or sonography with Doppler is highly recommended to distinguish between these different pathologies within the placenta.

Hydatidiform Mole

Hydatidiform mole refers to an abnormal conception in which usually no fetus is present. It occurs in about 1 in 2000 pregnancies in North America, although the incidence is much greater in certain other parts of the world for unknown reasons. Often, the presenting sign is a uterine size that is inappropriate for the date. With this condition, the uterus is filled with cystically dilated chorionic villi that resemble a bunch of grapes, known as *trophoblastic tissue* (Fig. 10-28). These villi absorb fluid and become

FIGURE 10-28 A sagittal sonographic image of the uterus that contains molar tissue.

swollen, and sonography demonstrates a characteristic pattern as well as absence of heart sounds. Usually, such a conception aborts spontaneously in the second trimester. If it does not, suction curettage is done, and no further treatment is required in most cases. Approximately 80% of molar pregnancies follow a benign course, but 15% to 25% may develop invasive disease. The use of sonography, clinical factors, and pelvic MRI is recommended to distinguish between an incomplete abortion and gestational trophoblastic disease.

Male Reproductive System

ANATOMY AND PHYSIOLOGY

The male reproductive system is composed of glands, ducts, and supporting structures. The glands of the male reproductive system include a pair of testes, a pair of seminal vesicles, a pair of bulbourethral glands, and one prostate gland. The testes are enclosed by a white, fibrous covering within the scrotum. They are responsible for the production of sperm and the secretion of hormones, mainly testosterone. The prostate gland lies just inferior to the bladder, and the urethra actually passes through this gland (Figs. 10-29 and 10-30). The prostate gland is responsible for secreting the majority of the seminal fluid and is normally about the size of a walnut.

FIGURE 10-29 The male reproductive system.

The ducts that connect the glands include a pair of epididymides, a pair of vasa deferentia, a pair of ejaculatory ducts, and one urethra. The testes are divided into lobules that contain seminiferous tubules, which converge into larger ducts and emerge at the head of the epididymis. The epididymides lie superior and lateral to the testes and serve as a passageway for sperm. They are also responsible for secreting a portion of the seminal fluid. The vasa deferentia extend from the epididymides and pass through the inguinal canal into the pelvic cavity. They pass superior to the bladder and continue down the posterior surface of the bladder to join the ducts emerging from the seminal vesicles. This junction forms the ejaculatory ducts. These ducts eventually empty into the urethra, which is responsible for delivering the seminal fluid to the exterior of the body.

IMAGING CONSIDERATIONS

Radiographic investigation of the male reproductive system is limited mainly to urethrography and intravenous urography. However, sonography is commonly used to evaluate testicular masses or an enlarged scrotum and to help differentiate among epididymitis, orchiditis, and testicular torsion. Nuclear medicine is also useful

FIGURE 10-30 The male urinary bladder, anterior cut away.

FIGURE 10-31 A coronal T2-weighted magnetic resonance imaging scan of the male pelvis depicting the bladder and the prostate gland.

in distinguishing between epididymitis and testicular torsion. Prostatic sonography via a rectal probe is used to evaluate nodules and guide the physician when performing biopsy of the prostate. MRI of the male pelvis is performed to evaluate the seminal vesicles, the prostate gland, and the scrotum (Fig. 10-31). MRI is useful in detecting and staging prostate cancer in men having a positive (+4) prostate-specific antigen (PSA) laboratory test. A specialized rectal coil is used in examining the prostate gland; however, high-field MRI units may be able to detect pathology without the use of the rectal coil. MRI is also useful in evaluating testicular cancer and can

determine if the cancer is present in one or both testicles. This differentiation is especially important in young men who plan to have children. The use of MRI, with or without contrast, is highly rated by the ACR as a pretreatment staging for prostate cancer. The use of endorectal coil MRI (erMRI) should be considered for those patients with a high value of PSA.

CONGENITAL ANOMALIES

Cryptorchidism

Near the end of gestation, the male testes normally descend through the inguinal canal into the scrotum. **Cryptorchidism** refers to undescended testes. The rate of malignancy is much greater in men with this condition, so treatment involves either bringing the testicle down and fixing it surgically or removing it. Sonography is often used to locate the testicle. Although more expensive than sonography, MRI may be of value in the diagnosis of this anomaly because of its superior ability to differentiate tissue.

NEOPLASTIC DISEASES

Prostatic Hyperplasia

Prostatic hyperplasia, a common benign enlargement of the prostate gland, is caused by the development of discrete nodules within the gland and is palpable through the rectum. Although enlargement may be determined by a digital rectal examination, the results may be misleading, so a laboratory blood test to assess serum PSA should be performed. Results may demonstrate a moderate elevation in PSA, depending on the degree of enlargement and urinary obstruction. The cause of prostatic hyperplasia is unknown, but the condition is thought to be caused by hormonal changes associated with aging, as it generally affects men after age 50 years. The benign nodules most frequently occur in the median lobe and in the central portions of the lateral lobes of the prostate gland. Because of these locations, the nodules often compress the portion of the urethra

FIGURE 10-32 A pelvic computed tomography image of a 68-year-old man demonstrating prostatic hyperplasia. Note the indentation into the urinary bladder.

FIGURE 10-33 An axial T2-weighted magnetic resonance imaging scan demonstrating enlargement of the posterior left portion of the prostate by prostate carcinoma.

passing through the prostate gland, thus interfering with urination.

Symptoms associated with this disorder include difficulty starting, stopping, and maintaining the flow of urine and inability to completely empty the bladder. Residual urine tends to infect the bladder, and this poses a risk of the kidneys being infected as well. In some cases, urinary tract obstructions may result from an overgrowth of the prostate gland. The most common treatment of prostatic hyperplasia is partial excision of the prostate gland, although nonsurgical treatment is available for some cases. A **transurethral resection of the prostate** (TURP) is performed by passing an endoscope through the urethra to core out the gland. Prostatic enlargement may be demonstrated on an intravenous urographic examination as a filling defect at the base of the bladder. Hyperplastic changes are also readily visible on MRI and CT examinations of the pelvic area (Fig. 10-32). Evidence does not conclusively suggest that development of prostatic hyperplasia increases an individual's risk of developing prostatic carcinoma.

Many men over age 50 years develop small, multiple calcifications within the prostate. These are termed **prostatic calculi,** which may be radiographically visible on plain abdominal or pelvic images. The development of these calculi is of no clinical significance.

Carcinoma of the Prostate

Adenocarcinoma of the prostate is a common cancer in men. It most frequently affects older men, with the incidence increasing with age. The cause of prostate cancer is unknown, but it generally affects the outer group of prostate glands and occurs more frequently in the posterior lobe of the prostate. This disease is most often diagnosed through physical examination and an elevation of acid phosphatase levels in blood. In cases of suspected prostatic disease, MRI or sonography may be used to determine the location and extent of disease (Fig. 10-33). Common signs and symptoms associated with prostate cancer include urinary tract obstructions; a hard, enlarged prostate on rectal palpation; and low back pain, which is often caused by metastatic spread to the pelvis and lumbar spine.

Some types of prostate cancers are fairly dormant, but others are very aggressive and yield a higher mortality rate. If it is diagnosed at an early stage, the initial treatment is surgical removal of the tumor. In addition, this neoplasm is highly testosterone dependent, so the testes are often removed along with the prostate. In some instances, female hormones may be administered to control the growth of the tumor by interfering with the action of testosterone. A new treatment modality involves planting radioactive seeds in the prostate, under the guidance of ultrasonography, to destroy the tumor.

Prostate cancer is staged A to D and graded I to III, depending on the extent of the disease. It tends to infiltrate surrounding structures early and extensively, particularly the skeletal system. Skeletal metastases occur in approximately 75% of all cases and manifest on plain radiographs as sclerotic lesions within bone (Fig. 10-34). Bone pain in an older man should particularly raise suspicion of prostate cancer. As the third leading cause of cancer-related deaths in men, it has a 5-year survival rate of approximately 33%.

The ACR recommends a technitium-99m (^{99m}Tc) bone scan of the whole body as the most effective method for monitoring recurrence of disease after a radical prostatectomy and rising

PSA levels among those men treated for prostate cancer. CT of the abdomen and pelvis with contrast is also highly recommended for monitoring for recurrence after surgery.

Testicular Masses

Testicular torsion occurs if a testicle twists on itself, inducing severe pain and swelling. Failure to correct this surgically in an immediate fashion may result in severe compromise of testicular vascularity. In patients with acute pain in the scrotum, it is very important to make sure that testicular blood supply is maintained. The use of ultrasound Doppler and nuclear medicine is highly recommended by the ACR to assess these patients for adequate blood supply to the testicle. Doppler ultrasound may also be used to detect the increased vascular flow associated with inflammation, which can accompany infection. Conversely, the inability to detect vascular flow within the testicle could indicate that the vascular supply is twisted and, as a result, proximal blood supply has been lost. Power Doppler is the most sensitive sonography application for the detection of low vascular flow; therefore, it is the best imaging choice for detecting the cause of scrotal pain. Likewise, the use of a nuclear medicine scan facilitates the detection of vascular flow associated with the uptake or lack of uptake of ^{99m}Tc (Fig. 10-35). Inflammation of the epididymis, or epididymitis, may similarly lead to scrotal swelling caused by the hyperemia. This inflammatory response by the epididymis and testis (**epididymo-orchitis**) may result from a bacterial infection such as urinary tract infection or gonorrhea or may be secondary to the placement of an

FIGURE 10-34 Skeletal metastatic disease of the pelvis and spine secondary to prostate cancer.

R   L

FIGURE 10-35 Torsion as seen on a nuclear medicine testicular scan, which reveals a relative absence of blood flow to the right testicle.

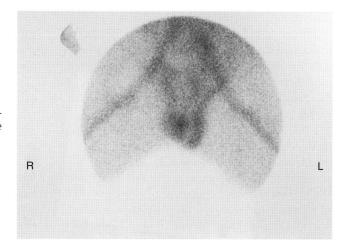

FIGURE 10-36 Epididymitis as revealed on a testicular scan, which shows increased uptake in the left testicle.

R   L

indwelling urinary catheter. In addition to scrotal edema, signs and symptoms include scrotal pain and erythema. The increased blood flow associated with or without trauma can be detected with Doppler or a nuclear medicine scan, which demonstrates increased uptake of ^{99m}Tc (Fig. 10-36).

Benign masses of the testes may be associated with epididymo-orchitis. Other common benign masses include hydroceles and spermatoceles. **Hydroceles** are common intrinsic scrotal masses, sometimes congenital in nature, caused by a collection of fluid in the testis or along the spermatic cord (Fig. 10-37). They may appear as a painless scrotal swelling, or they may demonstrate inflammation in combination with epididymitis and be quite painful. **Spermatoceles**, or spermatic cysts, are fluid-filled, painless scrotal masses within the testis adjacent to the epididymis (Fig. 10-38). Sonography may be used to differentiate between benign hydroceles or spermatoceles and solid, malignant neoplasms.

Malignant testicular tumors constitute approximately 1% of all cancers in males in the United States. Such tumors represent the most common malignancy among 15- to 34-year-olds, and the condition has a peak incidence around age 30 years and a second smaller peak around age 75 years. The cause of malignant tumors of the testes is unknown, but research has shown a

TRANS
RT
INF

FIGURE 10-37 A hydrocele is visualized as the dark collection of fluid surrounding the testicle, as seen on a sonogram of this 52-year-old man.

strong hereditary association. The most common signs include enlargement or palpable hardness of the testis. As with other cancers, testicular tumors are staged I to III, depending on the size and extent of the disease. All types of malignant testicular neoplasms are treated with surgical resection. Chemotherapy, radiation therapy, or both may be used in conjunction with surgery, depending on the type and staging of the disease. The four types of malignant germ cell tumors are (1) seminomas, (2) embryonal carcinomas, (3) teratomas, and (4) choriocarcinomas.

Testicular seminomas arise from the seminiferous tubules and account for approximately 40% of malignant testicular tumors (Fig. 10-39). Seminomas grow rapidly but tend to remain localized for a fairly long time before metastasizing. These neoplasms have an excellent prognosis because of their extreme radiosensitivity. If treated with radiation therapy, seminomas carry a 10-year survival rate of approximately 90%.

Testicular teratomas arise from primitive germ cells and account for approximately 25% of the malignant testicular masses (Fig. 10-40). These neoplasms are composed of various cell types such as connective tissue, muscle, and thyroid glandular tissue. Teratomas are associated with a poorer prognosis compared with seminomas and carry a 10-year survival rate of approximately 50% to 75%. Like seminomas, teratomas are highly malignant, spreading to the renal hilum via the lymphatics and via hematogenous spread.

Approximately 20% of malignant testicular tumors are **testicular embryonal carcinomas.** They are smaller than seminomas; however, they are very invasive and metastasize fairly quickly. Embryonal carcinomas carry a 10-year survival rate of approximately 35%.

Testicular choriocarcinomas make up the smallest portion of malignant testicular tumors, accounting for only 1% of malignant neoplasms of the testes. However, choriocarcinomas are very small and aggressive neoplasms. They are often nonpalpable and metastasize very early. Choriocarcinomas carry the worst prognosis, with a 10-year survival rate of approximately 10%.

Gynecomastia. Gynecomastia is the proliferation of breast tissue in the male patient. This usually presents as a palpable lump that has been detected in either young men or older men and is influence by hormonal stimulation. In some

FIGURE 10-38 A spermatocele, evidenced by a large fluid collection on the epididymis, as seen on a testicular sonographic scan of this 33-year-old man.

FIGURE 10-39 The hypoechoic mass seen in the superior aspect of the testicle on this testicular sonogram of a 31-year-old man is strongly suggestive of a seminoma.

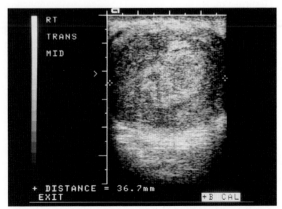

FIGURE 10-40 A large, echogenic heterogeneous mass in the right testicle is highly suspicious for a teratoma in the testicular sonogram of this 27-year-old man.

cases, the nipple will produce a clear discharge associated with the proliferation of this tissue. Gynecomastia is commonly a bilateral process, with one lump dominating, but rarely is associated with breast cancer. Breast ultrasonography is the recommended imaging modality to provide diagnostic confirmation of this entity.

Breast cancer in men is rare, with the National Cancer Institute reporting only 2190 new cases in 2011 in the United States. Male breast cancer affects older men and forms in the ducts and would require mammography to successfully image the invasion of the disease into surrounding soft tissue.

PATHOLOGY SUMMARY
The Reproductive System

Pathology	Imaging Modalities of Choice
PID (acute pelvic pain)	Sonography, MRI pelvis (with or without contrast)
Ovarian cysts (acute pelvic pain)	Sonography, MRI pelvis (with or without contrast)
Cystadenocarcinoma	Sonography
Carcinoma of the cervix	Staging: MRI pelvis (with or without contrast) and FDG-PET whole body and CT abdomen and pelvis with contrast
Leiomyoma of uterus (abnormal bleeding)	Sonography, SHG
Adenocarcinoma of endometrium (abnormal bleeding <5 mm endometrium on sonogram)	Staging: MRI pelvis (with or without contrast), CT chest (with or without contrast), CT abdomen with contrast, radiography of the chest
Fibroadenoma of breast	Mammography and sonography
Fibrocystic breast	Mammography and sonography
Carcinoma of breast	Mammography, sonography, and MRI
Pregnancy status	Sonography
Ectopic pregnancy	Sonography
Disorders of placenta	Sonography
Cryptorchidism (undescended testicle)	Sonography
Prostatic hyperplasia	Sonography of the pelvis, sonography of the kidney
Carcinoma of the prostate	MRI, ^{99m}Tc bone scan whole body
Testicular torsion	Sonography, nuclear medicine
Testicular mass	Sonography

^{99m}Tc, technetium-99m; *CT*, computed tomography; *FDG-PET*, 18F-fluorodeoxyglucose positron emission tomography; *MRI*, magnetic resonance imaging; *PID*, pelvic inflammatory disease; *SHG*, sonohysterography.

REVIEW QUESTIONS

1. Imaging studies performed on a nongravid woman include:
   a. Hysterosalpingography
   b. Transvaginal pelvic sonography
   c. Transabdominal pelvic sonography
   d. All of the above

2. Regular, yearly mammographic screening should occur in women ___ years of age or older.
   a. 20
   b. 30
   c. 40
   d. 50

3. The congenital disorder resulting in a complete duplication of the uterus, cervix, and vagina is:
   a. Bicornuate uterus
   b. Retroflexed uterus
   c. Unicornuate uterus
   d. Uterus didelphys

4. Which of the following cystic ovarian masses may form as a part of the normal menstrual cycle?
   1. Corpus luteum cysts
   2. Cystadenomas
   3. Follicular cysts
   a. 1 and 2
   b. 1 and 3
   c. 2 and 3
   d. 1, 2, and 3

5. A malignant neoplasm of the ovary is a:
   a. Cystadenocarcinoma
   b. Cystadenoma
   c. Leiomyoma
   d. Fibroadenoma

6. Which type of neoplastic disease is often diagnosed via a Pap test and confirmed by surgical biopsy?
   a. Adenocarcinoma of the endometrium
   b. Cervical carcinoma
   c. Fibroadenoma of the breast
   d. Leiomyoma of the uterus

7. In which anatomic region of the breast do the majority of breast masses occur?
   a. Lower inner quadrant
   b. Lower outer quadrant
   c. Upper inner quadrant
   d. Upper outer quadrant

8. The presence of excessive amniotic fluid is termed:
   a. Abruptio placentae
   b. Oligohydramnios
   c. Placenta previa
   d. Polyhydramnios

9. Prostatic hyperplasia most frequently occurs in men:
   a. Under age 30 years
   b. Between ages 30 and 50 years
   c. Over age 50 years
   d. None of the above; prostatic hyperplasia is a female condition

10. Benign masses of the testes include:
    1. Hydroceles
    2. Seminomas
    3. Spermatoceles
    a. 1 and 2
    b. 1 and 3
    c. 2 and 3
    d. 1, 2, and 3

11. Describe how breast parenchyma changes with age and parity and the effect these changes have on the radiographic visibility of potential masses.

12. Identify two purposes for requiring a female patient to have a full bladder for transabdominal sonographic examination.

13. Describe the benefits of routine mammography versus the risks of radiation exposure.

14. What would be the danger of leaving cryptorchidism untreated?

15. A 60-year-old man presents to his physician with complaints of frequent urination, particularly at night. Intravenous pyelography is ordered. The only visible abnormality is a filling defect at the base of his bladder. What is the likely cause?

11

Endocrine System

LEARNING OBJECTIVES

On completion of Chapter 11, the reader should be able to:
- Describe the anatomic components and function of the endocrine system.
- Identify and explain the various imaging modalities used in diagnosing and treating endocrine disorders.

- Specify the disorders, signs and symptoms, and prognosis of the endocrine pathologies discussed in this chapter.

OUTLINE

Anatomy and Physiology
Imaging Considerations
  Radiography
  Bone Mineral
    Densitometry
  Magnetic Resonance
    Imaging
  Computed
    Tomography
  Nuclear Medicine
    Procedures

Skeletal Disorders
  Osteoporosis
  Osteomalacia
  Paget Disease (Osteitis
    Deformans)
Pituitary Gland Disorders
  Acromegaly
  Diabetes Insipidus
  Hypopituitarism
Adrenal Gland Disorders
  Cushing Syndrome

  Addison Disease
  Adrenal Carcinoma
Pancreatic Disorders
  Diabetes Mellitus
**Thyroid and Parathyroid
Gland Disorders**
  Hyperthyroidism
  Hypothyroidism
  Thyroid Cancers
  Hyperparathyroidism
  Nephrocalcinosis

KEY TERMS

Acromegaly
Addison disease
Adrenal carcinoma
Adrenal glands
Cushing syndrome
Diabetes insipidus
Diabetes mellitus
Ductal adenocarcinoma
Glucagon

Gonads
Graves disease
Hormonal stimuli
Hormones
Humoral stimuli
Hyperparathyroidism
Hyperthyroidism
Hypopituitarism
Hypothalamus

ANATOMY AND PHYSIOLOGY

The endocrine system is responsible for metabolic activities within the human cells through the release of hormones. Endocrine glands are ductless glands that secrete **hormones** directly into the surrounding vascular and lymphatic systems or through neuroendocrine processes. The primary endocrine glands of the body include the **pituitary gland, pineal gland, adrenal glands, thyroid gland, parathyroid gland,** and **thymus gland**. The **pancreas, gonads,** and **hypothalamus** also produce hormones (Fig. 11-1). Hormones are synthesized and released in response to three types of stimuli: (1) **humoral stimuli,** which involve a direct response to changes in blood chemistry; (2) **neural stimuli,** such as in the case of the adrenal glands secreting epinephrine or norepinephrine in response to the sympathetic nervous system; and (3) **hormonal stimuli,** which involve a response to other hormones secreted in the body.

The **pituitary gland** comprises three separate lobes: (1) the anterior lobe, (2) the intermediate lobe, and (3) the posterior lobe. Each lobe functions as a separate gland; however, in humans, the intermediate lobe is rudimentary, consisting of only a few cells. The pituitary is considered the "master endocrine gland," and it is located below the hypothalamus at the base of the brain within the sella turcica of the sphenoid bone (Fig. 11-2). The hypothalamus is connected to

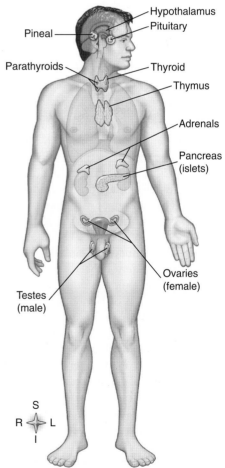

FIGURE 11-1 Principal endocrine glands.

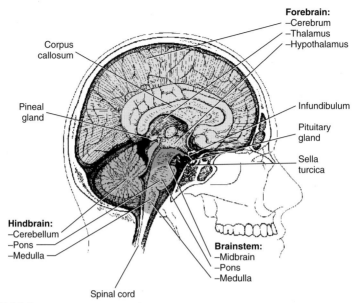

Forebrain:
–Cerebrum
–Thalamus
–Hypothalamus

Corpus
callosum

Pineal
gland

Infundibulum

Pituitary
gland

Sella
turcica

Hindbrain:
–Cerebellum
–Pons
–Medulla

Brainstem:
–Midbrain
–Pons
–Medulla

Spinal cord

FIGURE 11-2 Midsagittal section of brain demonstrating the pituitary and pineal glands.

the pituitary via the pituitary stalk, and the hypothalamus is responsible for controlling the function of the pituitary gland. Each lobe of the pituitary secretes specific hormones. The anterior lobe is responsible for secreting luteinizing hormone (LH), follicle-stimulating hormone (FSH), prolactin (PRL), adrenocorticotropic hormone (ACTH), growth hormone (GH), and thyroid-stimulating hormone (TSH). The intermediate lobe secretes melanocyte-stimulating hormone (MSH), and the posterior lobe is responsible for secreting oxytocin and antidiuretic hormone (ADH). The secretion of hormones by the anterior lobe occurs through the typical endocrine control mechanism by the release of hormones directly into the blood. However, the posterior lobe of the pituitary is an extension of the nervous system, with hormone secretion occurring via a neuroendocrine mechanism, in which the hormones are synthesized within the cell bodies of neurons within the hypothalamus.

The pineal gland is also controlled by the hypothalamus. It is located within the cranium, posterior to the third ventricle, superior to the colliculi of the midbrain, and inferior to the splenium of the corpus callosum (see Fig. 11-2). It

occasionally calcifies with age and is often quite visible on computed tomography (CT) images of the brain. This small endocrine gland is responsible for the production and excretion of melatonin. Melatonin is released when light exposure is inhibited; thus, the pineal gland is responsible for regulating the circadian rhythms. This hormone is often used to treat sleep disorders. The pineal gland also secretes gonadotropin-releasing hormone (GnRH), a hormone that stimulates the release of FSH and LH and is active in the onset of puberty.

The adrenal glands are pyramid-shaped glands located on the upper poles of the kidneys (Fig. 11-3). The inner portion of the adrenal gland, termed the *adrenal medulla*, acts as a part of the sympathetic nervous system and secretes the catecholamines epinephrine and norepinephrine. The effects of increased epinephrine production include increased cardiac output; increased heart rate; vasodilation of skeletal muscle; vasoconstriction of internal organs and skin; relaxation of smooth muscle in the gastrointestinal (GI) system, urinary bladder, and bronchials; and increased mental alertness. Epinephrine also increases glycogenesis in the liver and lipolysis in adipose tissue, as well as affecting the pancreatic hormone secretion by decreasing insulin production and increasing glucagon secretion. The outer portion, known as the *adrenal cortex*, is responsible for corticosteroid production. The adrenal cortex activity is primarily controlled by ACTH, which is secreted by the anterior pituitary. ACTH synthesizes three major types of corticosteroids: (1) mineralocorticosteroids, which are responsible for electrolyte balance; (2) glucocorticoids,

which are responsible for cell metabolism and for controlling blood sugar levels; and (3) low levels of gonadocorticosteroids or sex hormones. Mineralocorticoids such as aldosterone may affect extracellular fluid volume and blood volume, which ultimately affects blood pressure and cardiac output. Glucocorticoid secretions are greatly influenced by physical or psychological stress stimuli such as hypoglycemia, trauma, and acute or chronic anxiety. Hypoglycemia stimulates the secretion of cortisol, which, in turn, triggers a response in the liver to convert amino acids to glucose, thus increasing blood glucose levels.

The thyroid gland is located in the anterior neck just below the larynx (Fig. 11-4). It is divided into two lobes connected by an isthmus. This endocrine gland secretes two hormones: (1) thyroid hormone (TH) and (2) calcitonin. TH stimulates enzymes responsible for glucose oxidation and is actually a composition of two hormones: (1) thyroxine (T_4) and (2) triiodothyronine (T_3), both of which contain iodine as an integral part of the molecule. Unlike other hormones within the body, the thyroid hormone synthesis requires the presence of iodine. Levels of T_4 and T_3 are regulated by TSH, which is synthesized and stored within the anterior lobe of the pituitary. The thyroid gland is vital to maintaining normal blood pressure and

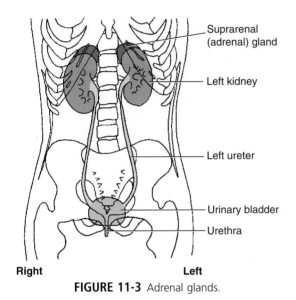

Right   **Left**

FIGURE 11-3 Adrenal glands.

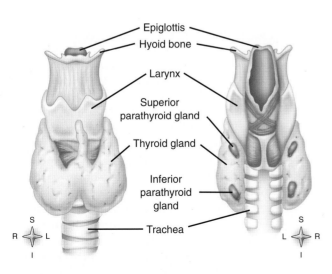

FIGURE 11-4 Thyroid and parathyroid glands.

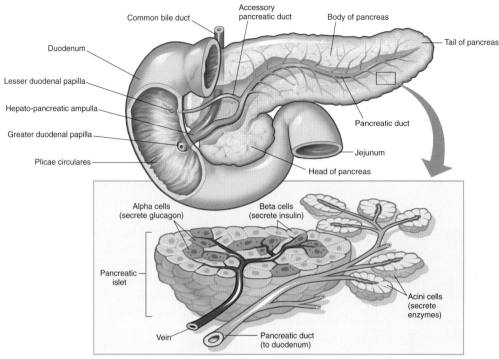

FIGURE 11-5 The pancreas.

in regulating tissue growth and development. Overactivity of the thyroid gland is termed **hyperthyroidism,** and underactivity is termed **hypothyroidism.** Either abnormal activity level may cause severe metabolic disturbances in the human body. Calcitonin is most important in childhood. It is an antagonist of parathyroid hormone (PTH) and serves to lower blood calcium levels by inhibiting osteoclast activity and stimulating calcium uptake in the bone matrix. The parathyroid glands are located on the posterior aspect of the thyroid gland. They are responsible for producing and secreting PTH, which also serves to control blood calcium levels. This hormone stimulates osteoclasts and increases calcium absorption in the kidneys and in the GI system. It is important to note that a reduction in bone density may occur and result in increased bone fragility if PTH secretion is sustained at a high level. However, new research in the use of therapeutic recombinant

parathyroid hormone (rPTH) shows promise in strengthening bone and increasing bone density in patients with osteoporosis.

The pancreas is located in the midabdomen just posterior to the stomach (Fig. 11-5) and functions both as an endocrine organ and an exocrine organ. The tail of the pancreas ends at the spleen, and the head is encircled by the duodenum. Specialized cells within the pancreas, termed the *islets of Langerhans* or *pancreatic islets,* are responsible for the production of important hormones. The α-cells are responsible for glucagon synthesis; the β-cells are responsible for balancing the secretion of insulin and glucagon, depending on food intake; and the δ-cells are responsible for secreting somatostatin, a hormone which influences the secretion of the α-cells and β-cells. **Glucagon** promotes the breakdown of glycogen to glucose within the liver, and glucose is ultimately released into the bloodstream. The α-cells of the pancreas secrete glucagon to increase blood sugar levels, and these cells are driven by humeral stimuli. Insulin, whose role is the opposite of glucagon's, acts to decrease blood sugar levels. **Insulin** is produced by the β-cells to inhibit the breakdown of glycogen to glucose.

IMAGING CONSIDERATIONS

Radiography

Radiographic examination is very helpful in diagnosing metabolic diseases of the skeletal system or endocrine disorders that ultimately affect the skeletal system, for example, Cushing disease. Skeletal disorders that result in a decrease in calcium in the bone matrix include osteoporosis and osteomalacia. Skull radiography is of limited use in evaluating metabolic disorders of the pituitary gland and is increasingly being replaced by magnetic resonance imaging (MRI), computed tomography (CT), or positron emission tomography (PET) in making a definitive diagnosis for pituitary disorders.

Bone Mineral Densitometry

Dual-energy x-ray absorptiometry (DXA) or bone mineral densitometry is an important modality in the evaluation of osteoporosis. DXA units readily show bone density by evaluating the bone mass of the distal radius, femoral neck, and lumbar spine. The results of bone densitometry are used in combination with routine laboratory tests of blood and urine to determine loss of bone mass. Bone mineral densitometry reports indicate the amount of bone mass present and compare the density of a particular individual to norms used in evaluation. A "T-score" is used to reflect standard deviations above or below the 30-year-old national reference population because it is assumed that this is the age of peak bone mass. Based on criteria established by the World Health Organization (WHO), a T-score greater than –1 is normal. T-scores less than –1 but greater than –2.49 are classified as osteopenia, and T-scores less than –2.5 reflect osteoporosis. The "Z-score" reports standard deviation above or below a population matched for age, gender, weight, and ethnicity. Z-scores less than –2 suggest bone disease.

Magnetic Resonance Imaging

MRI has largely replaced CT for imaging neuroendocrine disorders. According to the American College of Radiology (ACR), MRI is the only imaging modality that can reliably demonstrate pathologies of the hypothalamus. Pituitary disorders often result in an enlarged sella turcica, represented by the "empty sella syndrome," which can be confirmed with MRI. Gadolinium contrast-enhanced MRI is routinely used to demonstrate pituitary adenomas and is the modality of choice for visualizing microadenomas. MRI is also helpful in monitoring the progress of patients with pituitary adenomas. (See Chapter 8 for additional information on pituitary adenomas.)

Computed Tomography

Contrast-enhanced, high-resolution brain CT may also be used in the diagnosis and follow-up care of patients with pituitary disorders. It is frequently used when MRI is not available or may be contraindicated. The pineal gland is also clearly visible on CT evaluation. CT examinations of the neck are useful in the evaluation of neoplastic disease of the thyroid and parathyroid glands.

Most adrenal neoplasms in the cortex and the medulla are identified with abdominal CT, and biopsies of these tumors are frequently performed with CT-guided small-needle aspiration. Abdominal CT is also used in assessing enlargement of the adrenal glands of patients with Cushing disease.

Nuclear Medicine Procedures

In the case of thyroid disorders, nuclear medicine testing for iodine-123 (^{123}I) uptake is quite valuable in diagnosing thyroid gland function. It is used to detect nonpalpable nodules and to evaluate the remaining thyroid tissue after surgical resection or ablation.

The use of nuclear medicine imaging to localize medullary tumors in the adrenal glands using iodine-131 (^{131}I)-metaiodobenzylguanidine (MIBG) is gaining popularity. Patients are scanned over a 3-day period to look for an increased uptake, which indicates the presence of a pheochromocytoma. This radioisotope may also be used to treat this tumor of the medullary portion of the adrenal gland.

SKELETAL DISORDERS

Osteoporosis

A radiographically visible decrease in bone density is termed **osteopenia** and may occur as a result of osteoporosis or osteomalacia. Osteopenia is identified as a bone mass between 648 and 833 milligram per square centimeter (mg/cm^2). **Osteoporosis** is a commonly known metabolic bone disorder in which the structural integrity of the trabecular pattern of bone is destroyed and is identified as a bone mass less than 648 mg/cm^2. It may be classified as *primary osteoporosis* (type 1) or *secondary osteoporosis* (type 2). Primary osteoporosis may be further classified as *postmenopausal* or *senile*, and secondary osteoporosis is most commonly associated with an existing disease process or is the result of a medication. Osteoporosis may also be classified as *generalized* or *regional*. Postmenopausal osteoporosis is the most common form of the disease. Estimates are that more than half of the women in North America over age 60 years have osteoporosis, and it is a major cause of fractures of the hip, spine, and wrist in women over age 50 years. It is more common in white and Asian women. Although the formation of bone is normal, the bone reabsorption rate is abnormally high in individuals with osteoporosis. Thus, osteoporosis results in a thinning of cortical bone and an enlargement of the medullary canal without any change in the actual diameter of the bone. The normal equilibrium associated with osteoid production and withdrawal is quite complex and depends on a combination of dietary intake and absorption, hormonal interplay, and normal stress or muscular activity. In postmenopausal women, for example, the lack of the hormone estrogen creates a weakened bone matrix, contributing to the development of "porous" bones. As the condition becomes more severe, bones are subject to compression fractures, and they may literally cave in from the weakness. Risk factors for osteoporosis are listed in Box 11-1. As the vertebral bodies of the thoracic and lumbar spine are weakened, they collapse anteriorly, causing a kyphotic deformity of the spine, often termed "dowager's hump." These bony changes are well demonstrated by radiography of the spine (Fig. 11-6), in which decreased bone density stands out clearly against the cortex. Osteoporosis is a subtractive or destructive pathologic condition and requires a decrease in exposure technique. However, conventional radiography may be used to identify bone mass loss only when it is advanced or the bone has lost approximately 30% to 50% of its original mass. The best method for evaluating the early stages of osteoporosis is bone mineral densitometry of the hip and lumbar spine using DXA (Fig. 11-7).

Secondary osteoporosis may be caused by other diseases such as pathologies of the endocrine system, neoplastic disease, malnutrition, chronic renal failure, or hereditary diseases of the skeletal system, or it may be a result of drug therapy. Osteoporosis is, by far, the most common form of metabolic bone disease and can be differentiated from other causes of bone weakening by examining serum enzyme levels, especially alkaline phosphatase. For example, patients with osteoporosis have normal or elevated serum alkaline levels, whereas these serum levels are decreased in patients with osteomalacia. Elevated alkaline phosphatase is an indication of increased bone activity because it is found on the outside of osteoclast cells. Treatment of osteoporosis generally includes an increase in dietary intake of calcium, vitamin D, and magnesium in combination with moderate weight-bearing exercise.

BOX 11-1	**Risk Factors for Osteoporosis**

Genetic
Family history of osteoporosis
White or Asian race
Advanced age
Female sex

Anthropometric
Small stature
Fair or pale complexion
Thin build

Hormonal and Metabolic
Early menopause (natural or surgical)
Late menarche
Nulliparity
Obesity
Hypogonadism
Gaucher disease
Cushing syndrome
Weight below healthy range
Acidosis

Dietary
Low dietary calcium and vitamin D
Low endogenous magnesium
Excessive protein*
Excessive sodium intake
High caffeine intake
Anorexia
Malabsorption

Lifestyle
Sedentary lifestyle
Smoking
Alcohol consumption (excessive)

Concurrent Disease
Hyperparathyroidism

Illness and Trauma
Renal insufficiency, hypocalciuria
Rheumatoid arthritis
Spinal cord injury
Systemic lupus erythematosus

Liver Disease
Marrow disease (myeloma, mastocytosis, thalassemia)

Drugs
Corticosteroids
Dilantin
Gonadotropin-releasing hormone agonists

Loop diuretics
Methotrexate
Thyroid
Heparin
Cyclosporine
Depo-medroxyprogesterone acetate
Retinoids

*Low levels of protein intake also have been reported.
From: McCance KL, Huether SE, Brashers VL, et al: *Pathophysiology: The biologic basis for disease in adults and children*, ed 6, St. Louis, MO, 2009.

Osteomalacia

Osteomalacia is a condition caused by lack of calcium in tissues and failure of bone tissue to calcify. The mature bone exhibits an abnormal bone matrix consisting of soft osteoid instead of rigid bone. This normally results from a low-serum phosphate level because of inadequate intake or absorption of vitamin D, most commonly as a consequence of intestinal malabsorption of fats. Osteomalacia may be associated with hepatic disease, chronic pancreatitis, regional ileitis, and resections of the GI system because these conditions may inhibit the body from absorbing fat-soluble vitamin D. It is often also present in individuals with chronic renal failure secondary to the loss of renal parenchyma and the kidneys' inability to convert vitamin D into a form useful to the human body. If osteomalacia occurs before growth plate closure, it is known as **rickets** (Fig. 11-8).

With this condition, the bones are spongelike and demonstrate osteopenia on radiographic evaluation. Radiographically, osteomalacia appears similar to osteoporosis except for the presence of bands of radiolucency within the bone, termed **pseudofractures** or Looser zones. Common signs and symptoms include skeletal

FIGURE 11-6 A, Anteroposterior and **B,** lateral lumbar spine radiographs demonstrating osteopenia secondary to long-term steroid use.

pain, muscular weakness, low back pain, uremia, and bone fractures resulting from minimal trauma. Laboratory analysis to measure blood urea nitrogen (BUN), creatinine, serum calcium levels, and serum inorganic phosphate levels and other tests are necessary for differential diagnosis. Bone biopsy and measurement of serum fibroblast growth factor 23 (FGF-23) levels are the definitive methods of determining the presence of osteomalacia. This disorder may be treated by adjusting serum calcium and phosphate levels, inclusion of a dietary supplement of vitamin D,

administering calcium carbonate, chelating bone aluminum, renal dialysis, and controlling other disease processes such as hyperthyroidism and renal osteodystrophy.

Paget Disease (Osteitis Deformans)

Paget disease is a metabolic disorder of unknown cause; however, recent research indicates a genetic link and the possible role of viral infectious agents. It is fairly common in the older adult population, affecting men twice as frequently as

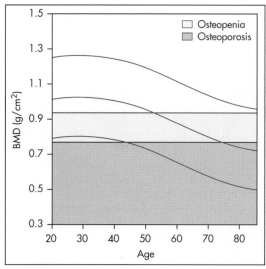

FIGURE 11-7 Lumbar spine bone mass density.

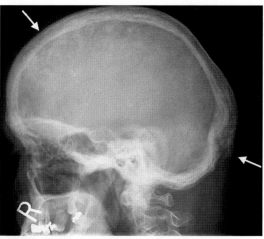

FIGURE 11-9 Lateral skull radiograph depicting an advanced proliferative phase of Paget disease. Note the changes within the inner and outer tables of the skull.

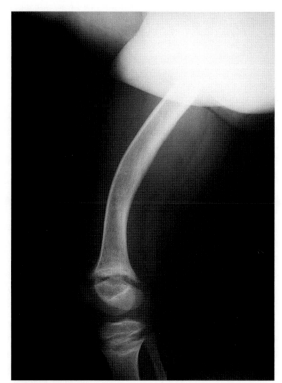

FIGURE 11-8 Radiograph of a femur of a child diagnosed with vitamin D–resistant rickets. Note the bowing of the extremity.

women. It usually begins in the fifth decade of life and may affect one or more bones, most commonly the pelvis, spine, skull (Fig. 11-9), and long bones (Fig. 11-10). Paget disease is characterized by two stages: (1) the *osteolytic stage,* in which the bone undergoes continuous destruction, and (2) the *osteoblastic stage,* in which bone is simultaneously replaced by abnormally soft and poorly mineralized material. The osteoid material that replaces normal bone tissue diminishes the trabeculae and is very bulky and porous, with exceptional vascularity. Although this osteoid matrix is thicker than normal bone, its softness often leads to weight-bearing, stress-induced deformities and fractures. This bony destruction and replacement produce a classic "cotton wool" appearance radiographically. As the skull enlarges, additional complications may occur because of impingement on the cranial nerves. These complications include hearing and vision disturbances. In addition, individuals with Paget disease have an increased risk of developing osteogenic sarcoma, a malignant neoplastic disease of the skeletal system. Radionuclide bone scans readily detect Paget disease, even in its very early stages. Radiographically, affected bones typically demonstrate cortical thickening, with a

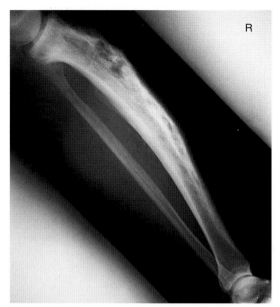

FIGURE 11-10 Radiograph of the tibia of the patient in Fig. 11-8 demonstrating the effect of advanced proliferative Paget disease on the tibia.

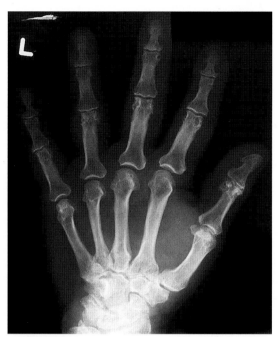

FIGURE 11-11 Radiograph of the hand of an individual diagnosed with acromegaly. Note the spadelike appearance of the hand.

coarse, thickened trabecular pattern. Mixed areas of radiolucent osteolysis and radiopaque osteosclerosis may be seen. Blood chemistry results indicate very high alkaline phosphatase levels with normal serum calcium and phosphorus. No known cure exists for this disease. Most cases are mild and asymptomatic; no treatment is necessary. In symptomatic cases, medications are administered to decrease bone reabsorption.

PITUITARY GLAND DISORDERS

Acromegaly

Acromegaly is an endocrine disorder caused by a disturbance in the function of the pituitary gland; this disorder primarily affects the skeletal system. It is more common in females than in males and most frequently occurs in individuals over age 40 years. This disorder is caused by excessive secretion of GH in adults, which is often the result of a pituitary adenoma. Acromegaly is a slowly progressive disease that may

be diagnosed years after the individual has symptoms. In adults, an increase in GH produces a thickening and coarsening of bone because the epiphyses have closed and bone cannot grow in length. Radiographic studies demonstrate an enlarged sella turcica and changes in the skull, often obliterating the diploë found between the inner and outer tables of cortical bone. However, MRI of the brain, with or without contrast enhancement, is the primary modality recommended by the ACR to evaluate the pituitary. Individuals with acromegaly have a prominent forehead and jaw, widened teeth, abnormally large, spadelike hands (Fig. 11-11), and a coarsening of facial features (Fig. 11-12). This disorder is frequently treated with a combination of surgery and radiotherapy to eradicate the adenoma. Although this is a slowly progressing disease, it may lead to premature death from associated cardiovascular and renal complications if it is not treated.

FIGURE 11-12 Skull radiograph depicting the changes caused by acromegaly.

Diabetes Insipidus

Central **diabetes insipidus** is one type of diabetes insipidus and is either neurogenic in origin because of a deficiency in vasopressin or nephrogenic in origin because of the insensitivity of the renal collecting tubules. This disorder results when the posterior pituitary gland secretes an insufficient level of ADH. In many cases, diabetes insipidus is secondary to interference with ADH synthesis and release such as that caused by a brain tumor, aneurysm, thrombus, or traumatic head injury affecting the hypothalamus, pituitary stalk, or posterior pituitary gland. CT and MRI are both helpful in demonstrating the presence of a lesion disturbing the balance of ADH.

Diabetes insipidus may also be genetic in nature, resulting from abnormalities of the vasopressin gene on chromosome 20. In some cases, a form of this disorder termed *nephrogenic diabetes insipidus* occurs as an acquired renal disorder associated with renal failure.

Symptoms of diabetes insipidus include frequent urination (polyuria) and increased thirst with frequent drinking. Decreased levels of ADH also create low urine osmolality in combination with high-normal plasma osmolality. Treatment of diabetes insipidus includes hormone replacement therapy (HRT).

Hypopituitarism

Hypopituitarism is the decreased level or absence of pituitary hormones originating from the anterior pituitary gland. The most common causes of this disorder are embryonic mutations of the prophet of pituitary transcription factor gene (*PROP-1*) or pituitary infarction, which may be caused by ischemic pituitary necrosis. It may also be associated with infarction caused by pregnancy (Sheehan syndrome), postpartum hemorrhage, shock, sickle cell disease, meningitis, syphilis, or head trauma. Signs and symptoms vary with the severity and types of hormones involved, and treatment includes the replacement of the hormone or hormones that are deficient. The ACR recommends enhanced and nonenhanced multiplanar MRI of the sellar region of the brain as the primary imaging modality. CT of the brain, with or without enhancement, may also be used if MRI is unavailable or contraindicated. Treatment includes hormone replacement therapy.

ADRENAL GLAND DISORDERS

Cushing Syndrome

Cushing syndrome results from a dysfunction within the adrenal cortex leading to hypersecretion of glucocorticoids from the anterior pituitary. In some patients undergoing steroid therapy, this syndrome may have an iatrogenic cause and will generally recede once the steroids are discontinued. Individuals with this disorder tend to have round, "moon" facies, with excess fat deposits in the neck and trunk regions of the body. The patient's skin is thin and does not heal well after injury. Female patients tend to have male characteristics because of an increased production of androgens, and their menstrual cycles are usually quite irregular. An analysis of plasma and urinary cortisol is the most frequent form of diagnostic testing, but enhanced or unenhanced MRI of the head may be used to assess the presence of pituitary adenomas, which may increase ACTH secretion and is one cause of Cushing syndrome. Treatment of Cushing syndrome depends on the point of origin, adrenal cortex versus pituitary gland, and focuses on correcting the hyperfunction. In some cases, radiotherapy may be used to treat pituitary adenomas, or surgical resection of the adrenocortical tumor may be required. If the condition is not treated, over half of the individuals with Cushing syndrome die within 5 years.

Addison Disease

Addison disease is a rare disease of primary adrenal insufficiency. It most frequently affects women between ages 30 and 60 years and generally results from an autoimmune destruction of the adrenal cortex, which impairs both glucocorticoid and mineralocorticoid production. It may also be caused by infection, neoplastic disease, or adrenal hemorrhage. Addison disease is characterized by elevated ACTH accompanied by inadequate corticosteroid synthesis. Signs and symptoms include weight loss, fatigue, weakness, nausea, diarrhea, low blood sugar, and low blood pressure leading to orthostatic hypotension. The most common diagnosis involves laboratory tests for levels of plasma cortisol and ACTH. Treatment includes the use of HRT in combination with a special diet. If left untreated, this disorder may progress to a life-threatening adrenal crisis.

Adrenal Carcinomas

Adrenal carcinomas are quite rare, but other types of cancers often metastasize to the adrenal glands. Lung cancers are the most common types of adrenal metastatic cancers, but cancers arising in the breast, kidney, pancreas, GI system, and lymphomas may also spread to the adrenal glands. Contrast-enhanced CT and MR studies are helpful in the diagnosis of adrenal masses. Sonography may also be employed. The risk of malignancy increases as the size of the tumor increases, so most masses are surgically removed.

PANCREATIC DISORDERS

Diabetes Mellitus

Diabetes mellitus is a syndrome that is associated with chronic hyperglycemia in combination with glucose intolerance and alterations in the metabolism of carbohydrates, fats, and proteins. Normal blood glucose levels range from 70 to 120 milligrams per deciliter (mg/dL), and fasting glucose levels greater than 126 mg/dL indicate the presence of this syndrome. The most common types of diabetes mellitus are type 1, caused by a defect in the primary β cells, and type 2, resulting in insulin resistance (Table 11-1).

Type 1 diabetes mellitus appears to be a genetic disorder, and although it accounts for only about 10% of cases of diabetes mellitus in the United States, it is one of the most common diseases in childhood. Type 1 diabetes can be further classified as type 1A and type 1B; type 1A is an autoimmune variation of the disease and is more common than type 1B. Type 1B is believed to be nonimmune in nature and generally occurs secondary to other pathologic processes. Type 1A diabetes is associated with a histocompatibility leukocyte antigen (HLA) marker, which has also been linked to other autoimmune endocrine diseases such as Graves and Addison diseases. Additionally, environmental factors such as viruses have also been linked to the development of type 1 diabetes.

Type 1 diabetes mellitus is often referred to as *juvenile diabetes* because most cases manifest before age 30 years. These young individuals produce little to no insulin because of an autoimmune destruction of the pancreatic β cells and are insulin dependent from a young age. Signs and symptoms of type 1 diabetes mellitus include weight loss, fluctuations in blood glucose levels, increased urination, excessive thirst, and an increased appetite. Ketoacidosis or increased levels of circulating ketones in the bloodstream, which are caused by the absence of insulin, are a common complication associated with this disease. The goal of treatment is to adequately control glucose levels without causing

TABLE 11-1	Epidemiology and Etiology of Diabetes Mellitus	
	Type 1 Diabetes: Primary β Cell Defect or Failure	**Type 2 Diabetes: Insulin Resistance with Inadequate Insulin Secretion**
Incidence		
Frequency	One of the most common childhood diseases (5% to 10% of all cases of diabetes mellitus)	Accounts for most cases (≈90% to 95%)
Change in incidences	Range from 29.5/100,000 (Finland) to 1.6/100,000 (Japan)	Prevalence rate in the United States (for age 18 years and older): 6.6%
	Increased incidences in British Isles, Finland, Norway, Denmark, Israel, Germany, and Poland; stable elsewhere	Prevalence for American Indian/Alaska Native; non-Hispanic black; Hispanic/Latino American; Asian American: 39.9%
		Incidence has risen in the United States since 1940
Characteristics		
Age at onset	Peak onset at age 11 to 13 years (slightly earlier for girls than for boys) Rare in children younger than 1 year and adults older than 30 years	Risk of developing diabetes increases after age 40 years; in general, incidence increases with age into the 70s; among Pima Indians, incidence peaks between ages 40 and 50 years, then falls
Gender	Similar in males and females	In the United States, more females than males
Racial distribution	Rates for whites 1.5 to 2 times higher than for nonwhites

Higher rates for those of Scandinavian descent than for those of central or southern European descent | Certain racial groups may be more likely to develop type 2 diabetes when exposed to a particular environment Common in migrant groups encountering a different environment (e.g., Polynesians moving from traditional to Western lifestyle) In the United States, risk is highest for American Indians; rates are higher for Pacific Islanders, Japanese, Puerto Ricans, Hispanics, and blacks than for whites |
Socioeconomic status	Conflicting data	A disease of the affluent in developing nations but more common among those of lower income and less education in the United States
Seasonal distribution	More new cases documented during fall and winter in the northern hemisphere	No known association
Childbirth association	No association documented	Effect of parity on subsequent development of type 2 diabetes varies among different populations
Obesity	Generally normal or underweight	Frequent contributing factor to precipitate type 2 diabetes among those susceptible; a major factor in populations recently exposed to Westernized environment Increased risk related to duration, degree, and distribution of obesity
Etiology		
Common theory	*Autoimmune:* genetic and environmental factors, resulting in gradual process of autoimmune destruction in genetically susceptible individuals *Nonautoimmune:* Unknown	Disease results from genetic susceptibility (although the precise gene or genes have not been determined) combined with environmental determinants and other risk factors Associated with long-duration obesity

Continued

TABLE 11-1	Epidemiology and Etiology of Diabetes Mellitus—cont'd	
	Type 1 Diabetes: Primary β Cell Defect or Failure	**Type 2 Diabetes: Insulin Resistance with Inadequate Insulin Secretion**
Heredity	Strong association with HLA-DQA and HLA-DQB genes Monogenic β-cell defect Risk to sibling: 5% to 10%; risk to offspring: 2% to 5%	Risk to first-degree relative (child or sibling): 10% to 15%
Presence of antibody	Islet cell autoantibodies (ICA) and/or autoantibodies to insulin, and autoantibodies to glutamic acid decarboxylase (GAD_{65}) and tyrosine phosphatases IA-2 and IA-2ß are present in 85% to 90% of individuals when fasting hyperglycemia is initially detected	Islet cell antibodies not present
Insulin resistance	Insulin resistance rare	Insulin resistance is generally caused by altered cellular metabolism and an intracellular postreceptor defect
Insulin secretion	Severe insulin deficiency or no insulin secretion at all	Typically increased at time of diagnosis, but progressively declines over the course of the illness

Data from: American Diabetes Association: Diagnosis and classification of diabetes mellitus, *Diabetes Care* 28(Suppl 1):S37–S42, 2005.

hypoglycemia. Therefore, treatment is varied and may include the use of immunosuppressive drugs, immunomodulation therapies, careful meal planning, exercise, and blood glucose checks multiple times per day in combination with daily insulin injections.

Type 2 diabetes mellitus is characterized as insulin-resistant diabetes with an inadequate secretion of insulin. It is much more common than type 1 in the United States, and the incidence of type 2 diabetes has doubled over the past 15 years. The risk of developing this type increases with age, especially after age 40 years. It is also more prevalent in women than in men and in blacks, Native Americans, Pacific Islanders, and Hispanics than in whites. Genetic susceptibility in combination with environmental factors is suspected to be the cause of this disease, as it is associated with obesity, hypertension, inactivity, and family history of the disease. Insulin resistance generally occurs as a result of

altered cellular metabolism versus a defect in the primary β cells of the pancreas.

Recently the medical community has identified **metabolic syndrome** as a precursor to type 2 diabetes mellitus. Metabolic syndrome is classified in individuals demonstrating three of the following five traits: (1) waist circumference greater than 40 inches in males and greater than 35 inches in females; (2) triglycerides 150 mg/dL or more; (3) high-density lipoprotein (HDL) cholesterol less than 40 mg/dL in males and less than 50 mg/dL in females; (4) blood pressure 130/85 mm Hg or greater; and (5) a fasting plasma glucose 100 mg/dL or greater. It is important to note that not all individuals with metabolic syndrome will develop type 2 diabetes mellitus, as individuals must also have genetic alterations that affect pancreatic β-cell function.

Individuals who have chronic type 2 diabetes for approximately 10 years also develop vascular complications. The risk for coronary artery disease (CAD), stroke, and peripheral vascular disease is increased for individuals with type 2 diabetes mellitus, and CAD is the most common cause of death for this patient population. The diagnosis and treatment of type 2 diabetes mellitus are similar to those for type 1.

THYROID AND PARATHYROID GLAND DISORDERS

Hyperthyroidism

Hyperthyroidism is most frequently caused by an autoimmune disorder termed **Graves disease**. In this disorder, the body creates antibodies that fight the thyroid TSH receptor, causing the thyroid gland to secrete excess amounts of this hormone. It is more common in females than in males, and a combination of genetic and environmental factors are linked to this disease. The normal hormonal regulatory mechanisms are inhibited by the production of thyroid-stimulating immunoglobulin antibodies leading to suppression of TSH.

Symptoms of this chronic disorder include an enlarged thyroid gland or goiter and changes to the eyes and skin. Patients may also exhibit nervousness and hyperactivity. Left untreated, hyperthyroidism may result in a critical event termed a *thyroid storm,* which is a life-threatening situation and must be treated within 48 hours. The diagnosis is made using laboratory tests to evaluate serum TSH levels in combination with a nuclear medicine ^{123}I thyroid uptake examination (Figs. 11-13 and 11-14). MRI of the brain, with or without contrast, with thin multiplanar sellar imaging may also be indicated. Treatments include antithyroid drugs, surgical resection of the thyroid gland, and, most commonly, the administration of radioactive iodine (^{123}I).

Hypothyroidism

Hypothyroidism is a common disorder of the thyroid gland and results from a deficiency of TH. This disorder has many causes and can affect individuals of any age or gender. However, primary hypothyroidism most commonly affects women over age 60 years. The disorder is commonly seen in patients diagnosed with autoimmune thyroiditis (Hashimoto disease). Deficiency of TH production results in an increase in TSH, which often results in a goiter. Hypothyroidism may also be iatrogenic in nature, resulting from treatment of a goiter through radioactive iodine therapy or surgical intervention. Although rarely seen in the United States, it may also be caused by iodine deficiency. Signs and symptoms of hypothyroidism occur slowly over many months and include a decreased energy level, cold intolerance, personality changes, and modest weight gain. This condition affects many organ systems throughout the body, including the neurologic system, reproductive system, hematologic system, cardiopulmonary system, renal system, GI system, musculoskeletal system, and skin. Laboratory tests provide useful information in the diagnosis of this disorder, and treatment generally involves HRT with synthetic hormones.

Thyroid Cancers

Although most neoplasms of the thyroid gland are benign, four types are malignant. These include (1) papillary, (2) follicular, (3) medullary, and (4) undifferentiated anaplastic cancers. Cancers of the thyroid are more common in younger individuals and in females. Females are two to three times more likely to develop malignant neoplasms of the thyroid, especially papillary carcinomas. A history of radiation exposure to the head, neck, or chest, especially in childhood, also increases the incidence of malignant thyroid lesions. Signs and symptoms of thyroid cancers include changes in voice and symptoms resulting from compression of the esophagus such as dysphagia, or compression of the trachea. Diagnosis is made using a nuclear medicine ^{123}I thyroid uptake examination (Fig. 11-15) in combination with serum laboratory analysis, and the diagnosis is generally confirmed by histologic assessment of tissue samples obtained from a sonographic-guided fine-needle aspiration biopsy.

FIGURE 11-13 A nuclear medicine ^{123}iodine thyroid uptake scan demonstrating elevated activity resulting from a goiter.

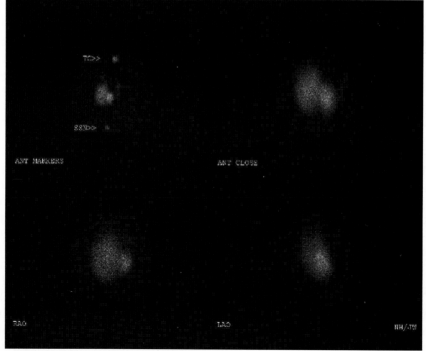

FIGURE 11-14 A nuclear medicine ^{123}iodine thyroid uptake scan demonstrating a hyperactive hot nodule.

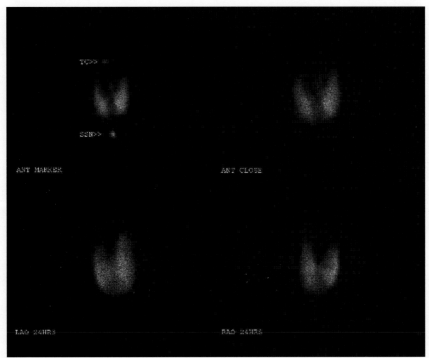

FIGURE 11-15 A nuclear medicine ^{123}iodine thyroid uptake scan demonstrating increased radioactive iodine uptake.

The most common treatment is the surgical removal of the thyroid gland followed by the administration of radioactive iodine (^{123}I) to ablate any remaining thyroid tissue and medication to suppress production of TSH.

Hyperparathyroidism

Hyperparathyroidism is a fairly common disease of the endocrine system that affects the skeletal system. This disease is often very mild and may go undetected for a long time. As with all metabolic bone diseases, the entire skeleton is affected in hyperparathyroidism, with some sites more affected than others.

The skeletal system is involved in the balance of serum calcium and phosphorus levels, and the body strives to keep this ratio constant. Hyperparathyroidism applies to any disorder that disrupts the calcium–phosphate ratio and results in an elevated level of PTH. Excess PTH secretion overstimulates the osteoclasts responsible for

bone removal, thus leading to bone destruction. This osteoclastic activity results in a decreased bone density, so a decrease in radiographic exposure is necessary to produce a high-quality radiographic image.

The three types of hyperparathyroidism are (1) primary hyperparathyroidism, (2) secondary hyperparathyroidism, and (3) hyperparathyroidism caused by ectopic production of a parathyroid-like hormone. Treatment varies with each specific cause of hyperparathyroidism and is very complex.

Primary hyperparathyroidism most frequently affects adults in their 30s or 50s and arises from an adenoma (Fig. 11-16), carcinoma, or hyperplasia of the parathyroid gland (Fig. 11-17). The excess production of PTH causes bone destruction, increased absorption of calcium by the intestines and kidneys, and an increase in urine calcium, which predisposes the individual to renal stones. The net effect of these reactions to the high level of PTH is an increase in serum

FIGURE 11-16 A nuclear medicine sestamibi parathyroid scan demonstrating an adenoma.

FIGURE 11-17 A nuclear medicine scan demonstrating hyperparathyroidism.

calcium with a decrease in serum phosphate. Individuals affected by primary hyperparathyroidism commonly have symptoms associated with hypercalcemia such as neuromuscular weakness and fatigue and may first demonstrate symptoms of renal colic as a result of renal stones or calcification of the kidneys (see later discussion of nephrocalcinosis). Radiographic investigation demonstrates subperiosteal bone reabsorption or osteopenia, especially in the diaphyses of the phalanges and clavicles. Bone reabsorption is also radiographically evident in teeth. Pathologic fractures may be present as a consequence of the softened bone matrix.

Secondary hyperparathyroidism (Fig. 11-18) represents a response to hypocalcemia, hyperphosphatemia, or hypomagnesemia. It is caused by a very complex metabolic disorder that is beyond the scope of this text and is most commonly seen in individuals with chronic renal disease caused by failure of glomerular filtration. Decreased renal function leads to a loss of the kidneys' ability to produce vitamin D and compromises their ability to excrete phosphate.

CT, sonography, and sestamibi nuclear medicine studies may be used in evaluating adenomas. Treatment usually requires surgical intervention in combination with medications such as bisphosphonates, corticosteroids, and calcimimetics.

Nephrocalcinosis

Disturbances of calcium metabolism, as in hyperparathyroidism, may result in **nephrocalcinosis,** a condition that is characterized by tiny deposits of calcium phosphate dispersed throughout the renal parenchyma. These deposits are readily seen on an intravenous urogram and even on plain radiographs of the abdomen. Calcium may also be deposited throughout the parenchyma as a result of tissue damaged by some other disease process or injury. If a metabolic cause exists, treatment of the specific metabolic condition indirectly treats nephrocalcinosis. Treatment designed to lower serum calcium levels is also important.

FIGURE 11-18 Radiograph of the hand of an individual with secondary hyperparathyroidism. Note the subperiosteal reabsorption of bone and calcification of the arteries of the hand.

PATHOLOGY SUMMARY
The Endocrine System

Imaging Modalities of Choice	Additive or Subtractive Pathology
Bone mineral densitometry	Subtractive
Bone mineral densitometry	Subtractive
Radiography	Both
MRI with and without contrast, CT	Additive
MRI with or without contrast, CT	
MRI with or without contrast, CT	
MRI with or without contrast	
^{123}I thyroid uptake, MRI with or without contrast	Increased activity
^{123}I thyroid uptake	Increased activity
CT, sonography, and sestamibi nuclear medicine studies	
Radiography	Additive
CT, MRI, and sonography	

CT, computed tomography; *^{123}I,* iodine-123; *MRI,* magnetic resonance imaging.

REVIEW QUESTIONS

1. Medical treatment designed to lower serum calcium levels is important in the management of:
   a. Cystitis
   b. Nephrocalcinosis
   c. Nephrosclerosis
   d. Polycystic kidney disease

2. *Osteopenia* is a term used to describe the radiographic appearance associated with a decrease in bone density and is associated with:
   a. Craniosynostoses
   b. Osteopetrosis
   c. Osteoporosis
   d. Scoliosis

3. Metabolic actions of the endocrine system in response to changes in blood chemistry best defines _____ stimuli.
   a. Hormonal
   b. Humoral
   c. Neural

4. Corticosteroid production occurs in the:
   a. Adrenal cortex
   b. Pancreas
   c. Pineal gland
   d. Thyroid gland

5. α-cells in the pancreas produce:
   a. Glucagon
   b. Gonadocorticosteroids
   c. Insulin
   d. Thyroxine

6. Acromegaly is a condition resulting from disorder of the _____ gland.
   a. Adrenal
   b. Pineal
   c. Pituitary
   d. Thymus

7. Graves disease is associated with:
   a. Hyperthyroidism
   b. Hyperparathyroidism
   c. Hypothyroidism
   d. Hypoparathyroidism

8. Type 1 diabetes mellitus is most common in:
   a. Adults
   b. Children

9. Describe the mechanism behind the development of osteoporosis.

10. Compare and contrast T- and Z-scores obtained from bone mineral densitometry examinations.

12

Traumatic Disease

LEARNING OBJECTIVES

On completion of Chapter 12, the reader should be able to:

- Differentiate among level I, II, and III trauma centers and the role each plays in the emergency medical system.
- Define common terminology associated with traumatic disease.
- Discuss the roles of various imaging modalities in the evaluation and treatment of traumatic injuries.

- Describe, in general, the radiographic appearance of each of the given pathologies.
- Classify skeletal fractures according to the various classifications discussed in this chapter and describe the healing process associated with skeletal trauma.
- Describe the general methods used for the treatment of skeletal fractures.

OUTLINE

KEY TERMS

Atelectasis
Avulsion fractures
Basilar skull fractures
Blowout fracture
Closed fracture
Closed reduction

Coma
Comminuted fracture
Compression fractures
Concussion
Contrecoup lesion
Contusions

Coup lesion	Linear fractures
Depressed fracture	Luxation
Dislocation	Nonaccidental trauma
Fatigue fractures	Noncomminuted fracture
Fracture	Occult fracture
Greenstick fracture	Open or compound fracture
Growth plate fractures	Open reduction
Hangman's fracture	Open reduction internal fixation
Hematoma	Pneumoperitoneum
Impacted fracture	Pneumothorax
Incomplete fractures	Slipped capital femoral epiphysis
Jefferson fracture	Stress fractures
Legg-Calvé-Perthes disease	Subluxation
Level I trauma centers	Torus fracture
Level II trauma centers	Traumatic brain injury
Level III trauma centers	Whiplash
Level IV trauma centers	

In the United States, injury is one of the leading causes of death and disability, and trauma is the most common cause of death for individuals between the ages of 1 and 44 years, accounting for over 48,000 deaths in 2008. Additional information can be obtained at the Centers for Disease Control and Prevention (CDC) National Center for Health Statistics Web site at www.cdc.gov/nchs/hus.htm. The annual medical cost associated with trauma injury is approximately $200 billion and is classified by several categories. Some examples are as follows:

- Death $4,360,000
- Incapacitating injury $220,300
- Nonincapacitating evident injury $56,200
- Possible injury $26,700
- No injury $2400

These costs are a measure of the dollars spent and income not received because of accidents, injuries, or fatalities. These costs also demonstrate the importance of prevention strategies initiated by the National Safety Council.

The American College of Surgeons (ACS) Committee on Trauma periodically reviews its guidelines to ensure optimal patient care by classifying medical centers and hospitals according to their ability to treat various injuries and by publishing guidelines for trauma management. Trauma results primarily from motor vehicle accidents (MVAs), unintentional accidents at home or in the workplace, gunshot wounds, stab wounds, physical altercations, domestic violence, and physical abuse. According to the Centers for Disease Control and Prevention (CDC), hospital emergency departments play a critical role in the U.S. health care system, from treatment of minor trauma to, more recently, the first-line defense against bioterrorism.

Deaths from traumatic injuries have a trimodal distribution (Fig. 12-1), with the first critical period occurring seconds after the injury. Death during this period results from lacerations of the brain and spinal cord or the heart and great vessels. The second critical period occurs during the first 4 hours after the injury, with death generally resulting from intracranial hemorrhage, lacerations of the liver and spleen, or significant blood loss from multiple injuries. The third critical period occurs weeks after the injury,

FIGURE 12-1 Distribution of trauma deaths.

when death results from infection and multiple organ failure.

A well-designed emergency medical system (EMS) provides for prehospital care, acute hospital care, and rehabilitative care. Medical facilities are classified as level I, level II, or level III trauma centers based on the availability of specialized medical personnel and equipment. When patients are triaged (medically screened to determine their relative priority for treatment), at the site of an accident, their injuries are classified as life-threatening, urgent, or nonemergent. Multiple injuries most likely occur in conjunction with severe head injuries. These patients must be treated with utmost care. Before a trauma victim is transported, a clear airway must be established, acute bleeding must be controlled, and the patient must be immobilized to avoid displacing fractures of the skeletal system. Immobilization of the spine is paramount to avoiding further injury to the spinal cord, and this is accomplished with the use of splints, backboards with head blocks, cervical collars, and special air splint suits.

The EMS ensures that the trauma victim is taken to the closest appropriate medical facility to receive the proper medical care for the injuries, but not necessarily to the closest hospital. Once the patient arrives at the proper medical facility, another careful assessment is necessary. This secondary triage assessment includes evaluation of the patient's state of consciousness, vital signs (blood pressure, pulse, temperature, and respiration), pupil size and reaction to light, and motor activity of the extremities. Cross-table lateral cervical spine radiography or computed tomography (CT) of the cervical spine is necessary to assess any damage to the cervical spine before the patient is moved. In addition, radiographs of the chest, abdomen, and skeletal system must be obtained to evaluate the extent of injuries. Although national vital statistics show that only 5% of all trauma victims have life-threatening injuries, these types of injuries are responsible for 50% of all in-hospital trauma-related deaths.

LEVEL I, II, AND III TRAUMA CENTERS

The primary hospitals in the trauma system are **level I trauma centers**. Such medical centers can provide total care for all injuries. Key elements of a level I trauma center include 24-hour in-house coverage by general surgeons and prompt availability of care in specialties such as orthopedic surgery, neurosurgery, anesthesiology, emergency medicine, radiology, internal medicine, and critical care. Other capabilities include cardiac, hand, pediatric, and microvascular surgeries and hemodialysis. The level I trauma center provides leadership in prevention, public education, and continuing education of the trauma team members, as well as serving as a research facility to help direct new innovations in trauma care. Level I trauma centers are generally located in large metropolitan areas and serve as both primary care and tertiary care institutions. Another stipulation for a health care institution to be classified as a level I trauma center is that it must treat 1200 admissions or 240 major trauma patients per year.

Level II trauma centers are the most common trauma facilities serving as community trauma centers. These institutions can handle the majority of trauma cases and transport patients to level I facilities only when necessary. Level II facilities include 24-hour immediate coverage by general surgeons, as well as coverage by the specialties of orthopedic surgery, neurosurgery, anesthesiology, emergency medicine, radiology, and critical care. More critical patients with needs such as cardiac surgery, hemodialysis, or microvascular surgery may be referred to a level I trauma center. These medical centers are generally community hospitals located in smaller cities and towns and provide a valuable service.

Level III trauma centers are usually located in remote rural areas and serve communities that do not have a level II center. A level III trauma center has a demonstrated ability to provide prompt assessment, resuscitation, stabilization of injured patients, and emergency operations. The key components of a level III trauma center include 24-hour immediate coverage by emergency medicine physicians and the prompt availability of general surgeons and anesthesiologists. The level III trauma center has formal transfer agreements for patients requiring more comprehensive care at a level I or level II trauma center.

As determined by the ACS Committee on Trauma, a level IV trauma center has a demonstrated ability to provide advanced trauma life support (ATLS) prior to transfer of patients to a higher-level trauma center. A level IV trauma center has basic emergency department facilities to implement ATLS protocols and 24-hour laboratory coverage. Transfer to higher-level trauma centers follows the guidelines outlined in formal transfer agreements.

IMAGING CONSIDERATIONS

Radiography

Conventional radiography is one of the first imaging modalities required in the management of a trauma victim. A cross-table lateral cervical spine radiograph may be obtained to evaluate the presence or absence of a fracture before the patient is moved. Portable chest, abdominal, and pelvic radiographs are also generally obtained as soon as the patient arrives in the emergency department.

Conventional radiography is still the primary means of evaluating skeletal trauma. Additional information about damage to the muscle, tendons, ligaments, and soft tissue structures is obtained using magnetic resonance imaging (MRI). CT and nuclear medicine studies may also be employed to identify subtle skeletal fractures.

Computed Tomography

The high-energy impact associated with most MVAs often results in injury to the neck and head, so CT is an important tool in assessing the trauma victim. CT is excellent for imaging acute cerebral hemorrhage and fractures of the skull and facial bones. Guidelines governing the use of CT in the case of head trauma include the Canadian rule, which suggests that injuries with a Glasgow Coma Scale (GCS) score of 13 to 15 should be evaluated by CT, as well as the more comprehensive New Orleans helical computed tomography (HCT) rule. The New Orleans HCT rule mandates CT examination of patients with a GCS score of 15 in combination with any one of the following: headache, vomiting, age above 60 years, drug or alcohol intoxication, persistent amnesia, visible trauma above the clavicle, or seizure. In lieu of the increased awareness of radiation dose, patient protection, and public safety campaigns such as Image Gently and Image Wisely, the ACR Appropriateness Criteria now include a relative radiation level (RRL) for imaging procedures for both adult and pediatric patients.

With the prevalent use of multidetector CT (MDCT), CT evaluation of the cervical spine has become a standard procedure in evaluating trauma patients. The National Emergency X-radiography Utilization Study (NEXUS) and Canadian C-Spine Review (CCR) concluded that CT demonstrates 99.6% sensitivity for the identification of cervical spine fractures. CT has replaced conventional radiography as the first-line approach to imaging the cervical spine, with

FIGURE 12-2 A computed tomography scan of coronal reconstruction of a C2 fracture.

the meta-analysis of research studies performed in 2005 indicating that CT demonstrates a much higher specificity of 98% compared with a specificity of 52% for conventional radiography of the cervical spine. Axial CT of the cervical spine is performed in conjunction with coronal and sagittal reconstruction to fully assess the areas of interest (Fig. 12-2). With more sensitive imaging techniques now available, CT and MRI have revealed a significant number of fractures and other injuries that are not diagnosed with radiography. CT evaluation can reduce hospital admission rates and results in more efficient surgical intervention by accurately identifying the presence and extent of injury in the trauma patient.

Blunt trauma to the abdomen is best evaluated with CT or abdominal sonography. Trauma to the urinary system occurs in about 10% to 15% of patients who experience blunt trauma to the lower abdomen and pelvis. In cases of hematuria, CT is preferred to conventional intravenous pyelography (IVP) or intravenous urography (IVU). Although the use of oral contrast agents for abdominal CT is debatable, intravenous contrast is routinely employed to allow evaluation of vascular injuries and to better visualize the spleen, pancreas, and kidneys. In addition, in cases of blunt abdominal trauma, CT is better able to visualize fractures of the transverse

processes of the lumbar spine, often missed on conventional spine radiography. CT, in combination with a conventional anteroposterior (AP) pelvic radiography, is also used to assess pelvic fractures commonly associated with abdominal injury (Fig. 12-3, *A*). In cases of pelvic fractures, it is also imperative to identify any possible trauma to the urinary bladder and to perform CT (see Fig. 12-3, *B*) to determine the extent of injury. Occasionally, emergent cystography may be performed to visualize any injury to the urinary bladder. In cases of penetrating trauma to the abdomen, angiography may also be used to identify the extent of injury. Sonography plays little or no role in the evaluation of genitourinary trauma. Several studies have documented the inability of sonography to detect injuries of the kidney or bladder in trauma patients.

TRAUMA OF THE VERTEBRAL COLUMN AND HEAD

The initial management of patients with head and spinal trauma is critical. Key items to assess at the scene of the accident include the mechanism of injury and changes in the patient's neurologic status. A neurologic assessment using the GCS should be conducted at the scene, and cervical spine injury should be assumed to be present until it is ruled out by radiologic investigation. A cervical spine fracture can be present in up to 20% of patients with a severe head injury.

The head and neck should be immobilized, and care must be taken if intubation is necessary. Hyperextension injuries of the head and neck or direct trauma to the neck may injure the carotid arteries. Bleeding must be controlled to prevent shock, which may worsen the head injury. Once the patient arrives in the emergency department, cervical spine radiographs or a CT scan of the cervical spine must be obtained. CT of the head may also be indicated, especially if the patient is comatose.

Many studies have been conducted regarding the effectiveness of airbags and seatbelts in preventing head and neck fractures in the event of an MVA. By far, those who do not use any

FIGURE 12-3 A, Anteroposterior pelvic view from a motor vehicle accident trauma victim demonstrates multiple fractures. **B,** Computed tomography sagittal reconstruction of the same patient as in *A*, demonstrating multiple fractures of the ilium.

protective device sustain the most injuries. Those who depend only on the airbags sustain the second largest number of injuries to the head and face, followed by those who use only a seatbelt. The most effective protection results from the use of both protective devices. In addition, individuals using only a lap-type seatbelt have a high incidence of lumbar spine injuries, and individuals wearing only a shoulder belt without a lap belt sustain more cervical spine injuries.

Injuries to the Vertebral Column

The causes of vertebral column injuries include direct trauma and hyperextension–flexion injuries (whiplash injuries). Radiographic indications of spinal column injuries include the interruption of smooth, continuous lines formed by the vertebrae stacked on one another (Fig. 12-4). Either a dull or sharp pain in the posterior neck is the primary manifestation of a whiplash injury. The pain may radiate down the arms or back. Muscle spasm as a result of trauma may cause a reversal or straightening of the normal spine curvatures.

Imaging of whiplash injuries is limited to soft tissue studies, with the exclusion of fractures and dislocations being the first priority. The loss of lordosis is the most common finding on radiographs of patients with whiplash injuries (Fig. 12-5).

Perhaps the most common condition of the vertebral column is generalized back pain, typically in the lumbar area. This may result from injury to the area or from degenerative disease. Such back pain may not always result from bone involvement. Disk disease may cause muscle spasm, with pain referral throughout the back or down the legs. Finally, back pain may be secondary to referred pain from the hip.

Compression fractures are the most frequent type of injury involving a vertebral body. Usually, the damage is limited to the upper portion of the vertebral body, particularly to the anterior margin. Such fractures generally occur in the thoracic and lumbar vertebrae (Fig. 12-6), with the most common site being T11-T12 in the thoracic spine and T12-L1 at the thoracolumbar juncture. Compression fractures are also associated with

FIGURE 12-4 A, A lateral cervical spine radiograph of an individual who was involved in a motor vehicle accident and has an endotracheal tube in place. **B,** The same radiograph as in A, but imaged in an inverted mode to assist in evaluation. This is one major advantage of digital imaging.

FIGURE 12-5 A lateral cervical spine radiograph of a patient involved in motor vehicle accident. Note the loss of the normal lordotic curvature indicates a whiplash injury.

osteoporosis and range from mild to severe. More severe fractures may cause significant pain, leading to inability to perform activities of daily living to life-threatening decline in the older patient. Cervical spine injuries may involve the odontoid process, usually at the junction of the odontoid and the body of the second cervical vertebra (see Fig. 12-2). A **hangman's fracture** (Fig. 12-7) is a fracture of the arch of the second cervical vertebra and is usually accompanied by anterior subluxation of the second cervical vertebra on the third cervical vertebra. A hangman's fracture, sometimes referred to as *traumatic spondylosis,* results from acute hyperextension of the head.

Jefferson fracture was first described as a "burst fracture" of the first cervical vertebra (atlas). It generally occurs as a result of a severe axial force that causes compression, as in a diving accident. The vertebral arch literally bursts. Radiographically, particular attention needs to be paid to the transverse longitudinal ligament by reviewing the lateral masses on the open-mouth odontoid projection. MRI is the preferred imaging modality to best examine the transverse longitudinal ligament.

Radiography or CT of the trauma patient with vertebral trauma is critical. Statistically, 5% to 10% of patients with one spinal fracture have

FIGURE 12-6 A lateral lumbar radiograph demonstrating compression fractures of the second and fourth lumbar vertebral bodies with no apparent fracture of the posterior elements of the spine.

FIGURE 12-7 A lateral cervical spine radiograph demonstrating a typical hangman's fracture with disruption of the spinal laminar line at C2 with the spinous process of C2 displaced posteriorly.

another fracture elsewhere in the vertebral column. Fractures and dislocations of the spine are classified as stable or unstable. The spine may be visualized as two columns, with the anterior column composed of vertebral bodies and intervertebral disks and the posterior column composed of the posterior elements (e.g., spinous processes, lamina). If either the anterior column or the posterior column of the spine is fractured or dislocated, the injury is classified as stable. However, if both columns are involved in the

injury, it is classified as unstable. In all cases, the patient should be immobilized until cross-table lateral radiographs or CT images have been obtained and cleared by a physician. To rule out possible fractures and dislocations, lateral cervical spine radiography must include all seven vertebrae in their entirety, including spinous processes and intervertebral disk spaces. At times, this may require assistance in depressing the patient's shoulders or the use of the specialized cervicothoracic lateral projection (Twining or swimmer's method) to clearly demonstrate the entire seventh cervical vertebra and the upper thoracic vertebra in a lateral projection. Additional trauma projections of the cervical spine such as the pillar projection or trauma oblique projection may be requested to better demonstrate the complex anatomy of the spine. Trauma cervical spine radiographs are analyzed to evaluate (1) the size, shape, and alignment of the vertebral bodies and spinous processes, (2) the position and integrity of the odontoid process of C2, (3) the orientation and clarity of the facet joints, (4) the relationship of C1 to the occipital bone, (5) the alignment of the spinolaminal lines, and (6) any prevertebral swelling.

FIGURE 12-8 An axial computed tomography scan demonstrating a comminuted fracture of a vertebral body and showing the location of each fragment.

FIGURE 12-9 A sagittal reconstruction computed tomography scan performed postoperatively after the repair of a comminuted fracture of L1.

Spinal injury often results in a loss of neurologic function that may be temporary or permanent, depending on the cause of the dysfunction. Compression of the spinal cord by contusion or hemorrhage leads to rapid swelling of the spinal cord. This causes a rise in intradural pressure and causes temporary neurologic dysfunction. This temporary loss of neurologic function usually resolves in several days. However, lacerations of the spinal cord or transection of the cord results in permanent damage because the severed nerves do not regenerate. Laceration of the spinal cord above the fifth cervical vertebra is almost always fatal, and lacerations below this region result in permanent paralysis. Patients with lacerations or transection of the cord develop immediate flaccid paralysis with loss of all sensation and reflex activity, which gradually changes to spastic paraplegia within days.

Fractures or dislocations of the vertebrae may impinge on the spinal cord and cause significant damage. The responsibility of the radiographer in terms of proper patient handling and obtaining diagnostic-quality images cannot be overemphasized. CT plays a vital role in the diagnosis and treatment of vertebral fractures, dislocations, and associated problems (Fig. 12-8). In certain situations, MRI may be used to evaluate the extent of ligamentous and soft tissue injury or injury to the spinal cord.

Stable injuries to the spine are treated with complete bed rest and steroids until swelling and pain subside. Unstable injuries are immobilized with traction until bone and soft tissue structures have healed. Cervical radiographs are often obtained to demonstrate proper alignment while the patient is in traction. Surgery may also be necessary for internal fixation of the fractures or to remove displaced fragments and decompress the spinal cord. CT of the spine is used preoperatively to serve as a road map for the surgeon because this imaging modality clearly demonstrates the size, number, and location of various fracture fragments. It may also be used postoperatively to demonstrate the success of the surgical procedure (Fig. 12-9).

Injuries to the Skull and Brain

The anatomy surrounding the delicate brain generally protects it well under normal conditions. The diploic arrangement of the calvaria, the mechanical buffering action of cerebrospinal fluid, and the tough dura mater all work to prevent brain injury. Despite this protection, sufficient force to the skull may cause injury to the brain. Head trauma is the major neurologic cause of mortality and morbidity in individuals under 50 years of age.

Head trauma may result in skull fractures, brain injury, or a combination of the two. The role of plain film radiography in evaluation of head trauma is rather limited, but CT allows rapid assessment of the nature of any brain injury. Assessment of the state of the brain after head injury is more crucial than that of the skull. For trauma victims, routine skull radiography may be delayed to allow treatment of the complications of brain injury readily diagnosed by CT. Skull fractures visualized by either modality are often seen with accompanying hematomas. If patients sustain an open skull fracture, they are at risk for development of meningitis or brain abscesses. Regardless of the imaging modality used, the technologist must constantly observe a patient with a head injury while performing an examination. Any change noted in the patient's condition should be reported immediately.

Cerebral Cranial Fractures. The term *cerebral cranial fractures* usually refers to fractures in the calvaria of the skull. Vascular markings in the skull, either venous or arterial, are routinely demonstrated as linear translucencies and may occasionally be mistaken for cerebral cranial fractures (Fig. 12-10). In most cases, a fracture appears more translucent than a vascular marking because a fracture traverses the full thickness of the skull. Although the edges of the fractures may branch abruptly, they may be seen to fit together, whereas venous channels have irregular edges that cannot be fitted together. The sutures between the individual cranial bones remain visible radiographically, even after they become fused. To an untrained eye these sutures may also resemble a fracture.

In most cases, the location of the skull fracture is more important than the extent of the fracture. If the fracture crosses an artery, an arterial bleed may occur, resulting in an epidural hematoma. A

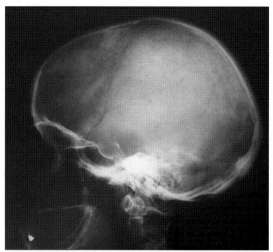

FIGURE 12-10 A lateral skull radiograph demonstrating normal vascular markings within the cerebral cranium.

fracture that enters the mastoid air cells or a sinus communicates with a potentially infected space and may lead to infection, possibly resulting in encephalitis or meningitis.

Fractures visible after skull trauma are generally classified as linear, depressed, or basilar skull fractures. **Linear fractures** appear as straight, sharply defined, nonbranching lines and are intensely radiolucent (Fig. 12-11). Up to 80% of all skull fractures are linear fractures. A **depressed fracture** appears as a curvilinear density because the fracture edges overlap (Fig. 12-12). These fractures are caused by high-velocity impact by small objects. Injury to the cerebral cortex may result, causing bleeding into the subarachnoid space. A depressed fracture is best demonstrated when the x-ray beam is directed tangentially to the fracture.

Basilar skull fractures are very difficult to demonstrate radiographically. The presence of air–fluid levels in the sphenoid sinus or clouding of the mastoid air cells is often the only radiographic finding suggesting a fracture. Therefore, it is important to include cross-table lateral skull radiography with the trauma skull radiographic series. CT and MRI are often used to better identify basilar area fractures and associated soft tissue damage within the skull (Fig. 12-13).

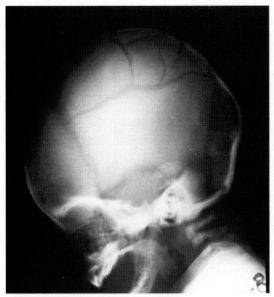

FIGURE 12-11 A lateral skull radiograph of a 3-month-old infant with a history of striking his head on a bathtub. The radiograph reveals a linear skull fracture of the parietal bone.

FIGURE 12-13 A computed tomography scan demonstrating basilar skull fracture with air fluid levels in the sphenoid sinus.

FIGURE 12-12 A lateral skull radiograph of a child who was struck in the head with a baseball bat. The radiograph demonstrates a depressed fracture of the occipital bone.

Brain Trauma. In addition to brain injury from a penetration wound (as could happen with a fracture), brain injury may also occur from acceleration and rapid deceleration of the head, which is termed a *closed head injury* or **traumatic brain injury** (TBI). With head trauma, the brain is traumatically shaken within the cranium and subjected to forces of compression, acceleration, and deceleration. Brain tissues are injured from compression, tension, and shearing, with the last perhaps most important (Fig. 12-14). The superficial cerebrum in the frontal, temporal, and occipital regions is most often affected.

TBI is a serious public health problem in the United States. Each year, traumatic brain injuries contribute to a substantial number of deaths and cases of permanent disability. Recent data from the CDC show that, on average, approximately 1.7 million people sustain a TBI annually. This incidence has increased significantly with athletics-related activities, and ongoing research is focusing on athletes from the junior high to professional levels.

FIGURE 12-14 A T2-weighted magnetic resonance imaging scan demonstrates a shearing injury of the corpus callosum (*arrow*) and a small subdural hematoma on the lateral margins of the brain in this young boy who had fallen and failed to regain consciousness.

After a blow to the head, an individual may experience temporary loss of consciousness and reflexes. This widespread paralysis of brain function is known as a **concussion** and is characterized by headache, vertigo, and vomiting. Higher mental functions may be impaired for several hours, with the patient remembering little of the events surrounding the concussion. A strong tendency toward spontaneous and complete recovery exists because no structural damage to the brain occurs. Recovery generally takes place in less than 24 hours. Treatment is conservative once assessment (usually by CT) has ruled out any hemorrhage or fracture. Bed rest and possible admission to the hospital are the usual means of dealing with concussion.

A brain contusion may also result from a direct blow to the head. This bruising of brain parenchyma is more serious than a concussion. A contusion formed on the side of the head where the trauma occurs is called a **coup lesion**, and one formed on the opposite side of the skull in reference to the site of trauma is a **contrecoup lesion** (Fig. 12-15). **Contusions** are characterized by neuron damage, edema, and punctate (pinpoint punctures or depressions) hemorrhaging. On CT, contusions appear as small, ill-defined

G.J. Wassilchenko

FIGURE 12-15 Coup and contrecoup brain injury following blunt trauma. **a,** Coup injury: impact against object. **b,** Contrecoup injury: impact within skull. These injuries occur in one continuous motion—the head strikes the wall (coup) and then rebounds (contrecoup).

foci of increased density (Fig. 12-16). Subdural or epidural hematomas may occur in conjunction with a contusion and result in increased intracranial pressure that may be life-threatening. Signs seen in the patient with a contusion include drowsiness, confusion, and agitation. Hemiparesis and unequal pupil size may also be seen. CT

FIGURE 12-16 An axial computed tomography scan of a young male patient demonstrates hemorrhagic contusions of the brain as a result of a car accident.

plays a major role in the diagnosis of hematomas resulting from contusions, providing ready visualization of hemorrhagic blood, as described in the following section. Treatment is generally conservative, centering on prevention of shock, control of edema, and drainage of any hematoma present.

Persistence of loss of consciousness for more than 24 hours is known as a **coma**. This is usually a serious condition and may be fatal. Comas result from trauma to the head as well as from nontraumatic metabolic malfunctions or circulatory problems that prevent sufficient blood flow to the brain. Diagnosis related to a coma may involve use of CT, MRI, positron emission tomography (PET), or fusion imaging and focuses on determining, if possible, the cause of the coma. Treatment then rests on success in treating and alleviating the cause of the coma.

Hematomas of the Brain. As noted earlier, brain trauma may result in hemorrhaging of blood from a ruptured artery or vein. Although venous bleeding occurs more slowly than arterial bleeding, both types of hemorrhaging and resultant edema of the brain cause an increase in intracranial pressure. Because the skull's structure does not allow expansion, the increased pressure displaces the brain toward its opening, the foramen magnum. This trauma to the brain results in serious neurologic consequences or even death if not treated promptly. CT plays the major imaging role in diagnosis of the hemorrhaging.

A **hematoma** is a collection of blood; four primary types of cerebral hematomas have been identified: epidural, subdural (Fig. 12-17), subarachnoid, and intracerebral. The highest mortality rate is associated with an *epidural (extradural) hematoma* (Fig. 12-18). Even when promptly recognized and treated, it has a mortality rate of up to 30%. An epidural hematoma results from a torn artery, usually the middle meningeal artery, with blood pooling between the bony skull and the dura mater. Most commonly, the artery or its branches are torn by a fracture of the thin, squamous portion of temporal bone. In more than 80% of cases, the skull fracture is visible radiographically. As an arterial bleed, it accumulates rapidly and quickly causes neurologic symptoms, including early coma. It is seen on CT scans as an increased density, generally occupying a small area with a sharply convex appearance. It is often accompanied by a fracture of the skull or facial bones. If not diagnosed and surgically treated quickly, the outcome is fatal as a result of brain displacement and herniation.

A *subdural hematoma* is positioned between the dura mater and the arachnoid meningeal layers (Figs. 12-19 and 12-20). It usually follows blunt trauma to the frontal or occipital lobes of the skull and results from tearing of the subdural veins connecting the cerebral cortex and the dural sinuses. As a venous hemorrhage, it bleeds much more slowly than an epidural hematoma. In the acute stage, it is seen on CT as a curvilinear area of increased density on parts or all of the cerebral hemispheres. It pushes the brain away from the skull and causes a mass effect (i.e., brain shift across the midline), with an accompanying shift of the ventricles. In the subacute stage (up to several days old), it appears on CT as a decreased or isodense fluid collection. In the

A

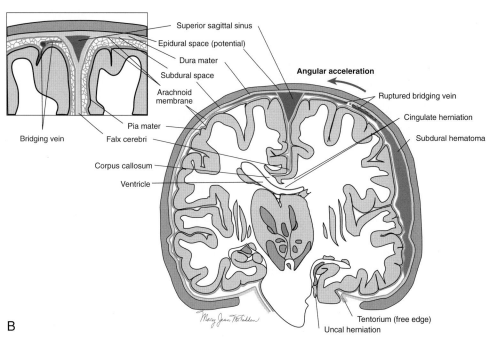

B

FIGURE 12-17 A, Epidural hematoma and **B,** subdural hematoma.

FIGURE 12-18 A noncontrast axial computed tomography view of this young male patient injured in an motor vehicle accident readily demonstrates a large epidural hematoma.

FIGURE 12-19 Computed tomography demonstration of a large subdural hematoma outside the brain tissue in the left frontoparietal area of this 76-year-old man.

chronic state (2 to 3 weeks old), the surface of the hematoma becomes concave. Delayed coma may occur with a subdural hematoma.

A *subarachnoid hematoma* accumulates between the arachnoid layer and the thin pia mater that invests the brain. It occurs most frequently at the vertex, where the greatest brain movement occurs in trauma, and it results from tearing of small vessels. In most head trauma cases, a subarachnoid hemorrhage is usually limited to one or two sulci, where it has a dense appearance (Fig. 12-21). Less commonly, the rupture of a major cerebral vessel results in a subarachnoid hematoma.

An *intracerebral hematoma* may result from trauma as well as from nontraumatic causes such as a ruptured hemangioma or stroke (cerebrovascular accident [CVA]). Common sites after trauma are the frontal, temporal, and occipital lobes of the brain. Small parenchymal vessels

tear as a result of coup and contrecoup forces. An intracerebral hematoma is seen on CT as an increased density within the brain causing significant mass effect (Fig. 12-22) and may have an accompanying subarachnoid component. These hematomas develop edema around them as time passes and are slowly reabsorbed if the patient survives.

Diagnosis of hematomas is made primarily through clinical history and neurologic signs and symptoms. As noted, CT and MRI play a major role in ready visualization of bleeding. Angiography may be used to visualize any defects in the cerebral vasculature. Treatment is often conservative unless active bleeding or significant mass effect is present, in which case an opening in the skull may be created surgically to allow drainage of blood and prevent complications. Prevention of infection and meningitis is important in the case of a fractured skull.

FIGURE 12-20 A, A T1-weighted sagittal magnetic resonance imaging (MRI) view demonstrates a large subdural hematoma as well as a temporal lobe infarct (*arrow*). The white versus gray appearance of the hematoma distinguishes subacute (fresh) from older blood. **B,** A T1-weighted axial MRI view with gadolinium demonstrates a large, bilateral subdural hematoma in this 67-year-old man. **C,** A T1-weighted coronal MRI view with gadolinium demonstrates the same bilateral subdural hematoma. The arrow indicates the right-sided temporal lobe infarct.

FIGURE 12-21 A, B, Axial magnetic resonance imaging (MRI) images demonstrating a subarachnoid hemorrhage as indicated by the sulci opacified by blood. **C,** A sagittal fluid-attenuated inversion recovery (FLAIR) MRI image of the same patient.

FIGURE 12-22 A massive intracerebral hematoma that occurred spontaneously in this 63-year-old woman. The patient died within a few hours after the bleed began.

SKELETAL TRAUMA

Fractures

A fracture is a discontinuity of bone caused by mechanical forces either applied to the bone or transmitted directly along the line of a bone. When a fracture occurs, blood vessels are broken as a result of the break in the endosteum and periosteum. As blood and lymph and tissue fluids infiltrate this area, swelling and pain result. Such soft tissue swelling is a major clue to diagnosis (Fig. 12-23). Digital imaging is an asset in evaluating the soft tissue structures surrounding a skeletal fracture because one image can be manipulated to demonstrate details of both soft tissue and bone.

Radiography is extremely important in the evaluation of skeletal trauma and serves several

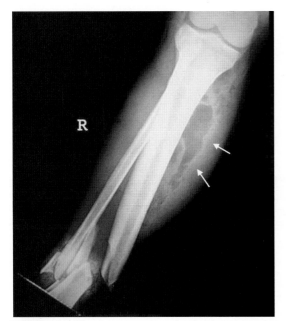

FIGURE 12-23 A computed radiography image of a comminuted fracture of the tibia and fibula with associated soft tissue edema.

FIGURE 12-24 A postreduction lateral wrist image showing proper alignment in the cast.

purposes. The most obvious of these is to diagnose the presence of a fracture or dislocation. If a fracture is present, for example, a determination can be made as to whether underlying bone is normal or whether the fracture is pathologic in nature. Before the fracture is stabilized, radiographs are taken to show the position of the bone ends. Fractures are in "good alignment" when no perceptible angulation or displacement is present in frontal and lateral projections. Postreduction radiographs indicate the success of the fracture reduction (Fig. 12-24). If the fracture is placed in a cast, the exposure factors do not need to be altered to radiograph through a dry fiberglass cast but must be increased differently to penetrate the wet fiberglass or plaster cast. Finally, subsequent radiographs are taken to assess continued alignment, healing, and any possible complications of fractures.

In any case of trauma, it is essential to have at least two projections of the part, preferably taken at right angles, or 90 degrees to each other. A minimum of two projections is also necessary to

adequately determine fracture alignment (Fig. 12-25). If long bones are involved, these radiographs should demonstrate the joint above and below the area of trauma because dislocation may be present and because the injury may transfer force to a point distal or proximal to the point of injury. An example is a fracture or dislocation of the fibular head concurrent with an ankle or distal tibial fracture, as in a Maisonneuve fracture.

Frequently, fractures are obvious on clinical examination, but radiographic changes in appearance may be subtle. Fractures usually appear as radiolucent lines, but they may be thin and easily overlooked. Occasionally, a fracture appears as a radiopaque line if the fragments overlap. A step in the cortex, as indicated by a break in the normal bone contour, is a second radiographic indication (Fig. 12-26). Other signs include interruption of the trabeculae, bulging or buckling of the cortex, soft tissue swelling, and joint effusion.

FIGURE 12-25 A, An anteroposterior projection of an open comminuted fracture of the forearm caused by a machine injury. **B,** A lateral projection of the same forearm demonstrating anterior and posterior displacement of the fractured bones.

Also, the relationship of the end of a bone to its shaft is an important sign, as in the loss of normal volar tilt to the distal radial articular surface with an impacted distal radial fracture. CT (Fig. 12-27) and nuclear medicine bone scan are often used in combination with conventional radiography to assess skeletal fractures. MRI is used as an adjunct to conventional radiography to assess soft tissues, muscles, ligaments, and tendons.

Skeletal trauma usually causes significant soft tissue injuries, including neurovascular damage, capsular and ligamentous tears, cartilage injury, and hemarthroses. Such injury may be assessed in several ways, but the primary modality for assessing damage is MRI. Stress radiography may also be used to determine ligamentous stability. Radiographs of both extremities are often used to compare epiphyseal appearance. Arteriography is used to assess any vascular damage as a result of skeletal trauma.

When performing radiography of the skeletal system, it is critical for the technologist to choose the appropriate exposure factors to produce a radiograph that demonstrates good soft tissue definition in addition to achieving good penetration of the bone anatomy. It is often helpful to the interpreting physician if the radiographer notes, through film markers or as written on the requisition, areas of point tenderness and a detailed patient history. This is a highly specific indication of a fracture that may be subtle. Larger body parts such as the hip, femur, and knee are less assessable for point tenderness; instead, inability to bear weight or significant decrease in range of motion may suggest a fracture. Again, an important role of the radiographer is to assess the patient with regard to symptoms, signs, range of motion, and mechanism of injury to provide the physician with as much information as possible, both on the radiographs and verbally or in writing with the patient's clinical history.

Bone tissue is unique in its ability to repair itself in that it reactivates processes that normally occur during embryogenesis (Fig. 12-28).

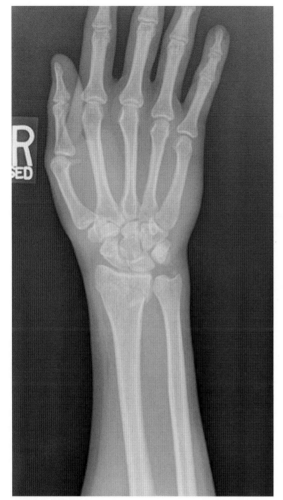

FIGURE 12-26 A posteroanterior projection of the wrist demonstrating a subtle fracture of the radius. Note the break in the bony cortex and discontinuity of the cortical bone.

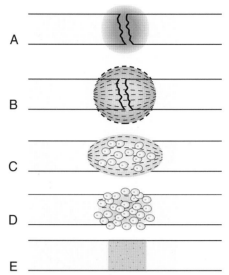

FIGURE 12-28 A schematic representation of the bone healing process. **A,** Bleeding at broken ends of the bone with subsequent hematoma formation. **B,** Organization of hematoma into fibrous network. **C,** Invasion of osteoblasts, lengthening of collagen strands, and deposition of calcium. **D,** Callus formation; new bone is built up as osteoclasts destroy dead bone. **E,** Remodeling is accomplished as excess callus is reabsorbed and trabecular bone is laid down.

FIGURE 12-27 A, A conventional anteroposterior projection of a shoulder demonstrating a fracture of the humeral neck sustained in a motor vehicle accident. **B,** A computed tomography coronal reconstruction of the same patient.

FIGURE 12-29 A femoral radiograph demonstrating advanced callus formation following a transverse fracture of the femur.

Initially, the break in the bone is filled by a large clot that temporarily bridges the fracture. Within 2 to 3 days, osteoblasts slowly begin to appear around the injured bone. Immobilization of the injured site is critical because any unnatural movement interferes with the deposition of the calcified matrix necessary for permanent union of the fracture. Provisional callus is mainly composed of cartilage and begins to form approximately 1 week after the fracture. As calcium continues to be deposited within the provisional callus, it is replaced by bony callus (Fig. 12-29), which is responsible for rigidly uniting the

fracture site. Although the break is rigidly united within 4 to 6 weeks, excess bone still encircles the external fracture site, and excess bone is still found within the marrow space at this time. Remodeling of the bone and total healing require months. Weight-bearing force on the fracture site tends to guide the modeling process, so in many cases, the patient may be instructed to begin using the affected limb in a limited fashion at this point in the healing process. If everything goes well during the healing process, the bone may repair to the point that the fracture site is no longer visible on subsequent radiographs. Proper healing greatly depends on the initial immobilization (casting, splinting, pinning, or plating), proper alignment or reduction of the fracture, and proper metabolic activity, which includes good vascularity and blood supply, proper nutrition, and normal hormone levels. Bacterial infections of the fracture site may inhibit callus formation, thus complicating the healing process.

Delayed union is a term referring to a fracture that does not heal within the usual time. If a fracture is not reduced properly or is not properly immobilized, malunion may occur. *Malunion* refers to a fracture that heals in a faulty position, thus impairing the normal function or cosmetic appearance of the affected body part (Fig. 12-30). The most serious complication is nonunion. *Nonunion* refers to a fracture in which healing does not occur and the fragments do not join (Fig. 12-31). This is often the result of lack of vascularization. Injuries to other soft tissue structures or organs can be associated with skeletal fractures such as a rib fracture that penetrates the lung and results in a pneumothorax. Additional complications of skeletal fractures include muscular ossification and fat emboli occurring in bones containing yellow bone marrow.

Fracture Classifications. Several means of classifying fractures exist (Fig. 12-32). One distinction is whether the fracture is open or closed. An **open** or **compound fracture** is one in which the bone has penetrated the skin (Fig. 12-33). This type of fracture leaves an open route for bacteria to enter from outside the body, which may lead to infection. As described earlier, the intrusion of

FIGURE 12-30 A magnetic resonance imaging scan after fracture of the wrist of a 55-year-old woman with a 2-month history of increasing pain and disability. The scan shows malunion of the distal radial fracture with loss of palmar inclination and reversal with subsequent dorsal inclination.

FIGURE 12-31 A, A knee radiograph of a 32-year-old man who sustained a gunshot wound to the left knee 3 years previously. Nonunion of the lateral femoral condyle is demonstrated. **B,** A magnetic resonance imaging scan of the same patient demonstrating nonunion of the posterior lateral femoral condyle with large subchondral defects.

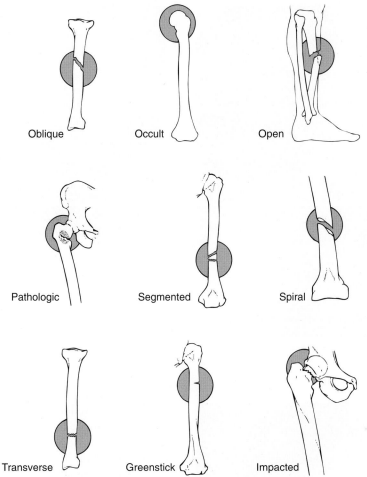

FIGURE 12-32 Examples of types of bone fractures.

bacteria may alter the healing process, so precautions must be taken to prevent infection from setting into bone or surrounding soft tissue structures. These fractures often require surgical intervention to irrigate and debride the area of interest. A **closed fracture** (formerly referred to as a *simple fracture*) is one in which the skin is not penetrated, which reduces the chances of infection (Fig. 12-34).

Fractures may be classified according to the mechanics of stress that produce the break or the appearance of the fracture line. Such classifications include torsion (twisting), transverse, linear,

and spiral fractures. When one of the fractured bone ends is jammed into the cancellous tissue of another fragment, it is called an **impacted fracture** (Fig. 12-35).

Fractures may also be classified according to their location, for example, intertrochanteric, transcervical (Fig. 12-36), supracondylar (Fig. 12-37), or transcondylar fractures. Fractures often do not fit into a specific classification because they may demonstrate mixed features.

Different types of treatments exist for skeletal fractures. The choice of treatment usually depends on the classification and severity of the

FIGURE 12-33 An open, comminuted fracture of the tibia and fibula with amputation.

FIGURE 12-34 A closed transverse fracture of the femur.

FIGURE 12-35 A radiograph of the pelvis of an older woman with trauma to her left hip. The radiograph demonstrates an impacted fracture of the left hip.

fracture. For closed and nondisplaced fractures, the most common treatment is splinting, casting, or both (Fig. 12-38). For a displaced fracture, it is necessary to improve the alignment of the fracture. This reduction may be either closed or open. **Closed reduction** requires that a local or general anesthetic be given to the patient for pain management. A splint or cast is then applied. **Open reduction** is required when orthopedic hardware is needed to maintain fracture reduction or when an open fracture needs to be irrigated. Generally, this is referred to as *open reduction internal fixation* (ORIF) (Fig. 12-39). Again, immobilization devices are often applied after surgery. It is imperative when imaging a patient with orthopedic hardware to include all of it on radiographs.

Comminuted Fractures. Sometimes, one or more fragments separate along the edges of the major fragment in addition to the major line of the fracture. Such fractures are said to be *comminuted* (Fig. 12-40). **Comminuted fractures** differ from multiple fractures as follows: In the case of a multiple fracture, each fracture is complete, leaving a fragment of intact shaft between them. Comminuted fractures do not represent a complete thickness of bone as do multiple

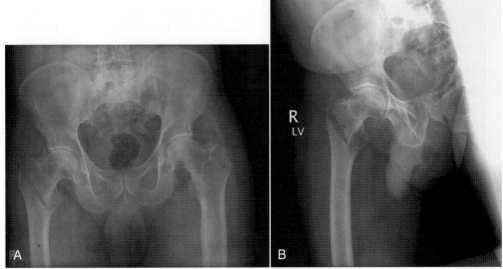

FIGURE 12-36 A, An anteroposterior (AP) projection of the pelvis demonstrating an intertrochanteric fracture of the femur. **B,** An AP projection of the affected hip in *A*.

FIGURE 12-37 Anteroposterior (*A*) and lateral (*B*) projections of a supracondylar fracture of the elbow.

fractures. Occasionally, the bone involved in a comminuted fracture may be extensively shattered, as might occur from a gunshot wound. Such fractures are also particularly apt to be open fractures (see Figs. 12-25 and 12-33).

A *butterfly fracture* is a comminuted fracture in which one or two butterfly wing–shaped or wedge-shaped fragments split off from the main fragments. A *splintered fracture* is a comminuted fracture with long, sharp-pointed fragments.

Complete, Noncomminuted Fractures. A complete, **noncomminuted fracture** is one in which the bone has separated into two fragments. The fracture may be recognized according to the direction of the fracture line. A *spiral* or *oblique fracture* is an example of this type. Such a fracture usually results from a rotary type of injury that twists the bone apart and is particularly common in the shafts of long bones (Fig. 12-41). A *transverse fracture* (Figs. 12-42, 12-43, and 12-44) is another type of complete, noncomminuted fracture. Demonstrated radiographically, such a fracture through normal bone is invariably ragged along the fracture line. A *pathologic*

FIGURE 12-38 A, Oblique and **B,** lateral views of a closed reduction of Colles fracture with application of a cast.

FIGURE 12-39 A, A radiograph of an open reduction internal fixation of a tibial fracture and **B,** fracture of the radius and ulna (*B*).

PT UNable to flex foot

FIGURE 12-40 A comminuted fracture of the calcaneus as depicted by conventional radiographs. **A,** An anteroposterior axial projection. **B,** A lateral projection. **C,** An axial computed tomography scan of the same patient.

FIGURE 12-41 A humerus radiograph of an individual who sustained a twisting injury of the humerus. The radiograph demonstrates a spiral fracture of the humerus.

FIGURE 12-42 A hand radiograph of a 32-year-old man involved in an industrial accident, demonstrating transverse fractures of the second and third metacarpals.

fracture is commonly a transverse fracture occurring in abnormal bone that is weakened by various diseases such as a bone cyst or metastatic bone neoplasm (Fig. 12-45). It may result from the disease process itself or from a relatively minor trauma. Often, pathologic fractures may be the first indication of the presence of pathology. *Multiple fractures* are another type of complete, noncomminuted fracture in which two or more complete fractures occur involving the shaft of a single bone (Fig. 12-46).

Avulsion Fractures. Avulsion fractures occur when a fragment of bone is pulled away from the shaft. Such fractures usually occur around joints because of ligament, tendon, and muscle tearing, as associated with a sprain or dislocation (Fig. 12-47), or may affect the spinous processes of

FIGURE 12-43 An anteroposterior projection of a transverse fracture of the femur.

FIGURE 12-44 An anteroposterior projection of a transverse fracture of the humerus sustained in a motor vehicle accident. Note the backboard visible on the image.

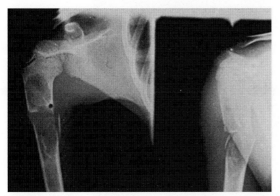

FIGURE 12-45 A humerus radiograph demonstrating a pathologic fracture through a bone cyst. The patient had complained of pain and denied a history of trauma associated with this fracture.

FIGURE 12-46 A forearm radiograph of an individual involved in a motor vehicle accident. The radiograph revealed multiple fractures of the forearm.

FIGURE 12-47 A wrist radiograph obtained after trauma to the wrist that resulted in perilunate dislocation with an associated avulsion fracture of the distal radius.

the vertebral column. A *chip fracture* is an avulsion fracture of a small fragment or chip of bone from the corner of a phalanx or other long bone. These are very common in the fingers and are often tiny. A mallet finger is an example of this (Fig. 12-48).

Incomplete Fractures. Incomplete fractures are those in which only part of the bony structure gives way, with little or no displacement. A common example is the **greenstick fracture,** in which the cortex breaks on one side without separation or breaking of the opposing cortex (Fig. 12-49). The effect is similar to that of trying to break a green twig, hence its name. Greenstick fractures are found almost exclusively in infants and children under the age of 10 years because of the softness of the cancellous bone. A **torus fracture,** commonly referred to as a *buckle fracture,* is a greenstick fracture in which the cortex

FIGURE 12-48 A radiograph demonstrating an old mallet finger injury on the dorsal lip of the fifth distal phalanx associated with arthritic changes in the distal interphalangeal joint.

FIGURE 12-49 A forearm radiograph of a child who sustained a fall. The radiograph demonstrates a greenstick fracture of the middle portion of the ulna. Note the incomplete break of the cortex of the ulna.

FIGURE 12-50 A forearm radiograph of a 14-year-old girl who fell on her hand, resulting in a torus fracture of the distal radius.

bulges outward, usually in the metaphysis, producing only a slight irregularity (Fig. 12-50). Such fractures are commonly found in the distal forearm or tibia-fibula after a fall.

Incomplete fractures may also occur in demineralized bone, as occurs with osteoporosis. The bone in question breaks only part of the way through, resulting in a sharp angular deformity without displacement.

Penetrating fractures are a type of incomplete fracture resulting from penetration by a sharp object such as a bullet or a knife. Frequently, a comminution exists at the site of the injury.

Growth Plate Fractures. Growth plate fractures involve the end of a long bone of a child

(Fig. 12-51). The fracture may be limited to growth plate cartilage and is thus not directly visible unless displacement occurs, or it may extend into the metaphysis, epiphysis, or both. Crush injuries of the growth plate may also occur. These growth plate fractures are classified according to severity and involvement of the epiphysis. This system is known as the *Salter-Harris system;* fractures are numbered I through VI, with I being least severe and VI being most severe. Comparison projections are often used with such fractures to compare growth plate appearances, and MRI may be used to further evaluate epiphyseal separations. Healed injuries of this type may result in an alteration of the length of the involved bone.

FIGURE 12-51 A lower leg radiograph demonstrating an epiphyseal-metaphyseal fracture of the tibia with a transverse diaphyseal fracture of the distal fibula.

Because of possible length discrepancies, frequent radiographic examinations may be required, often up to years after the injury.

Slipped capital femoral epiphysis (SCFE) is another example of a growth plate injury. SCFE is a posterior and inferior slippage of the proximal femoral epiphysis on the metaphysis through the physeal plate. It frequently affects adolescents, especially after a growth spurt. It is more common in obese children and more prevalent in boys than in girls. SCFE is generally idiopathic in nature and related to obesity, physeal orientation, and hormonal changes experienced during puberty, which may affect physeal strength. Physical examination usually yields intermittent limping and generalized groin, thigh, or knee pain. An injury is not necessarily associated with SCFE. Radiographic examination is the most common method of diagnosis. Bilateral AP and lateral hip projections or AP and frogleg pelvis projections are obtained so that comparisons can be made (Fig. 12-52). Severity of SCFE is

FIGURE 12-52 Anteroposterior pelvic radiograph demonstrating slipped capital femoral epiphysis in the hip of an 11-year-old girl.

classified according to stability and whether surgical intervention is required. The most widely accepted treatment is in situ fixation using a single central screw (Fig. 12-53). Unstable SCFE may require corrective osteotomy. Avascular necrosis is a complication that may occur as a result of SCFE.

Stress and Fatigue Fractures

Stress fractures usually occur as a result of an abnormal degree of repetitive trauma. They are generally found at the point of muscular attachments, as in the tibia or fibula of a runner. Stress fractures may not be clearly visible on plain radiographs, especially initially on injury, but may be diagnosed with a nuclear medicine bone scan or MRI of the affected area (Fig. 12-54). **Fatigue fractures** occur at sites of maximal strain on a bone, usually in connection with unaccustomed activity. Most frequently, fatigue fractures are

FIGURE 12-53 Radiographs demonstrating postsurgical intervention with a single central screw to correct the slipped capital femoral epiphysis in the patient in Fig. 12-51.

FIGURE 12-54 A, An ankle radiograph of a 55-year-old woman complaining of pain in the medial aspect of the distal tibia. The radiograph appears normal, with no evidence of fracture. **B,** A magnetic resonance imaging scan of the same patient demonstrating a stress fracture of the distal tibia.

FIGURE 12-55 A, A right wrist radiograph of a 31-year-old man who sustained an injury by falling while ice skating. No definite fracture or dislocation is demonstrated. **B,** A magnetic resonance imaging scan of the right wrist of the same patient as in *A,* demonstrating an occult, oblique, intraarticular distal radial fracture beginning just proximal to the styloid and extending to the middle third of the radius.

found in the metatarsals, particularly the second metatarsal—the classic "march" fracture. Other common names for fatigue fractures include *stretch fractures* and *insufficiency fractures.*

Occult Fractures and Bone Bruise

In an **occult fracture,** clinical signs are manifested without radiologic evidence. Follow-up examination within 10 days reveals bone reabsorption or displacement at the fracture site (Fig. 12-55). The most common sites for occult fractures are the carpal scaphoid and the ribs. A bruise to the bone may be revealed on MRI examination (Fig. 12-56) and is presumed to represent hemorrhage and edema, usually beneath an adjacent joint surface. A common area for a bone bruise is the distal femur with an associated knee injury such as a meniscal or ligamentous injury. Nuclear

FIGURE 12-56 A magnetic resonance imaging scan of the right knee of a 17-year-old boy who suffered a rotary injury while playing basketball. The image demonstrates extensive bone bruising of the lateral meniscocondylar notch and femoral condyles.

medicine bone scan may also be helpful in assessing subtle rib fractures.

Fractures in Specific Locations

Some fractures occur in selected areas and are usually easily recognized. One of these is *Colles fracture* (Fig. 12-57), which is a fracture through the distal inch of the radius. The distal fragment is usually angled backward on the shaft, with impaction along the dorsal aspect. An avulsion fracture of the ulnar styloid process occurs in more than half of all Colles fractures. This is the most common wrist fracture, and it usually results from falling on an outstretched hand. The external skin contour in Colles fracture displays a "dinner fork" deformity. *Smith fracture* is the opposite of Colles fracture, with displacement of the distal fragment toward the palmar aspect of the hand. A direct blow or fall with the wrist in hyperflexion is the usual mechanism of injury.

A *boxer's fracture* occurs when the fifth metacarpal (and occasionally the fourth metacarpal) fractures as a result of a blow to or with the hand (Fig. 12-58). It is the most common type of metacarpal fracture and may be immobilized with or without reduction, as it is difficult to maintain the reduction in this type of fracture. *Bennett*

FIGURE 12-57 A radiograph of the wrist of an older woman who fell on an outstretched hand. The radiograph demonstrates a classic Colles fracture.

FIGURE 12-58 A radiograph demonstrating a boxer's fracture of the fifth metacarpal head of the right hand.

FIGURE 12-59 A forearm radiograph of an individual who fell off a cliff, landing on an outstretched hand with the elbow partially flexed. The radiograph demonstrates a Monteggia fracture of the forearm.

fracture is a fracture and dislocation of the first carpometacarpal joint. This fracture results in an avulsion fracture of the base of the first metacarpal in association with a dislocation of the trapezium from the pulling action of the abductor pollicus longus tendon in the hand. The injury occurs when the thumb is forced backward while in partial flexion and is commonly seen in basketball players and skiers. It may be repaired with a closed pinning technique if the fracture displacement is less than 3 mm or with an open reduction in cases of displacement greater than 3 mm. *Monteggia fracture* is a fracture of the proximal third of the ulnar shaft, with anterior dislocation of the radial head (Fig. 12-59). *Galeazzi fracture* occurs at the proximal radius, with a dislocation of the distal radial-ulnar joint

(DRUJ). With both proximal and distal injuries to the forearm, it is important to ensure that both joints are included on the radiograph.

In the ankle, the most common injuries are to the malleoli. *Pott fracture* involves both malleoli, with dislocation of the ankle joint (Fig. 12-60). A trimalleolar fracture involves the medial and posterior malleoli of the tibia and the lateral malleolus of the fibula (Fig. 12-61). Less common fractures may seem more like minor sprains, requiring the radiologist to examine every aspect of the bone anatomy. *Maisonneuve fracture* (Fig. 12-62) is a less frequent ankle injury. It consists of a severe ankle sprain or disruption of the syndesmosis between the distal tibia and fibula with a fracture of the proximal third of the fibula. This fracture may

FIGURE 12-60 Ankle radiographs (**A,** anteroposterior projection; **B,** lateral projection) depicting Pott fracture of the ankle. Note the bimalleolar fracture and dislocation of the joint. The injury was sustained in a motor vehicle accident between a car and semi-truck.

be easily overlooked because the more painful ankle injury may cause the proximal fibular injury to be missed. Most disruptions or ligamentous injuries involving the ankle syndesmosis require surgical intervention.

As mentioned earlier, radiographic signs of some fractures are subtle at best. Such is sometimes the case with the elbow. The elbow "fat pad sign" may be an indicator of a nonvisualized, underlying fracture of the bones of the elbow. In the elbow, normally a small accumulation of fat is present adjacent to the anterior surface of the distal humerus and the anterior surface of the proximal radius. These radiolucencies are normally visible radiographically on a lateral projection of the elbow. A similar pad is found along the posterior surface of the distal humerus but is normally not visualized radiographically. If the joint capsule is distended by fluid as a result of a fracture, the posterior fat pad becomes displaced from bone and is visible on the lateral projection of the elbow. Visualization of a posterior fat pad is considered a sign of a possible underlying fracture or dislocation. The anterior fat pad may also be displaced, giving a sail-shaped appearance (Fig. 12-63). This is a prime example of how soft tissue demonstration can assist in making a diagnosis. Fractures of the elbow may include supracondylar fractures (especially in children), radial head fractures from a fall on an outstretched hand (FOOSH injury), or an olecranon fracture. These may require treatment from splinting to open reduction internal fixation (ORIF).

FIGURE 12-60, cont'd **C** to **E,** Postreduction images obtained after surgical repair of the fracture.

FIGURE 12-61 Ankle radiograph demonstrating a trimalleolar fracture.

FIGURE 12-62 A, A left ankle radiograph of a patient sustaining a twisting injury demonstrates a widening ankle mortise on the medial aspect with marked soft tissue swelling indicative of a Maisonneuve fracture. **B,** A left tibia–fibula radiograph of the same patient demonstrating a Maisonneuve fracture with minimal angulation and external rotation of the proximal fragment.

FIGURE 12-63 Lateral elbow demonstrating a positive anterior fat pad sign.

Visceral Cranial Fractures

Visceral cranial fractures are fractures of the facial bones and generally result from a blow to the face. As discussed earlier, facial or head trauma may also indicate a possible cervical spine fracture or injury. In addition, soft tissue injury of the eyes, nose, and mandible is often accompanied by bone fractures. CT has largely replaced the use of conventional radiographs in evaluating fractures of the maxillofacial bones and orbits (Fig. 12-64).

A *zygomatic arch fracture* may initially be difficult to recognize because of the edema. However, a fracture may be indicated by clinical signs, which include black eyes, flattening of the cheek, and a restriction of the movement of the mandible. Careful examination by palpation is performed by the physician because a fracture of the zygomatic arch may be present without accompanying facial fractures. A depressed fracture of the zygomatic arch may also be difficult to demonstrate radiographically (Fig. 12-65). If radiographs are requested, an oblique submento-vertical projection (tangential projection) may be used to best demonstrate the extent of the fracture. A parietoacanthial projection (Waters method) is also of value in examining the fractures of the zygomatic arch.

A *tripod fracture* occurs when the zygomatic or malar bone is fractured at all three sutures: frontal, temporal, and maxillary (Fig. 12-66). The patient with a tripod fracture complains of restricted jaw movement because the mandible's coronoid process is trapped by the zygoma. This fracture results in a free-floating zygoma and may cause facial disfigurement if not diagnosed and properly treated.

The mandible is highly prone to fracture because of the prominence of the chin; therefore, any patient who has sustained a head or facial injury should be clinically examined for a *mandibular fracture*. Anatomically, the mandible is strongest at the center and weakest at the ends, with the most common site for fracture at the angle, followed by the condyles. It is not uncommon for such fractures to be bilateral because of the transmitted force and shape of the mandible. Mandibular fractures (Fig. 12-67) are generally detected by the patient's inability to open mouth and pain when moving the mandible. These fractures also cause a misalignment of the patient's teeth. Care must be taken to demonstrate all areas of the mandible (body, ramus, and symphysis) when ruling out mandibular fractures. The mandible is the slowest healing bone in the body and will show clinical union much sooner than radiographic union.

Fractures of the maxilla are serious because of the adjacent nasal cavity, paranasal sinuses, and orbit and the close proximity of the brain. The maxilla also transmits cranial nerves and major blood vessels. Maxillary fractures may be divided into three major classifications: horizontal, pyramidal, and transverse. A *horizontal* fracture of the maxilla (LeFort I) refers to a separation of the body of the maxilla from the base of the skull above the palate and below the zygomatic process. This type of fracture results in a freely

FIGURE 12-64 Axial and coronal computed tomography (CT) examinations of the maxillofacial bones after trauma to the face. **A,** A coronal CT scan of a patient complaining of a nosebleed after being hit in the face. The CT scan demonstrates blood in the nasal and sinus cavities, with associated facial bone fractures and displacement of the nasal septum. **B,** An axial projection of the same patient as in *A*. **C,** A coronal CT scan of a patient sustaining a direct blow to the left orbit resulting in a blowout fracture of the floor of the left orbit. Note the blood in the maxillary sinus. **D,** An axial CT scan of the same patient as in *C.*

FIGURE 12-65 A submentovertical projection of the zygomatic arch demonstrating a depressed fracture of the zygomatic arch resulting from a direct blow to the left cheek.

FIGURE 12-66 A computed tomography image demonstrating a tripod fracture of the right zygomatic bone.

FIGURE 12-67 A, Posteroanterior and anteroposterior axial and **B,** Towne method projections of the mandible demonstrating a mandibular fracture.

FIGURE 12-68 Three-dimensional computed tomography reconstructions of a patient involved in a motor vehicle accident demonstrating bilateral zygomatic arch fractures, comminuted fracture of every wall of the right maxillary sinus, the medial and posterior walls of the maxillary sinus, bilateral orbital floor fractures, fractures of the lateral walls of both orbits, fracture of the left pterygoid plate, and both temporoparietal regions.

movable jaw. A *pyramidal* fracture (LeFort II) involves vertical fractures through the maxilla at the malar and nasal bones, forming a triangular separation of the maxilla. A *transverse* fracture (LeFort III) is the most extensive and serious type of maxillary fracture; it extends across the orbits and results in separation of the visceral and cerebral cranium (Fig. 12-68).

A **blowout fracture** results from a direct blow to the front of the orbit that transfers the force to the orbital walls and floor. This fracture occurs in the thinnest, weakest portion of the orbit, the orbital floor just above the maxillary sinuses (see Fig. 12-64, *C* and *D)*. If this condition is not diagnosed and treated, impairment of extraocular movements develops. A modified parieto-acanthial projection (modified Waters method) provides the most information in terms of conventional radiographic diagnosis of blowout fractures because the petrous ridges are projected below the floor of the orbit. CT is the best modality for imaging the orbits.

The nasal bone is the most frequently fractured facial bone. The fracture is usually transverse and depresses the distal portion of the nasal bones. A *nasal bone fracture* may be accompanied by a fracture of the ascending process of the maxillae (anterior nasal spine) or of the nasal septum. The nasal septum is composed of the vomer and the perpendicular plate of the ethmoid bone. *Epistaxis,* or nosebleed, is usually present with a nasal bone fracture. As discussed earlier, CT is the best method of assessing fractures of the facial bones (see Fig. 12-64, *A* and *B);* however, radiographs of nasal bone fractures may be obtained in addition to a clinical examination to confirm a fracture or ascertain fracture displacement (Fig. 12-69).

Dislocations

A joint **dislocation,** or luxation, results when a bone is out of its joint and not in contact with its normal articulation (Fig. 12-70). Common sites for joint dislocations are the shoulder, hip, and acromioclavicular joints. A **subluxation** is a partial dislocation, often occurring with fracture (Fig. 12-71). The ankle and the vertebral column, especially the cervical spine, are common sites of subluxations.

Shoulder joints most commonly dislocate anteriorly (Fig. 12-72). Such dislocations are readily detectable radiographically because the humeral head usually locates below the glenoid fossa and coracoid process. Often an avulsed greater tuberosity is present with anterior dislocations. A Hills-Sachs deformity is a compression fracture of the humeral head. It occurs on the superior and posterior head of the humerus

FIGURE 12-69 A lateral nasal bone radiograph of a man who was struck in the face. The radiograph demonstrates nasal bone fracture.

because of impaction of the humeral head against the glenoid labrum during dislocation. If undetected by the clinician, this defect may increase the risk of subsequent dislocations of the same shoulder. It is detected radiographically with the West Point method. Posterior dislocations of the shoulder (Fig. 12-73) are more difficult to diagnose, as they may appear normal on an AP radiograph. A transscapular (Y) projection, as well as a posterior oblique projection, is useful in locating the humeral head in a suspected posterior dislocation. Other than trauma, seizure disorders and electric shock are the major causes of

FIGURE 12-70 An anteroposterior projection of a dislocated knee prosthesis.

FIGURE 12-71 An anteroposterior view of a hand demonstrating a metacarpal fracture and subluxation of the proximal interphalangeal joint, third digit.

shoulder dislocations. In fact, a posterior dislocation may be the first sign of a seizure disorder.

With traumatic dislocation of the hip, the femoral head is most commonly displaced posteriorly to lie against the sciatic notch (Fig. 12-74). It may also displace anteriorly and lie adjacent to the pubis or obturator foramen. Congenital hip dislocations are not caused by trauma, are usually unilateral, are more common in female patients, and are recognized by a shortening of the extremity. If the condition is not recognized until the child begins to walk, conservative therapies may be replaced by surgical intervention.

Acromioclavicular joint separations (Fig. 12-75) are more common in children than in adults. The typical imaging sequence for this diagnosis involves radiographs taken with or without weights with the patient in the upright position. Determining the alignment between the acromial end of the clavicle and the acromion process of the scapula allows assessment of a joint separation. These radiographs are commonly performed bilaterally for comparison.

Battered Child Syndrome

Battered child syndrome is a term associated with a physical form of child abuse and was first described in 1860, but the term was not used until Henry Kempe did so in 1962. Battered child syndrome is also referred to as *nonaccidental trauma* (NAT). Physical child abuse often coexists with both emotional and sexual abuse. This syndrome affects boys and girls equally, generally under age 4 years. Approximately 16.1% of cases involve children under age 3 years. In addition, about 20% of the children who survive physical abuse suffer permanent injuries. An accurate incidence of child abuse is difficult to ascertain, but statistics from the National Child Abuse and Neglect Data System indicate that in the United States, approximately 1537 children died of neglect or abuse in 2010. It has been shown that family history is a strong predictor of child abuse because adults who were abused as children often abuse their own children, primarily because they do not know how to handle

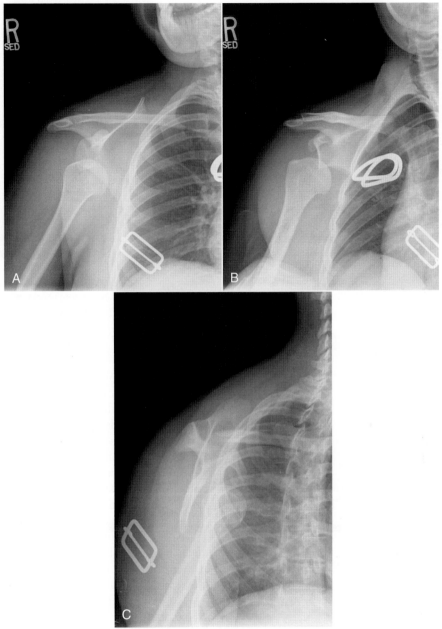

FIGURE 12-72 A, Anteroposterior, **B,** oblique, and **C,** transscapular projections of the shoulder demonstrating an anterior dislocation of the humeral head. Note the location of the humeral head below the glenoid fossa and coracoid process of the scapula.

FIGURE 12-73 A shoulder radiograph demonstrating a posterior dislocation of the humerus with the humeral head overlapping the rim of the glenoid fossa. The humeral head is also displaced slightly superolaterally.

FIGURE 12-75 A weight-bearing acromioclavicular radiograph demonstrating a dislocation as evidenced by uneven alignment of the acromial end of the clavicle and the acromion process of the scapula.

FIGURE 12-74 A pelvic radiograph of a 25-year-old man whose right knee struck the dashboard in a motor vehicle accident, resulting in a posterior dislocation of the right femoral head.

their anger. Statistics also indicate a higher incidence of abuse in homes with single parents, homes with young parents, families in which substance abuse is prevalent, or families living in poverty. Radiographs are often used as evidence in cases of suspected child abuse.

Physical signs of battered child syndrome include bruises, burns, abrasions, and fractures in various stages of healing. Active children who are not abused often have bruises over the bony areas of the body such as knees and elbows. However, bruises or injury around the eyes, cheeks, mouth, buttocks, or thighs, bite marks, certain bone fractures, and cigarette burns are suspicious. In most cases, the explanation for the injury is inconsistent with the actual injury.

Radiographic skeletal surveys to include bones of the upper extremities, lower extremities, skull, spine, and ribs should be performed on initial inspection of the child if abuse is suspected. In some cases, the bone survey may be repeated 2 weeks later to better identify new fractures not visible on the initial series. Radiographic signs of child abuse include hematomas and single or multiple fractures of varying ages, especially in areas where self-infliction of injury is difficult (Fig. 12-76). Often fractures may indicate that an extremity has been twisted or turned until it breaks, or multiple rib fractures indicate repeated traumatic injuries, generally inflicted by a parent or guardian.

FIGURE 12-76 A pediatric chest radiograph revealing numerous rib fractures with adjacent soft tissue masses resulting from hemorrhage surrounding the fracture sites.

Shaken baby syndrome is a severe type of physical abuse that affects the child's head and neck. Shaking of the child causes whiplash injury to the neck as well as brain trauma such as a subdural or subarachnoid hematoma, with no evidence of trauma to the external cranium. Shaken baby syndrome is associated with a high morbidity and mortality rate, with more than 25% of cases resulting in death. CT and MRI of the brain are excellent modalities for diagnosing this syndrome.

All emergency room personnel should be familiar with signs of child abuse and are legally and ethically required to report suspected cases of child abuse to the proper authorities. In addition, children may be admitted to the hospital or transferred to a specialized crisis intervention facility for further evaluation.

Avascular Necrosis

Avascular necrosis is a term used to denote bone death resulting from inadequate blood supply. It frequently affects the hip, knee, shoulder, or carpal scaphoid and is most common in men between ages 30 and 60 years. It may occur idiopathically or may follow trauma to a joint (posttraumatic avascular necrosis), especially in cases of joint dislocation involving a tear of the joint capsule. The symptoms are nonspecific but may include pain up to 1 year or more after the trauma. If the lower extremity is affected, a limp may also be present.

MRI is the modality of choice for evaluating avascular necrosis of bone because it can demonstrate abnormalities associated with early-stage necrosis. Additional information is obtained with a nuclear medicine bone scan or CT. Conventional radiography is not sensitive enough to demonstrate early signs of avascular necrosis but does demonstrate the later stages of the disease. The radiographic appearance of avascular necrosis at a later stage includes sclerosis in combination with a collapse of the affected bone and narrowing of the joint space. Treatment consists of analgesics for pain and exercise to maintain range of motion. If the condition is diagnosed early, surgical intervention to provide cortical bone grafts or core decompression may help provide support and relieve pressure to allow revascularization of the bone.

Legg-Calvé-Perthes Disease

Legg-Calvé-Perthes disease is a common form of avascular necrosis affecting the femoral head. The cause of this disorder is unknown, and the disease process is fairly quiet. *Perthes* refers specifically to ischemic necrosis of the head of the femur. It tends to occur in boys between ages 5 and 10 years. It may be idiopathic or may follow injury or trauma to the affected hip. Clinically, these patients have a limp that is accompanied by little or no pain.

Radiographically, the bone in the center of the epiphysis is fragmented, and the head of the femur is flattened (Fig. 12-77) and contains both areas of sclerotic bone and osteolytic regions. MRI images normally demonstrate low signal intensity from the affected hip in Legg-Calvé-Perthes disease (Fig. 12-78). In many

FIGURE 12-77 An anteroposterior pelvic radiograph of a young man demonstrating Legg-Calvé-Perthes disease of the left femoral head. Note the asymmetry of the femoral heads.

FIGURE 12-78 A magnetic resonance imaging scan of the patient in Fig. 12-74. The image demonstrates low signal intensity in the left femoral epiphysis, consistent with Legg-Calvé-Perthes disease.

cases, the patient develops a secondary degenerative osteoarthritis (see Chapter 2). This condition is treated with casting, traction, and bed rest or with surgical osteotomy and internal fixation.

TRAUMA OF THE CHEST AND THORAX

Approximately 25% of all trauma deaths occurring annually result from chest injuries. Diagnosis of the cause of the respiratory distress and the extent of the injury must be made quickly. For patients with acute respiratory distress with suspected hemothorax or pneumothorax, a chest tube may be inserted in the fourth or fifth intercostal space without waiting for a chest radiograph. Portable chest radiography is then performed to further evaluate the thorax after placement of the "blind" chest tube. Bone injuries such as rib fractures, clavicular fractures, scapular fractures, and sternal fractures may result in penetration of the lungs and damage to the heart and the great vessels. Pulmonary contusion may also result from other penetrating, compressive, or decelerating trauma to the chest. Radiographically, changes in the lungs from contusion appear 4 to 6 hours after the trauma. The radiographic appearance changes frequently during the first 24 to 48 hours, so multiple chest radiographs may be necessary to assess the damage to the lung tissue because pulmonary contusions are usually much larger than apparent on the initial chest radiograph.

Blunt trauma to the chest may also result in injury to the descending thoracic aorta. Patients may have upper back pain, a cough or wheezing, and hemoptysis. A traumatic injury to the thoracic aorta may be visualized as a widened mediastinum on chest radiography, CT (Fig. 12-79), MRI, and transesophageal sonography.

Pneumothorax

A **pneumothorax** occurs when free air is trapped in the pleural space and compresses lung tissue. This air may enter the pleural space from perforation of the visceral pleura, allowing gas to enter from the lung, from penetration of the chest wall, or by generation of gas by gas-forming organisms in an empyema.

Common causes of a pneumothorax (Fig. 12-80) include penetrating chest trauma such

FIGURE 12-79 A computed tomography scan demonstrating traumatic aortic injury at the level of the isthmus with an enlarged mediastinal hematoma displacing the trachea anteriorly. Right and left pleural effusions are also present.

FIGURE 12-81 Large emphysematous blebs as seen on computed tomography. Spontaneous blowout of these could result in a pneumothorax.

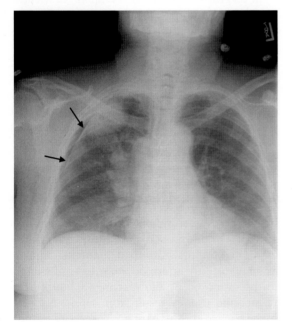

FIGURE 12-80 An anteroposterior chest image obtained from mobile radiography equipment demonstrating a traumatic pneumothorax and atelectasis of the right upper lobe of the lung.

as stab wounds, gunshot wounds, fractured ribs, or a thoracocentesis needle, and a spontaneous blowout of a bleb (a flaccid vesicle such as a blister) resulting from some other pulmonary disease (Fig. 12-81). A pneumothorax may occur spontaneously from trauma or as the result of some pathologic process. The typical manifestation of a spontaneous pneumothorax is sudden, one-sided chest pain followed by dyspnea. This tends to occur more frequently with tall, hyposthenic male patients.

Radiographically, a pneumothorax appears as a strip of radiolucency devoid of vascular lung markings, with separation of the visceral and parietal pleura. It is best demonstrated on an erect expiration posteroanterior (PA) chest radiograph obtained in conjunction with routine PA and lateral inspiration chest radiographs. Occasionally, wrinkles in the patient's skin produce artifacts that may mimic a pneumothorax. Such an artifact is called a *pseudopneumothorax*.

A *tension pneumothorax* occurs when air enters the pleural space but cannot leave the space because of a check valve mechanism in the fistula. This results in a complete collapse of the lung and a shift of the mediastinum to the

FIGURE 12-82 Tension pneumothorax of the right lung after a stab wound in this 25-year-old man. The collapsed lung has almost no air in it and is seen as a soft tissue density adjacent to the heart.

side opposite the pneumothorax (Fig. 12-82). A tension pneumothorax requires immediate medical attention to prevent life-threatening circulatory collapse.

Treatment of a pneumothorax depends on the amount of lung collapse and the type of pneumothorax. A collapse of 30% or less is usually treated by bed rest and needle aspiration. Immediate treatment of a tension pneumothorax might involve insertion of a needle into the chest wall to equalize air pressure. Otherwise, many pneumothoraces are treated with decompression by a closed-tube thoracostomy attached to a water-seal drain.

Atelectasis

Atelectasis means incomplete expansion of the lung as a result of partial or total collapse. In trauma situations, this often occurs in combination with a penetrating wound to the chest. Atelectasis itself is not a disease, but it is a sign of an abnormal process. One common manifestation is

bibasilar atelectasis, which is also seen after trauma to the thorax occurs during surgical procedures. A chest radiograph reveals the airless area of the lung, which may be segmental or lobar. If an entire lobe is affected, the mediastinum shifts to the affected side because of loss of volume of the affected lung. The chest radiograph also demonstrates a decrease in the intercostal interspace, elevation of the hemidiaphragm of the affected side, and depression or elevation of the hilum, depending on which lobe is affected. If the atelectasis is segmental, the radiographic shadow is triangular, with the apex of the triangle pointing toward the hilum of the affected lung.

Compression atelectasis occurs when blood, pleural effusions, pneumothoraces, or other space-occupying lesions cause collapse (Fig. 12-83). Air that is completely absorbed from alveoli beyond an obstructed bronchus results in *absorption atelectasis*. *Platelike atelectasis* describes the radiographic appearance of one or more linear opacities, usually at the lung bases and parallel to the diaphragm (Fig. 12-84).

Treatment of acute atelectasis is accomplished with appropriate respiratory therapy such as coughing and deep breathing. Bronchoscopy may also be used to allow suctioning of secretions that are causing an obstruction. Thoracocentesis is used to relieve the compression caused by an effusion.

ABDOMINAL TRAUMA

Traumatic injuries to the abdomen result from gunshot wounds, stab wounds, and blunt abdominal trauma. Although abdominal injuries account for only approximately 15% of trauma deaths, most occur more than 48 hours after trauma and usually result from sepsis. As mentioned earlier in this chapter, the severity of injuries sustained in an MVA are greatly reduced by wearing both shoulder and lap belts, whether the individual is in the front seat or back seat of a motor vehicle; however, chest and abdominal contusions and abdominal trauma may result from a rapid deceleration into the seatbelt, even

FIGURE 12-83 A, Absorption atelectasis caused by the obstructive effects of carcinoma of the bronchus supplying the upper lobe of the right lung. **B,** The lateral projection of the same patient clearly demonstrates atelectasis of the right upper lobe secondary to bronchogenic carcinoma.

FIGURE 12-84 A, Platelike atelectasis seen as a linear opacity in the base of the left lung as indicated by the arrow in this posteroanterior projection. **B,** A lateral projection of same patient also clearly demonstrates platelike atelectasis.

FIGURE 12-85 Axial computed tomographic images demonstrating a ruptured spleen resulting from blunt trauma from a motor vehicle accident. The patient was unrestrained and thrown from the vehicle.

when it is worn properly. Many patients with serious abdominal injuries from MVA initially have very minimal symptoms and physical findings. Abdominal trauma may cause serious injury not only to the gastrointestinal (GI) tract but also to abdominal organs such as the liver, spleen, kidneys, and pancreas; the retroperitoneum; the aorta; and the pelvic organs. Blunt trauma from steering wheel injuries often damages the liver and the spleen because the energy of deceleration and compression frequently damages the parenchyma of these structures (Fig. 12-85).

Supine and erect abdominal radiographs and erect chest radiographs are most desirable after abdominal injury. Chest radiography is important to assess diaphragmatic injury. In addition, free air is best demonstrated radiographically with the patient in the erect position. Often, free air is well demonstrated on a chest radiograph because of the proximity of the central ray to the diaphragm. Free air ascends and accumulates under the diaphragm on one or both sides, and as little as 1 cc of air can be demonstrated radiographically on the erect projection. Much larger amounts of air must be present to be visualized on a supine radiograph. However, placing the patient erect is not always possible because of the patient's condition. Left lateral decubitus radiographs of the abdomen may be substituted for the erect projection, with any free air present

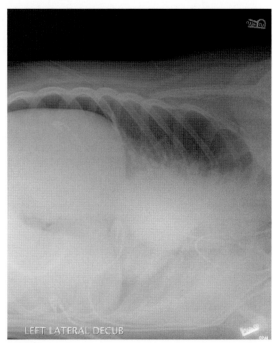

LEFT LATERAL DECUB

FIGURE 12-86 Decubitus abdominal radiograph demonstrating free air over the dome of the liver.

accumulating over the lateral aspect of the liver and the lateral aspect of the pelvis (Fig. 12-86). Optimally, the patient should remain on the left side for approximately 5 to 10 minutes before the exposure to allow sufficient time for the air to ascend.

FIGURE 12-87 An intravenous urogram demonstrating a right kidney fractured in a football injury.

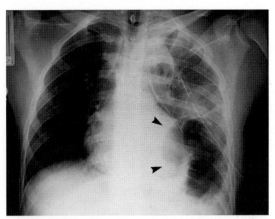

FIGURE 12-88 A chest radiograph demonstrating a traumatic diaphragmatic hernia resulting from a motor vehicle accident.

Supine abdominal radiographs help identify foreign objects such as bullets, separation in the bowel loops, or loss of the psoas muscle shadow as a result of fluid or blood within the peritoneum and air around the right kidney or psoas muscle margins. The initial inspection of the abdominal trauma may be followed by specific studies involving the urinary tract (Fig. 12-87). IVUs may be indicated if injury to the urinary system is suspected; however, CT examination of the abdomen after an injection of an iodinated contrast agent provides a much clearer view of the renal anatomy and organ injury.

CT has also proven to be the best means of diagnosing GI trauma and is capable of visualizing lacerations, hematomas, and ruptures. Even small amounts of intraabdominal hemorrhage can be readily detected with CT. The duodenum is the portion of the GI tract most often damaged by blunt trauma. Because of its relationship to the spine, the duodenum may be compressed between the abdominal wall and the spine, resulting in a duodenal hematoma. Often CT evaluation of liver and spleen injuries helps in opting for surgical versus nonsurgical management of these injuries.

Penetrating abdominal wounds such as gunshot wounds may produce free air if the bowel has been injured. Some of the common conditions seen radiographically after trauma are fractures of the spine, pelvis, or ribs; subcutaneous emphysema; obliteration of normal fat planes and visceral margins; accumulation of peritoneal fluid such as blood; and the presence of free peritoneal air (Fig. 12-88).

Intraperitoneal Air

In the normal person, the peritoneum is a closed cavity (except for the female reproductive system) containing only small amounts of serous fluid. The presence of free air in this cavity, a **pneumoperitoneum**, is usually abnormal and may indicate perforation of the GI tract. Large amounts of air likely indicate colon perforation, whereas small amounts of air are more indicative of duodenal perforation.

FIGURE 12-89 An abdominal radiograph of a 5-year-old child with a passive pneumoperitoneum resulting from perforation of the stomach during anesthesia. Note how the free air outlines the outer border of the bowel, liver, and spleen.

The common causes of a pneumoperitoneum (Fig. 12-89) include traumatic rupturing of the stomach or intestines or nontraumatic bowel perforations. In response to perforation, an intense inflammatory response develops and may eventually wall off the perforation into an abscess.

On an AP radiograph, with the patient in a supine position, the "football sign" may be demonstrated as an indicator of a pneumoperitoneum. This is a lucent, oval gas collection that corresponds to the anterior peritoneal cavity. The pattern of gas resembles the shape of a football, with the seam of the football being the falciform ligament outlined by free air. Visualization of this sign requires a relatively large amount of free air to be present.

PATHOLOGY SUMMARY
Traumatic Disease

Pathology	Imaging Modalities of Choice
Initial triage	Radiography, CT
Vertebral column—bony	CT, radiography
Vertebral column—soft tissue	MRI
Cerebral and visceral cranium	CT, MRI, radiography
Appendicular skeleton	Radiography, CT, MRI
Battered child syndrome	Radiography
Avascular necrosis	Radiography, MRI, CT
Legg-Calvé-Perthes disease	Radiography, MRI
Chest and thorax	Radiography, CT
Abdomen	Radiography, CT, sonography
Pelvis	Radiography, CT

CT, Computed tomography; *MRI,* magnetic resonance imaging.

REVIEW QUESTIONS

1. A contusion formed on the side of the head where trauma occurs is called a:
   a. Concussion
   b. Contrecoup lesion
   c. Coup lesion
   d. Spondylosis
2. A fracture of the skeletal system in which the bone has penetrated the skin is termed:
   a. Closed
   b. Comminuted
   c. Noncomminuted
   d. Open
3. Fractures that occur at sites of maximal strain on a bone, usually in connection with unaccustomed activity, are classified as _____ fractures.
   a. Avulsion
   b. Fatigue
   c. Growth plate
   d. Stress
4. A fracture that heals in a faulty position is termed a:
   a. Callus
   b. Delayed union
   c. Malunion
   d. Nonunion

5. Shoulder dislocations are most commonly displaced:
   a. Anteriorly
   b. Posteriorly
   c. Interiorly
   d. Exteriorly
6. Avascular necrosis commonly affects the:
   1. Shoulder
   2. Hip
   3. Fingers
   a. 1 and 2
   b. 1 and 3
   c. 2 and 3
   d. 1, 2, and 3
7. "Incomplete expansion of a lung as a result of partial or total collapse" describes:
   a. Atelectasis
   b. Empyema
   c. Pleurisy
   d. Pneumothorax
8. Penetrating chest trauma could lead to a:
   a. Coma
   b. Coup lesion
   c. Pneumoperitoneum
   d. Pneumothorax
9. Demonstration of a pneumothorax is best accomplished by making the exposure with the patient in the:
   a. Erect, lateral position
   b. Lateral decubitus position
   c. Erect posteroanterior (PA) position on expiration
   d. Erect PA position on inspiration
10. Which portion of the gastrointestinal system is most frequently damaged by blunt trauma to the abdomen?
    a. Cecum
    b. Duodenum
    c. Ileum
    d. Jejunum
11. Define the term *shaken baby syndrome,* and explain its effect on the central nervous system.
12. Spinal cord compression results in neurologic dysfunction that may be temporary or permanent. Explain the mechanism for each type of dysfunction described in the text.
13. Differentiate among the four types of hematomas to the brain, and specify which type has the highest mortality rate. Why?
14. What imaging modality or modalities best demonstrate stress or fatigue fractures? Why?
15. Describe the difference between comminuted and noncomminuted fractures of the skeletal system.

CHAPTER 1

1. C
2. B
3. B
4. B
5. B
6. C
7. B
8. D
9. D
10. A
11. D
12. B

CHAPTER 2

1. B
2. B
3. B
4. A
5. C
6. A
7. D
8. B
9. B
10. C
11. D
12. D
13. B
14. B
15. D

CHAPTER 3

1. C
2. C
3. B
4. B
5. C
6. C
7. A
8. D
9. B
10. B

CHAPTER 4

1. D
2. A
3. B
4. B
5. B
6. E
7. B
8. C
9. C
10. B
11. D
12. C
13. B
14. D
15. B

CHAPTER 5

1. A
2. C
3. C
4. C
5. C
6. C
7. D
8. D
9. D
10. A

CHAPTER 6

1. B
2. B
3. B
4. D
5. F
6. C
7. D
8. D
9. B
10. C

CHAPTER 7

1. D
2. A
3. D
4. A
5. B
6. C
7. C
8. E
9. B
10. D
11. D
12. B
13. A
14. B

CHAPTER 8

1. A
2. B
3. B
4. C
5. B
6. A
7. B
8. B
9. B
10. D

CHAPTER 9

1. C
2. A
3. D
4. B
5. A
6. D
7. D
8. A
9. B
10. B

CHAPTER 10

1. D
2. D
3. D
4. B
5. A
6. B
7. D
8. D
9. C
10. B

CHAPTER 11

1. C
2. C
3. B
4. A
5. A
6. C
7. A
8. B

CHAPTER 12

1. C
2. D
3. B
4. C
5. A
6. A
7. A
8. D
9. C
10. B

2-D echocardiography Cross-sectional sonographic imaging of the heart demonstrating the heart chambers, valves, major vessels, and cardiac output.

achalasia A neuromuscular abnormality of the esophagus that results in failure of the lower esophageal sphincter to relax.

achondroplasia A hereditary, congenital disturbance that causes inadequate bone formation and results in a peculiar form of dwarfism.

acoustic neuroma A tumor of the peripheral nerve sheath.

acquired immunodeficiency syndrome (AIDS) An acquired viral infection that paralyzes normal human immune mechanisms.

acromegaly A disease marked by progressive enlargement of the head, hands, and feet caused by abnormal secretion of growth hormone.

acute Having a quick onset and lasting a short period of time with a relatively severe course.

Acute glomerulonephritis An acute inflammation of the capillaries of the renal glomeruli.

acute lymphocytic leukemia A rapidly progressing form of leukemia in which there are too many very young (immature) white blood cells, called *lymphoblasts*, in the bloodstream and bone marrow.

acute monoblastic leukemia A type of acute myeloid leukemia.

acute myelocytic leukemia A cancer of the myeloid line of blood cells, characterized by the rapid growth of abnormal white blood cells that accumulate in bone marrow and interfere with the production of normal blood cells.

Addison disease Deficiency in the secretion of adrenocortical hormones.

adenocarcinoma Carcinoma derived from glandular tissue.

adenocarcinoma of the prostate A cancer originating from glandular tissue in the prostate gland accounting for the majority of prostate cancers.

adrenal carcinoma A neoplastic disease of the adrenal gland, a small endocrine gland located above the kidney.

adrenal glands A pair of triangular-shaped endocrine glands located superior to the kidneys responsible for producing steroid hormones, epinephrine, and norepinephrine.

adventitia The outermost layer of connective tissue covering major organs and vessels within the body.

adynamic ileus A failure of bowel peristalsis, often seen after abdominal surgery, which may result in bowel obstruction.

agglutination Clumping that occurs when a specific immune serum is added to a bacterial culture.

Albers-Schönberg disease A form of osteosclerotic osteopetrosis; a benign skeletal anomaly that involves increased bone density in conjunction with fairly normal bone contour.

alcohol-induced liver disease Liver damage caused by alcohol consumption resulting in hepatitis and cirrhosis of the liver.

anal agenesis Congenital disorder characterized by lack of an anal opening to the exterior.

anemia A condition in which level of hemoglobin in blood is less than 12 g per 100 mL.

anencephaly Congenital absence of the cranial vault.

aneurysm A localized ballooning or outpouching of a vessel wall as a result of weakening from atherosclerotic disease, trauma, infection, or congenital defects.

aneurysmal bone cyst A solitary benign osteoplastic serum or blood-filled lesion of the bone.

ankylosing spondylitis A form of rheumatoid arthritis of unknown cause that affects the spine in a progressive fashion, eventually fusing the spine into a rigid block of bone.

annulus fibrosus The outer layer of an intervertebral disk.

anomaly Any marked deviation from the norm, especially as a result of congenital or hereditary defects.

anthracosis Pneumoconiosis caused by inhalation and deposition of coal dust.

antibody The formation of protein substances by the human body in response to an antigen.

antigen Foreign substances introduced into the body, such as bacteria, or substances formed within the body that stimulate the formation of antibodies.

appendicitis   An inflammation of the appendix.

arteries   Blood vessels which carry blood away from the heart.

arthritis   Inflammation in which lesions are confined to the joints.

asbestosis   Pneumoconiosis caused by inhalation and deposition of asbestos dust.

ascites   An accumulation of fluid in the peritoneal cavity.

aspiration pneumonia   Pneumonia caused by entrance of foreign particles (e.g., vomitus) aspirated into the lower respiratory tract.

asthma   Chronic inflammation of the bronchi resulting in hyper-responsiveness and airway obstruction.

astrocytoma   A glioma composed of astrocytes, which are star-shaped neuroglial cells with many branching processes.

asymptomatic   Showing or causing no identifiable symptoms.

atelectasis   Loss of air in a lung resulting from a partial or total collapse of a lung.

atherosclerosis   A common form of arteriosclerosis in which deposits of fibrofatty plaque or thickenings form within the intima or intermedia of large and medium-sized arteries.

atheroma   A mass of plaque occurring in atherosclerosis.

atherothrombotic brain infarction   An area of necrotic brain tissue resulting from an obstruction of blood circulation due to a thrombus.

atresia   Congenital absence or abnormal closure of a normal anatomic opening.

atrial septal defect   An abnormal opening between the right and left atria of the heart which allows mixing of oxygenated and unoxygenated blood within the atria.

atrophy   A reduction in size or wasting of cells, tissues, or organs as a result of poor nutrition or nonuse.

autoantibody   Antibody acting against its own tissue or organism.

autoimmune disorder   Disease in which antibodies form against and injure the patient's own tissues, in contrast to the normal process in which antibodies form in response to foreign antigens.

avulsion fracture   A fracture in which a fragmented bone is pulled away from the shaft, usually occurring around a ligament or tendon and often with muscle tearing, as is associated with a sprain or dislocation.

basilar skull fracture   A fracture of bones comprising the base of the skull and may include the occipital bone, sphenoid, ethmoid, and temporal bones.

benign neoplasm   A localized tumor of well-differentiated cells that does not invade surrounding tissue or metastasize to distant areas within the body.

bicornuate uterus   A uterus with paired uterine horns extending to the uterine tubes.

bladder carcinoma   A malignant neoplasm originating from the epithelial lining of the bladder wall.

bladder diverticula   A pouch in the wall of the urinary bladder.

bladder trabeculae   Roughening of the normally smooth bladder wall.

blood–brain barrier   The special functioning of the cerebral capillaries that prevents the passage of unwanted substances into the brain.

blowout fracture   A fracture of the orbital floor resulting from a direct blow to the front of the orbit, with the force of the blow transferred to the orbital walls and floor.

brain abscess   A collection of immune cells, pus, and fluid within the brain in response to a bacterial or fungal infection.

breast carcinoma   A malignant neoplasm originating from the ductal or glandular tissue within the breast.

Bright disease   An inflammatory reaction of the renal parenchyma caused by an antigen–antibody reaction in the glomeruli.

bronchial carcinoid tumor   A neuroendocrine malignant tumor situated in the submucosal tissues of large bronchi.

bronchiectasis   Chronic dilatation of the bronchi, with inflammation and destruction of bronchial walls and cilia.

bronchitis   Inflammation of one or more bronchi.

bronchogenic carcinoma   Carcinoma of the lung that arises from the epithelium of the bronchial tree.

bursitis   Inflammation of the bursae of the tendons, with the subdeltoid bursa as the most common site.

callus   An unorganized meshwork of woven bone formed after a fracture, ultimately replaced by hard, adult bone.

cancellous bone   Bone that has spongy, lattice-like structure filled by bone marrow.

capillaries Small blood vessels connecting venules and arterioles which allow the exchange or water, gases, and nutrients within the blood.

carbohydrate intolerance The inability to digest and process sugars and starches into a source of energy due to an enzyme deficiency.

carcinoma A malignant growth composed of epithelial cells that tends to invade surrounding tissues and give rise to metastases.

carcinoma of the gallbladder A malignant neoplasm of the gallbladder of glandular origin.

cardiomegaly The appearance of an enlarged heart, as indicative of many cardiovascular disorders.

central venous pressure (CVP) line Specialized catheter inserted usually via the subclavian vein to the level of the right atrium to compensate for loss of peripheral infusion sites or to allow for fluid infusion in significant amounts.

cerebrovascular accident (CVA) A loss of blood supply to the brain from a cerebral bleed or a thrombus or embolus.

cervical carcinoma A slow-growing, malignant neoplasm in the tissue within the neck of the uterus most commonly caused by human papillomavirus infection.

cervical dysplasia Abnormal cellular changes within the epithelial cells of the cervix or uterine neck.

cervical spondylosis Degenerative joint disease affecting the cervical vertebrae, vertebral disks, and surrounding ligaments and connective tissue.

cholecystitis An acute inflammation of the gallbladder most frequently caused by obstruction.

cholelithiasis The presence of gallstones.

chondrosarcoma A malignant bone tumor composed of atypical cartilage.

chronic Presenting slowly and persisting over a long period of time.

Chronic Bronchitis A chronic inflammation of the bronchi.

chronic lymphocytic leukemia A type of B-cell lymphoma, which presents primarily in the lymph nodes.

chronic myelocytic leukemia A form of leukemia characterized by the increased and unregulated growth of predominantly myeloid cells in the bone marrow and the accumulation of these cells in the blood.

chronic obstructive pulmonary disease (COPD) Designation applied to conditions that result in pulmonary obstruction, most commonly chronic bronchitis and pulmonary emphysema.

cirrhosis Liver condition in which the parenchyma and architecture are destroyed and replaced by fibrous tissue and regenerative nodules.

closed fracture A fracture that does not produce an open wound.

closed reduction Manipulation of bone fragments to reduce a dislocation or fracture without surgical intervention.

clubfoot Deformity of the foot involving the talus.

coarctation of the aorta A narrowing or compression of the aorta.

coccidioidomycosis Systemic fungal infection caused by a fungus that thrives in semiarid soil and is particularly endemic in the southwestern United States and northern Mexico.

coin lesion Small solitary round nodules in the lung tissue.

colostomy An opening from the colon to the exterior abdomen created by a surgical procedure to allow excretion of feces.

coma A state of unconsciousness from which the patient cannot be aroused.

comminuted fracture A fracture in which the bone is splintered or crushed.

compact bone Dense, outer portion of bone.

complete noncomminuted fracture A fracture in which the bone separates into two fragments.

compression fracture A fracture produced by compression.

concussion Brief loss of consciousness as a result of a blow to the head.

congenital Existing at, and usually before, birth and resulting from genetic or environmental factors.

congestive heart failure Condition existing when the heart is unable to propel blood at a sufficient rate and volume to prevent congestion of circulatory subsystems.

contrecoup lesion A contusion formed on the opposite side of the skull in reference to a trauma site.

contusion An injury in which the tissue is bruised but not broken.

cor pulmonale Hypertension in the pulmonary artery and an enlargement of the right ventricle of the heart.

coronary artery disease (CAD) Disease of the arteries of the heart often resulting from deposition of atheromas in the arteries supplying blood to the heart muscle.

corpus luteum ovarian cyst A cyst that develops in the yellow endocrine body formed in the ovary at the site of a ruptured ovarian follicle.

coup lesion A contusion formed on the side of the head on which trauma occurs.

craniopharyngioma A cystic, benign tumor that usually grows above the sella and upward into the third ventricle of the brain.

craniosynostosis Premature or early closure of the sutures of the skull.

Craniotubular dysplasia An overgrowth of bone of the face and skull resulting in sclerosis and major skeletal deformities.

Crohn disease A chronic granulomatous inflammatory disease of unknown cause involving any part of the gastrointestinal tract, but commonly involving the terminal ileum; also known as *regional enteritis*.

crossed ectopy A condition in which one kidney lies across the body midline and is fused to the other kidney.

cryoablation A process that uses extreme cold to remove tissue.

cryptorchidism Failure of one or both testes to descend into the scroum.

Cushing syndrome A syndrome resulting from excessive production of glucocorticoids.

cystadenocarcinoma Malignant neoplasm of the ovary; generally occurs in women over the age of 40 years.

cystic fibrosis Congenital disorder affecting exocrine gland function, with respiratory effects, including excessive secretions, obstruction of the bronchial system, infection, and tissue damage.

cystic teratomas (dermoid cysts) Cystic masses arising from unfertilized ova, containing hair, fat, or bone, and located in an ovary.

cystitis Inflammation of the bladder as a result of its infection.

degenerative Refers to deterioration of the body usually associated with the aging process.

depressed fracture A fracture of the skull in which a fragment is depressed inward.

developmental dysplasia of the hip An abnormal development of the hip joint which results is a misalignment of the femoral head and the acetabulum of the pelvis.

diabetes insipidus Increased urination and thirst resulting from inadequate secretion of the antidiuretic hormone.

diabetes mellitus A carbohydrate metabolism disorder caused by inadequate production or use of insulin.

diagnosis The name of a disease an individual is believed to have.

diaphysis Shaft of a long bone.

diastole The phase of the heart cycle in which the myocardium is relaxing.

diffusion The exchange of oxygen and carbon dioxide within the alveoli of the lungs.

diploë The spongy bone tissue found between the two tables of the cranial bones.

disease Any abnormal disturbance of the normal function or structure of a body part, organ, or system; may display a variety of manifestations.

dislocation The displacement of any part out of contact with its normal articulation.

dissecting aneurysm An aneurysm resulting from hemorrhage that causes longitudinal splitting of the arterial wall.

diverticulitis Inflammation of a diverticulum.

diverticulosis The presence of diverticula in the absence of inflammation.

diverticulum A pouch or sac of variable size occurring normally or created by herniation of a mucous membrane through a defect in its muscular coat.

ductal adenocarcinoma A malignant tumor originating in the ductal epithelium.

ductus arteriosus The blood vessel connecting the pulmonary artery to the proximal descending aorta in the fetus which should normally close at birth.

dysphagia Difficulty in swallowing.

dysplasia Abnormal tissue development. *Escherichia coli* species of ameba normally found in the upper intestinal tract.

ectopic kidney A kidney that is out of its normal position, usually lower than normal.

ectopic pregnancy A pregnancy in which the fertilized ovum is implanted outside of the uterus.

embolization Interventional angiography procedure in which devices such as coils are used to intentionally clot off vessels, often before surgery to prevent excessive bleeding.

emphysema A lung condition characterized by an increase in the air spaces distal to the terminal bronchioles and with destruction of alveolar walls.

encephalitis   Inflammation of the brain.

endemic   Term describing disease of high prevalence in an area where the causative organism is commonly found.

endochondroma   A benign growth of cartilage arising in the metaphysis of a bone.

endocardium   The inner membrane layer of tissue lining the heart.

endometrial carcinoma   A malignant neoplasm arising from the inner lining of the uterus.

endometriosis   A condition in which endometrial tissue implants in aberrant pelvic locations.

endoscopy   The use of lighted instruments with optic connections to visualize disease of the esophagus and stomach, or rectum and distal colon (e.g., sigmoidoscopy).

ependymoma   A glial tumor that is firm and whitish and arises from the ependyma, the ventricle lining.

epicardium   The inner layer of pericardium surrounding the heart which forms an outer layer of connective tissue covering the heart.

epidemiology   The investigation of disease in large groups.

epididymo-orchitis   A testicular condition that may result in benign masses of the testes.

epiphysis   An ossification or growth center in the bones of children.

erythrocytes   Red blood cells.

Escherichia coli   A gram-negative bacterium found in the large intestine that may produce a toxin causing intestinal illness.

esophageal varices   Varicose veins of the esophagus that occur in patients with portal hypertension.

etiology   The study of the cause and origin of disease.

Ewing sarcoma   A primary malignant bone tumor arising in medullary tissue, occurring more often in cylindric bones.

exostosis   A benign bone growth, projecting outward from the bony cortex.

expectoration   Expulsion of mucus or phlegm from the throat.

exudate   Pus, celluar debris, or clear fluid that leaks out of the blood vessels into the surrounding tissues.

fatigue fracture   A fracture which occurs due to repeated or unusual stress.

fatty liver disease   A buildup of lipids that are deposited in liver tissue.

fibroadenoma   Adenoma containing fibrous tissue.

fibrocystic breast   A benign, generally bilateral breast condition characterized by various-sized cysts located throughout the breasts.

Foley catheter   A catheter that is placed through the urethra and retained in the urinary bladder by a balloon that is inflated with air or fluid.

follicular ovarian cyst   A cyst arising from the ovum.

foramen ovale   An opening between the right and left atria of the fetal heart which should normally close at birth.

fracture   The breaking or rupturing of bone caused by mechanical forces either applied to the bone or transmitted directly along the line of a bone.

fusiform aneurysm   An arterial aneurysm in which the entire circumference of the vessel wall is affected.

gallstone ileus   A condition in which gallstones erode from the gallbladder, creating a fistula to the small bowel that may cause a bowel obstruction.

ganglion   Cystic swelling that develops in connection with a tendon sheath, usually on the back of the wrist.

gastroenteritis   General grouping of a number of inflammatory disorders of the stomach and intestines.

gastroesophageal reflux disease   An incompetent cardiac sphincter allowing the backward flow of gastric acid and contents into the esophagus.

gated cardiac blood pool scan   A gated nuclear medicine procedure of the heart that demonstrates heart motion and the ejection of blood from the heart.

genetic mapping   A map assigning deoxyribonucleic acid (DNA) fragments to chromosomes.

genome   The entirety of an organism's hereditary information, including both the genes and the non-coding sequences of DNA and ribonucleic acid (RNA).

giant cell tumor   A neoplastic growth of the skeletal system consisting of numerous multinucleated osteoclastic giant cells; also called *osteoclastoma*.

glioblastoma multiforme   The highest grade glioblastoma, a malignant brain neoplasm arising from the astrocytes (glial cells).

glioma A tumor composed of tissue that represents neuroglia, commonly occurring in the cerebral hemispheres of the posterior fossa.

glucagon Secretion of the alpha cells of the pancreas to break down glycogen and increase sugar in the bloodstream.

gluten-sensitive enteropathy An autoimmune hereditary disorder involving increased sensitivity to the gliadin fraction of gluten, an agent found in wheat, barley, and rye products.

gouty arthritis An inherited, metabolic disorder with excess amounts of uric acid produced and deposited in the joint and adjacent bone, most commonly in the metatarsophalangeal joint of the great toe.

granulomatous colitis Chronic inflammation of the colon characterized by granulations associated with an infective process.

Graves disease An autoimmune disease affecting the thyroid gland and the most common cause of hyperthyroidism.

greenstick fracture A fracture in which the cortex breaks on one side without separation or breaking of the opposing cortex.

growth plate fracture A fracture that involves the end of a long bone of a child and that may be limited to growth plate cartilage or extend into the metaphysis, epiphysis, or both.

gynecomastia Abnormal breast tissue development in males due to a hormone imbalance.

hangman's fracture A fracture of the arch of the second cervical vertebra, usually accompanied by anterior subluxation of the second cervical vertebra on the third cervical vertebra; also known as *atraumatic spondylosis;* such fractures usually result from acute hyperextension of the head.

haplotype A combination of DNA sequences at adjacent locations on the chromosome that are transmitted together.

hemangioma A benign tumor of dilated blood vessels.

hematocrit A common laboratory test that determines the body's total number of red blood cells.

hematogenous spread Spread through the blood.

hematoma A localized collection of blood in an organ, space, or tissue as a result of a break in the wall of a blood vessel.

hemocytoblast The stem cell for blood cell formation.

hemophilia (A, B, C) A genetic mutation disorder that inhibits proper blood clotting due to a variety of factors.

hemorrhagic stroke A stroke in which a blood vessel in the brain breaks or ruptures.

hemothorax Pleural effusion containing blood.

hepatitis An inflammation of the liver resulting from a variety of causes.

hepatocellular adenoma A benign tumor of the liver most frequently associated with oral contraceptives.

hepatocellular carcinoma A primary malignant tumor of the liver.

hepatomegaly Enlargement of the liver as might be seen with viral hepatitis.

hereditary Genetically transferred from either parent to child and derived from ancestors.

hernia The protrusion of a part of an organ (e.g., bowel loop) through a small opening in the wall of a cavity.

herniated nucleus pulposus Herniation of the nucleus pulposus of the disk through a rupture in the annulus fibrosus.

hiatal hernia Protrusion of any structure, especially some portion of the stomach, into the thoracic cavity through the esophageal hiatus of the diaphragm.

Hirschsprung disease Absence of neurons in the bowel wall, typically in the sigmoid, preventing relaxation of the colon and normal peristalsis; congenital megacolon.

HIV protease An enzyme that converts immature, noninfectious human immunodeficiency virus (HIV) to its infectious state within the cell.

Hodgkin lymphoma A malignant condition of lymphoid tissue associated with Reed-Sternberg cells.

Hormonal Stimuli A hormonal agent that directly influences the activity of the body.

horseshoe kidney A condition in which the lower poles of the kidney are joined across midline by a band of soft tissues, resulting in a rotation anomaly on one or both sides.

hospital-acquired infection Refers to diseases acquired in or from a health care environment.

human immunodeficiency retrovirus (HIV) The virus associated with acquired immunodeficiency syndrome.

humoral stimuli Hormone release by endocrine glands as a result of changing levels of certain ions in body fluids such as blood or bile.

hydatidiform mole Represents an abnormal conception in which the fetus is absent and the uterus is filled with cystically dilated chorionic villi that resemble a bunch of grapes.

hydrocele A benign testicular mass consisting of a collection of fluid in the testis or along the spermatic cord.

hydrocephalus A congenital or acquired condition resulting from accumulation of cerebrospinal fluid in the ventricles of the brain and leading to ventricular enlargement, compression of brain tissue, and increased intracranial pressure.

hydronephrosis An obstructive disease of the urinary system that causes a dilatation of the renal pelvis and calyces with urine.

hypercapnia A condition of high carbon dioxide blood levels usually associated with hypoventilation or lung disease.

hyperostosis frontalis interna A thickening of the inner side of the frontal bone due to a benign tumor.

hyperparathyroidism Abnormally increased activity of the parathyroid glands, causing excess hormone production; this overstimulates osteoclasts, which are responsible for bone removal.

hyperplasia Overdevelopment.

hyperthyroidism Excessive secretion of hormones by the thyroid glands that increases metabolism.

hypertrophic pyloric stenosis A congenital anomaly of the stomach in which the pyloric canal is greatly narrowed because of hypertrophy of the pyloric sphincter.

hypertrophy Increase in number of cells and tissue resulting in an increased organ size without the presence of a tumor.

hypopituitarism Decreased secretion of pituitary hormones.

hypoplasia Less than normal development.

hypothyroidism Diminished secretion of hormones by the thyroid glands that decreases metabolism.

hypoxemia A condition in which arterial blood is insufficiently oxygenated.

hysterosalpingography A radiographic examination for screening of the nongravid woman; injection of contrast into the uterus and the flow into the uterine tubes reveals their patency, which may affect the ability to become pregnant.

iatrogenic Pertains to any adverse condition that occurs in a patient as a result of medical treatment.

idiopathic Having no identifiable causative factor.

ileostomy An opening from the ileum to the exterior abdomen created by a surgical procedure to allow excretion of intestinal waste.

impacted fracture A fracture in which fragments of one end of a broken bone are wedged or driven into the other end of the bone.

imperforate anus Congenital disorder characterized by absence of anal opening to the exterior.

incidence A statistical measure that refers to the number of new cases of a disease found in a given time period.

incomplete fracture A fracture in which only part of the bony structure gives way, with little or no displacement.

infarct An area of ischemic necrosis.

infection An inflammatory process caused by exposure to some disease-causing organism.

inflammatory Refers to the body process of destroying, diluting, or walling off a localized injurious agent.

insulin A hormone secreted by the β-cells of the pancreas to help maintain proper blood sugar levels.

intima The spread and multiplication of a pathogenic organism or malignant cells.

intussusception The prolapse of a segment of bowel into a distal segment.

Invasion The prolapse of a segment of bowel into a distal segment.

involucrum A shell or sheath of new supporting bone laid down by periosteum around a sequestrum of necrosed bone.

ischemia A local and temporary impairment of circulation caused by obstruction of circulation.

ischemic stroke A stroke in which a blood clot blocks a blood vessel in the brain.

jaundice Yellowish discoloration of the skin and whites of the eyes caused by bilirubin accumulation in the body tissues.

Jefferson fracture A burst fracture of the vertebral arch resulting from a severe axial force that causes compression, as in a diving accident.

juvenile rheumatoid arthritis A form of rheumatoid arthritis which affects children.

Kaposi sarcoma A sarcoma present in the connective tissues of about one fourth of all patients with acquired immunodeficiency syndrome (AIDS).

lacunar infarction Small vessel disease that results in a thrombotic stroke.

left ventricular failure Congestive heart failure that results when the left ventricle cannot pump an amount of blood equal to the venous return in the right ventricle.

Legg-Calvé-Perthes disease Osteonecrosis of the head of the femur due to poor blood supply.

legionnaire's disease Severe bacterial pneumonia named for its outbreak at an American Legion convention in Pennsylvania in 1976.

leiomyoma A benign tumor derived from smooth muscle.

lesion General term used to describe the various types of cellular changes that can occur in response to a disease.

leukemia A malignant disease of the leukocytes and their precursor cells in blood and bone marrow.

leukocytes White blood cells.

Level 1 trauma center The primary hospitals in the trauma system capable of providing total care for all injuries.

Level 2 trauma center Hospitals which provide care for all but the most critical patients who may need cardiac surgery, microvascular surgery, or hemodialysis.

Level 3 traoma center Hospitals that provide quick assessment, resuscitation, and stabilizations of patients prior to transferring them to a higher level trauma center.

Level 4 trauma center Hospitals that offer basic emergency department facilities.

linear fracture A fracture that extends lengthwise through a bone.

Luxation A dislocation of vertebrae.

lymphatic spread Spread through the lymphatic system.

lymphocytes White blood cells important in building immunity.

lymphoma Neoplastic growth in the lymphatic system.

malignant neoplasm A lesion that grows, spreads, and invades other tissues.

malrotation Unnatural position of the intestines caused by failure of normal rotation during embryologic development.

manifestation Observable changes resulting from cellular changes in the disease process.

mastalgia Breast pain.

mastitis Inflammation of the breast, most often caused by *Staphylococcus* bacteria.

mechanical bowel obstruction Refers to a bowel obstruction that occurs as a result of blockage of the bowel lumen.

media The middle, muscular layer of a vessel wall.

mediastinal emphysema (pneumomediastinum) The presence of air or gas in the mediastinum as a result of leakage of air from the bronchial tree.

medical jaundice Jaundice resulting from hemolytic disease, in which excessive amounts of red blood cells are destroyed, or when the liver is damaged as a result of cirrhosis or hepatitis.

medullary canal Inner spongy or cancellous portion of a long bone where bone marrow is produced.

medullary sponge kidney A congenital anomaly of the urinary system in which the only visible abnormality is the dilatation of the medullary and papillary portions of the collecting ducts, usually bilaterally.

medulloblastoma Soft, infiltrating tumors of neuroepithelial tissue that are highly malignant.

meningioma A hard, usually vascular tumor that occurs mainly along meningeal vessels and the superior longitudinal sinus.

meningitis Inflammation of the meninges caused by a bacterial or viral agent.

meningocele Hernial protrusion of the meninges through a defect of the skull or vertebral column.

meningomyelocele Protrusion of the spinal cord and meninges through a defect of the vertebral column, as is commonly associated with spina bifida.

metabolic syndrome A combination of medical disorders that, when occurring together, increase the risk of developing cardiovascular disease and diabetes.

metabolism The normal physiologic function of the body.

metaphysis The growing portion of bone.

metaplasia Conversion of a specific type of tissue into a different kind of tissue.

metastatic spread The spread of cancer cells.

Metastatic liver Disease The spread of another primary cancer to the liver.

miliary tuberculosis Type of tuberculosis caused by hematogenous spread of the disease, with a characteristic appearance similar to millet seeds, which are small, white grains.

M-mode echocardiography Dynamic, one-dimensional sonographic images of the heart.

morbidity rate The incidence in the population of illness sufficient to interfere with an individual's normal daily routine.

morphology The form and structure of disease.

mortality rate The number of deaths from a particular disease averaged over a population.

multiple myeloma A malignant neoplasm of plasma cells characterized by skeletal destruction, pathologic fractures, and bone pain.

multiple sclerosis A chronic, slowly progressive disease of the central nervous system, characterized by demyelination of the nerve sheath.

murmur An abnormal extra heart sound indicating a structural or functional defect of the heart.

Mycoplasma pneumonia The most common form of primary atypical pneumonia, occurring most frequently in young adults.

myelocele Protrusion of the spinal cord through the normally closed bony neural arch of the spine.

myeloid tissue Tissue within the bone marrow.

myocardium The muscular layer of the heart.

neoplastic Pertaining to new, abnormal tissue growth.

nephroblastoma (Wilms tumor) A rapidly developing malignancy of the kidneys, usually affecting children before age 5 years.

nephrocalcinosis A condition characterized by precipitation of calcium in the tubules of the kidney, resulting in renal deficiency.

nephroptosis Prolapse of a kidney.

nephrosclerosis Intimal thickening of predominantly the small vessels of the kidney as a result of reduced blood flow through arteriosclerotic renal vasculature.

nephrostomy tube A tube inserted through the abdominal wall into the renal pelvis to drain urine.

neural stimuli The release of hormones due to nerve stimulation of an endocrine gland.

neurofibroma A tumor of peripheral nerves caused by abnormal proliferation of Schwann cells.

neurogenic bladder A bladder dysfunction caused by interference with the nerve impulses concerned with urination.

noncomminuted fracture A fracture in which the bones do not break into multiple pieces or fragments.

nongravid Not pregnant.

non-Hodgkin lymphoma A malignancy of the lymphoid cells found in the lymph nodes, bone marrow, spleen, liver, and gastrointestinal system.

nucleus pulposus The inner soft portion of an intervertebral disk.

occult fracture A fracture that gives clinical signs of its presence without radiologic evidence; follow-up within 10 days reveals bone reabsorption or displacement at the fracture site.

oligodendroglioma A glioma, which is a slow-growing astrocytic tumor that is usually relatively benign.

oligohydramnios The presence of too little (less than 300 mL) amniotic fluid at term, generally associated with renal disorders in the fetus.

open or compound fracture A fracture in which the bone ends penetrate the soft tissue and skin, creating an opening to the exterior of the body.

open reduction Manipulation of bone fragments to reduce a dislocation or fracture with surgical intervention.

open reduction internal fixation The surgical placement of orthopedic hardware to repair a skeletal fracture.

osteoarthritis Noninflammatory degenerative joint disease occurring mainly in older persons, producing gradual deterioration of the joint cartilage.

osteoblastoma Tumors of the bone arising from osteoblasts.

osteoblasts The bone-forming cells responsible for bone growth, ossification, and regeneration.

osteochondroma A benign tumor of adult bone capped by cartilage.

osteoclastoma A tumor that is usually benign and characterized by osteolytic areas, most commonly found around the knee and wrist of young adults and composed of numerous, multinucleated osteoclasts; also called *giant cell tumor.*

osteoclasts Cells that are associated with absorption and removal of bone.

osteogenesis imperfecta A congenital disease in which the bones are abnormally brittle and subject to fractures.

osteoid osteoma A benign tumor of bonelike structure that develops on a bone and sometimes on other structures.

osteoma A benign neoplasm of the bone.

osteomalacia A condition marked by softening of the bones, caused by lack of calcium in tissues and failure of bone tissue to calcify.

osteomyelitis Infection of bone, most often caused by *Staphylococcus*, which may localize or spread to bone to involve marrow and other bone tissues.

osteopenia A softening of bone demonstrated radiographically as a decreased bone density, as in osteoporosis or osteomalacia.

osteopetrosis A hereditary disease characterized by abnormally dense bone, likely resulting from faulty bone reabsorption.

osteophytes Osseous outgrowths (spurs).

osteoporosis Metabolic bone disorder resulting in demineralization of bone, most commonly seen in women after menopause.

osteosarcoma A primary malignancy of bone usually arising in the metaphysis, most commonly around the knee.

Paget disease A metabolic disorder of unknown cause, most common in the elderly, characterized by an early, osteolytic stage and a late, osteoblastic stage.

palliative Treatment designed to relieve pain without the goal of curing the disease.

pancreatic cancer A disease in which malignant cells grow from the epithelial cells of the pancreas.

pancreatitis Acute or chronic, asymptomatic or symptomatic inflammation of the pancreas caused by autodigestion by pancreatic enzymes.

paralytic ileus A failure of bowel peristalsis, often seen after abdominal surgery, which may result in bowel obstruction.

patent ductus arteriosus Abnormal persistence of an open ductus arteriosus after birth, resulting in recirculation of arterial blood through the lungs.

pathogenesis Development of disease.

pathologic fracture A fracture that occurs in abnormal bone weakened by a disease process.

pathology The study of structural and functional manifestations of disease.

peau d'orange Orange-peel appearance of multiple small depressions on the skin surface as a result of hair follicles becoming visible from skin edema, as might occur with breast cancer.

pelvic inflammatory disease (PID) A bacterial infection of the female genital system, most often caused by bacteria.

peptic ulcer Ulceration of the mucous membrane of the esophagus, stomach, or duodenum.

percutaneous transluminal angioplasty (PTA) Use of a specialized catheter, typically equipped with an inflatable balloon, to perform vessel repair from within the artery or vein during angiography.

permanent catheterization Interventional angiography procedure, in which a catheter is placed in the subclavian or jugular vein and tunneled under skin to allow for improved dialysis access.

pessary A device inserted into the vagina to provide proper support to a uterus that lacks proper support.

phlebitis Inflammation of a vein, often associated with venous thrombosis.

physical mapping A form of genetic mapping based on direct analysis of DNA, in which the physical distance between DNA fragments are measured. This is used to assign DNA fragments to specific chromosomes.

Pituitary adenoma A benign tumor of the pituitary gland.

placenta accreta Abnormal adhesion of the placenta to the uterine wall.

placenta previa The condition in which the placenta develops in the lower half of the uterus, on or encroaching on, and completely or partially covering, the internal cervical os.

platelike atelectasis Radiographic appearance seen in atelectasis, in which one or more linear opacities are seen, usually at the lung bases and parallel to the diaphragm.

pleural effusion A collection of excess fluid in the pleural cavity.

placental abruption Condition in which a normally implanted placenta prematurely separates from the uterus.

Placental percreta A condition in which the placenta extends into the myometrium.

pleural effusion An accumulation of fluid in the pleural cavity or space.

pleurisy Inflammation of the pleura with exudation into the pleural cavity and on its surface.

pneumococcal pneumonia The most common bacterial pneumonia, generally affecting an entire lobe of a lung.

pneumoconioses A group of occupational diseases characterized by permanent deposits of particulate matter in the lungs and by resultant pulmonary fibrosis.

Pneumocystis carinii **pneumonia**   Life-threatening infection of the lungs most commonly associated with AIDS.

pneumonia   The most frequent type of lung infection, resulting in an inflammation of the lung with compromised pulmonary function.

pneumoperitoneum   The presence of air or gas in the peritoneal cavity.

pneumothorax   An accumulation of free air or gas in the pleural space that compresses the lung tissue.

polycystic kidney disease   A familial kidney disorder in which innumerable tiny cysts that are present congenitally gradually enlarge during aging to compress and eventually destroy normal tissues.

polycystic ovaries   Ovaries that contain multiple small cysts.

polydactyly   The presence of more than five digits.

polyhydramnios   An excess of amniotic fluid; it may be associated with anencephaly or gastrointestinal disturbances in the fetus.

polyp   A small mass of tissue arising from the mucous membrane to project inward into the lumen of the bowel.

Pott disease   A fracture of the lower part of the fibula involving both malleoli with dislocation of the ankle joint.

prevalence   A statistical measure that refers to the number of cases of a disease found in a given population.

prognosis   The prediction of course and outcome for a given disease.

progressive disseminated histoplasmosis   A respiratory disease endemic in the Mississippi and Ohio river valleys caused by a fungal infection.

prostatic calculi   Stones within the prostate gland.

prostatic hyperplasia   Abnormal benign cell growth within the prostate gland.

pseudocyst   An abnormal or displaced space resembling a cyst.

pseudofracture   A band of bone material of decreased density may form alongside the surface of the bone.

psoriatic arthritis   An inflammatory arthritis associated with psoriasis of the skin.

pulmonary embolus   A mass of foreign matter present in a pulmonary artery or one of its branches.

pulmonary tuberculosis   A contagious bacterial infection of the lungs caused by *Mycobacterium tuberculosis*.

pyelonephritis   Bacterial infection of the kidney and its pelvis.

pyuria   The presence of pus in urine, created by its drainage from renal abscesses into the kidney's collecting tubules.

radiofrequency ablation   A process that uses radiofrequency waves to remove tissue.

Reed-Sternberg cells   A specific type of cells that help differentiate Hodgkin lymphomas from other types of lymphatic diseases.

reflux esophagitis   The backward flow of gastric acids into the esophagus.

regional enteritis   A chronic granulomatous inflammatory disease of unknown cause involving any part of the gastrointestinal tract, but commonly involving the terminal ileum.

Reiter syndrome   A group of symptoms associated with complications of urethritis.

renal agenesis   The absence of the kidney on one side, with an unusually large kidney on the other side.

renal calculi   Kidney stone.

renal colic   Severe, agonizing pain that refers along the course of a ureter toward the genital and loin regions in response to the movement of a renal calculus.

renal cyst   A fluid-filled growth within the kidney.

renal failure   The end result of a chronic process that gradually results in lost kidney function.

respiratory distress syndrome (RDS)   A respiratory disorder of infants born at less than a 37-week gestation caused by incomplete maturation of the surfactant-producing system.

respiratory failure   Failure of the lungs to ventilate.

reticuloendothelial system   Specialized cells found in the liver, bone marrow, and spleen, whose function is phagocytosis.

reverse transcriptase   An enzyme that converts viral RNA into a DNA copy that becomes integrated into the host cell DNA.

Rh factor   The factor first discovered in the blood of the rhesus monkey; contained by approximately 85% of the population who are said to be "Rh-positive."

rheumatic fever   An illness that results from an untreated strep throat condition.

rheumatoid arthritis   A chronic, systemic disease primarily of joints, characterized by an overgrowth of synovial tissues and articular structures and progressive destruction of cartilage, bone, and supporting structures.

Rh-negative   Blood type that does not include the Rh (Rhesus) antigen factor.

Rh-positive   Blood type that does include the Rh (Rhesus) antigen factor.

rickets   Osteomalacia that occurs before growth plate closure, caused by deficiency of vitamin D, especially in infants and children.

saccular aneurysm   A localized sac affecting only a part of the circumference of an arterial wall.

sarcoma   A type of tumor, often highly malignant, composed of a substance similar to embryonic connective tissue.

schwannoma   A benign nerve sheath neoplasm or tumor.

scoliosis   Abnormal lateral curvature of the spine.

seeding   Traveling of cancerous cells to a distant site or distant organ.

sequelae   Conditions resulting from a disease.

sequestrum   A piece of dead, devascularized bone that separates from living bone during the process of necrosis.

sickle cell anemia   An inherited blood disorder in which the red blood cells are distorted to a crescent shape, resulting in anemia and other manifestations.

sign   An objective manifestation of disease perceptible to the managing physician, as opposed to subjective symptoms perceived by the patient.

silicosis   Pneumoconiosis caused by inhalation of silica dust, as is common among miners, grinders, and sand blasters.

simple unicameral bone cyst   A benign, fluid-filled bone neoplasm.

single-nucleotide polymorphisms   A DNA sequence variation occurring when a single nucleotide in the genome differs between members of a biologic species or paired chromosomes in an individual.

sinoatrial (SA) node   The heart's "pacemaker"; this is a bundle of nerve fibers located in the upper portion of the right atrium near the superior vena cava; from this node an electrical current is transmitted through the myocardium, resulting in a heartbeat.

sinusitis   Inflammation of a sinus, which may be purulent or nonpurulent and acute or chronic.

situs inversus   Complete reversal of the viscera of the thorax and the abdomen.

slipped capital femoral epiphysis   A separation of the femoral head and shaft occurring through the epiphyseal plate.

sonohysterography   A sonographic examination of the uterus and fallopian tubes, in which normal saline is injected into the uterus.

spermatocele   A cystic dilatation of the epididymis.

spina bifida   A developmental anomaly characterized by incomplete closure of the vertebral canal, through which the choriomeninges may or may not protrude.

spondylolisthesis   Forward displacement of one vertebra over another (commonly occurring at the L5–S1 junction), usually caused by a developmental defect in the pars interarticularis.

spondylolysis   A condition marked by a cleft or breaking down of the body of a vertebra between the superior and inferior articular processes.

staghorn calculus   A large renal calculus that assumes the shape of the pelvicalyceal junction, resembling the horn of a stag.

Staphylococcus aureus   Gram-positive micrococcaceae commonly present on skin and mucous membranes.

steatosis   An excess of fatty acids within the liver leading to fatty infiltration of the liver.

stent   A specialized device placed to provide patency, usually in a vessel or duct.

stress fracture   A fracture that occurs at a site of maximal strain on a bone, usually connected with some unaccustomed activity (also known as a *march, stress,* or *insufficiency fracture*).

subarachnoid hematoma   A hematoma that accumulates between the brain's arachnoid layer and its pia mater.

subcutaneous emphysema   The presence of air or gas in the subcutaneous tissues of the body.

subdural empyema   A collection of pus below the dura layer of the meninges.

subdural hematoma   A hematoma positioned between the dura mater and the arachnoid meningeal layer.

subluxation   An incomplete or partial dislocation.

supernumerary kidney   A relatively rare anomaly consisting of the presence of a third, small rudimentary kidney.

suprapubic catheter   A urinary catheter that is placed into the urinary bladder through the skin in the suprapubic area to allow drainage of urine.

surgical jaundice   Jaundice that occurs as a result of biliary system blockage, which prevents bile from entering the duodenum.

sylvian triangle   An anatomic landmark in cerebral angiography, created by the middle cerebral artery and its branches.

symptom   Any subjective evidence of a disease as perceived by a patient.

syndactyly   A webbing or fusion of digits.

syndrome   A group of signs and symptoms that occur together and characterize a specific abnormal disturbance.

systole   The phase of the heart cycle during which the myocardium is contracting.

tendonitis   Inflammation of a tendon.

tenosynovitis   Inflammation of a tendon and its sheath.

testicular choriocarcinoma   A malignant germ cell tumor of the testicle.

testicular embryonal carcinoma   A malignant germ cell tumor of the testicle.

testicular seminoma   A malignant germ cell tumor of the testicle.

testicular teratoma   A malignant germ cell tumor of the testicle.

tetralogy of Fallot   A combination of four congenital cardiac defects: pulmonary stenosis, ventricular central defect, overriding aorta, and hypertrophy of the right ventricle.

thalassemia   A genetic disorder resulting in abnormal hemoglobin molecules within blood, resulting in severe anemia.

thrombocytes   Platelets.

thrombolysis   An interventional angiography procedure in which urokinase, a high-intensity anticoagulant, is dripped over a period of hours directly onto a clot to dissolve it.

thrombophlebitis   The presence of inflammation and blood clots within a vein.

thrombus   A blood clot that obstructs a blood vessel.

torus fracture   A fracture in which the cortex folds back on itself, with little or no displacement of the lower end of the bone.

trabecula   The spongy substance found within a bone; it gives a characteristic appearance to bone details.

trabecular pattern   The arrangement of supportive strands of connective tissue of the alveolar bone in relation to the bone marrow spaces within the cancellous bone.

transesophageal echocardiography (TEE)   A type of echocardiographic procedure in which the patient swallows a mobile, flexible probe. The heart's structure can then be readily visualized without having structures such as the skin, rib cage, and chest muscles interfere.

transient ischemic attack (TIA)   A temporary episode of neurologic dysfunction that can precede a cerebrovascular accident.

transitional vertebra   A vertebra that assumes the characteristics of the vertebrae on each side of a major spine division.

transjugular intrahepatic portosystemic stent (TIPSS)   An interventional angiography procedure in which a catheter is used to connect the jugular vein to the portal vein to reduce the flow of blood through a diseased liver.

transposition of great vessels   Congenital malformation of the cardiovascular system, in which the aorta arises from the right ventricle and the pulmonary artery from the left ventricle.

transudates   Fluid substances that pass through a tissue membrane.

transurethral resection of the prostate   A cystoscopic surgical procedure in which a portion of the prostate is removed.

traumatic   Pertaining to the effects of a wound or injury, whether physical or psychological.

traumatic brain injury   Damage to the brain from an external mechanical force such as rapid acceleration or deceleration associated with neurologic deficits.

tuberculosis   Any of the infectious diseases of man and animals caused by *Mycobacterium tuberculosis*, generally affecting the lungs in the human body.

type 1 diabetes mellitus   A childhood autoimmune disease in which T cells destroy beta cells in the pancreas, inhibiting the production of insulin.

type 2 diabetes mellitus   A metabolic disease resulting in a hyperglycemia due to insulin resistance usually occurring in adults.

ulcerative colitis   A chronic, recurrent ulceration of the colon mucosa of unknown cause.

unicornuate uterus   A uterus whose uterine cavity is elongated and has a single uterine tube emerging from it.

uremia   The retention of urea in blood, as characteristic of renal failure.

ureteral diverticula   An outpouching in the ureteral wall.

ureteral stent   A tube used to maintain patency of the ureter, with the proximal end placed in the renal pelvis and the distal end placed in the urinary bladder.

ureterocele   Cystlike dilatation of the terminal portion of the ureter as a result of stenosis of the ureteral meatus.

urethral valves   Congenital presence of mucosal folds that protrude into the posterior urethra, which may cause significant obstruction to urine flow.

urinary tract infection (UTI)   The most common of all bacterial infections, a UTI is an infection in the urinary tract usually caused by a gram-negative bacillus, which invades by an ascending route through the urethra to the bladder to the kidney.

uterine fibroids   Benign growths within the muscle layer of the uterus.

uterus didelphys   Complete duplication of the uterus, cervix, and vagina.

valvular stenosis   Narrowing of a valve.

venous thrombosis   The formation of blood clots within a vein.

ventilation   The process of air movement into and out of the lungs.

ventricular septal defects   An abnormal opening between the right and left ventricles of the heart allowing the mixing of oxygenated and deoxygenated blood.

vesicoureteral reflux   The backward flow of urine out of the bladder and into the ureters.

viral pneumonia   Pneumonia caused by a virus, spread by an infected person to a nonimmune individual.

virulence   The ease with which an organism overcomes body defenses.

volvulus   An intestinal obstruction caused by a twisting of the bowel about its mesenteric base.

von Willebrand disease   An inherited blood disorder resulting in a tendency to hemorrhage.

whiplash   Hyperextension–flexion injury of the spine.

AMERICAN COLLEGE OF RADIOLOGY, RESTON, VIRGINIA

Figs. 2-9, 2-11, 2-14, 2-18, 2-22, 2-23, 2-26A, 2-28, 2-38, 2-41, 2-44, 2-47, 2-48, 2-50, 2-51, 3-7, 3-11, 3-27, 3-30, 3-31, 3-34, 3-36A, 3-38, 3-40, 3-42, 3-48, 4-2, 4-3, 4-6, 4-7, 4-38, 4-41, 5-26, 5-30, 5-31, 5-33 to 5-36, 5-38, 5-39, 5-40, 5-41, 5-43, 5-46, 5-48, 5-51, 5-52, 5-54, 5-56, 5-58, 5-59, 5-62 to 5-65, 5-68, 5-70 to 5-72, 5-74, 6-25, 7-11, 7-13, 7-33, 7-36, 7-56, 7-57, 8-7 to 8-11, 8-25, 9-6, 9-7, 10-14, 11-8, 11-10 to 11-12, 12-4, 12-5, 12-6, 12-9, 12-28, 12-34, 12-46, 12-49, 12-50, 12-58, 12-70, 12-72, 12-73, 12-75, 12-77, 12-81, 12-82, 12-88

AMERICAN COLLEGE OF SURGEONS COMMITTEE ON TRAUMA, CHICAGO, ILLINOIS

Fig. 12-1

AMERICAN HOSPITAL ASSOCIATION: TRENDWATCH

Figs. 1-3, 1-4

BONTRAGER KL: *TEXTBOOK OF RADIOGRAPHIC POSITIONING AND RELATED ANATOMY*, ED 6, ST. LOUIS, MO, 2005, MOSBY

Figs. 2-1 to 2-4, 3-1, 4-1, 4-5, 5-1 to 5-8, 6-1, 6-2, 7-1 to 7-4, 7-44, 8-1 to 8-6, 8-24, 10-1, 10-3, 10-29, 10-30, 11-2, 11-3

CENTERS FOR DISEASE CONTROL AND PREVENTION (CDC)

Figs. 1-1, 1-2, 1-5

CUTTER, MG, DREXLER, E, MCCULLOUGH, LB, MCINERNEY, JD, MURRAY, JC, ROSSITER, B, & ZOLA, J: *MAPPING AND SEQUENCING THE HUMAN GENOME: SCIENCE, ETHICS, AND PUBLIC POLICY*. COLORADO SPRINGS, CO: BSCS AND THE AMERICAN MEDICAL ASSOCIATION, 1992

Fig. 1-6

NATIONWIDE CHILDREN'S HOSPITAL, COLUMBUS, OHIO

Figs. 4-32, 4-34, 4-36, 5-27A & B, 5-28, 8-26 and 8-27

CROWLEY LV: *INTRODUCTORY CONCEPTS IN PATHOLOGY*, CHICAGO, IL, 1972, MOSBY

Fig. 1-9

DAMJANOV I: *ANDERSON'S PATHOLOGY*, VOL 2, ED 10, ST. LOUIS, MO, 1996, MOSBY

Figs. 8-24, 10-27, 12-16

HAINES DE: *FUNDAMENTAL NEUROSCIENCE*, PHILADELPHIA, 1997, CHURCHILL LIVINGSTONE

Fig. 8-28

STANDRING S: *GRAY'S ANATOMY*, ED 40, PHILADELPHIA, CHURCHILL LIVINGSTONE, 2009

Fig. 3-10

MCCANCE KL, HUETHER SE: *PATHOPHYSIOLOGY: THE BIOLOGIC BASIS FOR DISEASE IN ADULTS AND CHILDREN*, ED 6, ST. LOUIS, MO, 2010, MOSBY

Figs. 1-7, 1-8, 1-10, 2-20, 2-33, 2-34, 2-35, 4-27, 4-29A, 4-30, 4-31, 4-33, 4-35, 4-37, 4-42, 4-50, 5-6, 5-25, 5-29, 5-32, 5-37, 5-47, 5-57, 5-73, 6-14, 8-41, 8-56, 9-1, 9-4, 9-12, 11-7, 12-14, 12-27, 12-31

PERKINS, DG: *MOSBY'S COLOR ATLAS AND TEXT OF NEUROLOGY*, LONDON, 1998, MOSBY-WOLFE

Fig. 8-56

THE OHIO STATE UNIVERSITY WEXNER MEDICAL CENTER, COLUMBUS, OHIO

Figs. 2-5, 2-7, 2-8, 2-10, 2-12, 2-15, 2-24, 2-25, 2-26B, 2-27, 2-29, 2-30, 2-31, 2-36, 2-37, 2-39, 2-40, 2-42, 2-43, 2-45, 2-46, 2-52, 2-53, 3-2, 3-3, 3-8, 3-9, 3-12 to 3-26, 3-28, 3-29, 3-33, 3-35, 3-36B, 3-39, 3-40, 3-41, 3-43 to 3-46, 3-49, 3-50, 3-51, 4-8, 4-15 to 4-18C, 4-28B, 4-29B, 4-39, 4-43, 4-44, 4-47, 4-53 to 4-56, 4-59, 5-9, 5-10, 5-12, 5-13, 5-14, 5-15, 5-17 to 5-19, 5-24, 5-40, 5-42, 5-44, 5-45, 5-53, 5-66, 5-67, 6-3, 6-5 to 6-7, 6-10, 6-13, 6-16, 6-17, 6-19, 6-20, 6-23, 7-5 to 7-9, 7-12, 7-14 to 7-17, 7-19, 7-21 to 7-23, 7-30, 7-31, 7-35, 7-37, 7-38, 7-40, 7-41, 7-43, 7-45, 7-46, 7-47, 7-49 to 7-51, 7-59, 8-12, 8-14 to 8-23, 8-29, 8-32, 8-33, 8-34, 8-37, 8-38, 9-2, 9-5, 9-8 to 9-11, 10-5, 10-10 to 10-12, 10-14 to 10-18, 10-20, 10-22, 10-23, 10-24 to 10-26, 10-28, 11-6, 11-9, 11-13 to 11-17, 12-2 to 12-4, 12-7, 12-8, 12-12, 12-20, 12-22 to 12-26, 12-32, 12-33, 12-35 to 12-39, 12-41, 12-42, 12-43, 12-47, 12-51, 12-52, 12-58, 12-59, 12-60, 12-62 to 12-64, 12-66 to 12-71, 12-74, 12-78, 12-79, 12-84, 12-85, 12-86, 12-87

RIVERSIDE METHODIST HOSPITAL, COLUMBUS, OHIO

Figs. 2-6, 2-16, 2-17, 2-19, 2-21, 2-24A, 2-32, 2-39, 2-41, 2-49, 3-4, 3-6, 3-37, 3-52, 3-55, 4-4, 4-9 to 4-14, 4-26, 4-40, 4-45, 4-46, 4-48, 4-49, 4-51, 4-52, 4-57, 4-58, 5-11, 5-16, 5-20 to 5-23, 5-43, 5-49, 5-50, 5-55, 5-60, 5-61, 5-69, 5-75, 6-4, 6-8, 6-9, 6-11, 6-12, 6-15, 6-18, 6-21, 6-22, 6-24, 6-26, 6-27, 7-10, 7-18, 7-20, 7-24, 7-25 to 7-29, 7-32, 7-34, 7-39, 7-42, 7-48, 7-52 to 7-54, 7-58, 8-13, 8-30, 8-31, 8-35, 8-36, 8-39 to 8-40, 8-41 to 8-55, 8-57, 8-58, 9-3, 10-2, 10-4, 10-6 to 10-9, 10-13, 10-19, 10-21, 10-24, 10-25, 10-27, 10-31 to 10-40, 12-10, 12-11, 12-13, 12-15, 12-17 to 12-19, 12-21, 12-27, 12-30, 12-40, 12-41, 12-44, 12-45, 12-48, 12-53 to 12-57, 12-61, 12-65, 12-80, 12-83

THIBODEAU GA, PATTON KT: *ANATOMY & PHYSIOLOGY* ED. 5, ST. LOUIS, 2003, MOSBY

Figs. 11-1, 11-4, and 11-5

Aletaha D, Neogi T, Silman AJ, et al: 2010 rheumatoid arthritis classification criteria: arthritis & rheumatism. *Am Coll Rheumatol* 62(9):2569–2581, 2010.

American Academy of Pediatrics: Diagnostic imaging of child abuse. *Pediatrics* 105(6), 2000.

American College of Radiology: ACR Appropriateness Criteria: http://www.acr.org/SecondaryMainMenuCategories/quality_safety/app_criteria/pdf/. Accessed January 16, 2012.

American College of Radiology: Practice guideline for the performance of HSG: http://www.acr.org/SecondaryMainMenuCategories/quality_safety/guidelines/dx/genit/hysterosalpingography.aspx. Accessed November 2, 2012.

American College of Surgeons: Trauma centers by state or regional designation/certification and ACS verification status by level of trauma care: www.amtrauma.org/tiep/reports/ACSclassification. Accessed June 28, 2006.

American College of Surgeons (ACS) Trauma Committee: *Injury prevention saves lives*, Chicago, IL, 2000, ACS.

American College of Surgeons: American College of Surgeons consultation/verification program reference guide of suggested classification: http://www.facs.org/trauma/vrc1.pdf. Accessed May 25, 2012.

American Hospital Association: *TrendWatch*, Washington D.C., 2011.

American Hospital Association: *TrendWatch*, Washington D.C., 2011.

American Stroke Association: Guidelines for the early management of patients with ischemic stroke: a scientific statement from the Stroke Council of the American Stroke Association. *Stroke* 34:1056, 2003.

Ba-Sslaamah A, Uffmann M, Saini S, et al: Clinical value of MRI liver specific contrast agents: a tailored examination for a confident non-invasive diagnosis of focal liver lesions. *Eur Radiol* 19:342–357, 2009.

Batchelor J, McGuiness A: A meta-analysis of GCS 15 head injured patients with loss of consciousness or post traumatic amnesia. *Emerg Med J* 19(6):515, 2002.

Black R: *Rose and Black's clinical problems in nephrology*, Boston, MA, 1996, Little, Brown and Co.

Bontrager K, Lampignano J: *Textbook of radiographic positioning and related anatomy*, ed 6, St. Louis, MO, 2005, Mosby.

Bontrager KL: *Textbook of radiographic positioning and related anatomy*, ed 3, St. Louis, MO, 1993, Mosby.

Boss B: Chapter 17: Alterations of neurologic function. In McCance Kl, Huether SE, editors: *Pathophysiology: the biologic basis for disease in adults and children*, ed 5, Toronto, Canada, 2006, Mosby.

Braunwald E: *Heart disease*, ed 5, Philadelphia, PA, 1997, Saunders.

Brenner BM: *Brenner and Rector's the kidney*, ed 5, vols 1 and 2, Philadelphia, PA, 1996, Saunders.

Bull RK, Edwards PD, Kemp PM, et al: Bone age assessment: a large scale comparison of the Greulich and Pyle, and Tanner and Whitehouse (TW2) methods. *Arch Dis Child* 81:172, 1999.

Bullock B: *Pathophysiology, adaptations and alterations in function*, ed 4, Philadelphia, PA, 1996, Lippincott-Raven.

Centers for Disease Control and Prevention (CDC): *2003 National Hospital Discharge Survey, Advance Data from Vital and Health Statistics*, No. 359, Hyattsville, MD, 2005, U.S. Department of Health and Human Services.

Centers for Disease Control and Prevention (CDC): *Health insurance coverage: estimates from the 2010 National Health Survey*, Hyattsville, MD, 2011, Division of Health Interview Statistics, U.S. Department of Health and Human Services.

Centers for Disease Control and Prevention (CDC): *Injury prevention and control: traumatic brain injury*, Hyattsville, MD, 2012, U.S. Department of Health and Human Services.

Centers for Disease Control and Prevention (CDC): *National hospital ambulatory medical care survey 2000, advance data from vital and health statistics*, No. 326.31, Hyattsville, MD, 2001, U.S. Department of Health and Human Services.

Centers for Disease Control and Prevention (CDC): *National vital statistics reports*, vol 59, No. 8, Hyattsville, MD, 2011, U.S. Department of Health and Human Services.

Centers for Disease Control and Prevention (CDC): HIV in the United States, March 2012: http://www.cdc.gov/hiv/resources/factsheets/PDF/HIV_at_a_glance.pdf. Accessed May 15, 2012.

Centers for Medicare and Medicaid Services: *TrendWatch chartbook 2011*, 2010, Office of the Actuary.

Clemons JL, Aguilar VC, Tillinghast TA, et al: Patient satisfaction and changes in prolapsed and urinary symptoms in women who were fitted successfully with a pessary for pelvic organ prolapsed. *Am J Obstet Gynecol* 190(4):1025–1029, 2004.

Cobrin G: Capsule endoscopy. *Cancer* 107:22, 2006.

Cotran R, Rennke H, Kumar V: The kidney and its collecting system. In editor: *Robbins basic pathology*, ed 7, St. Louis, MO, 2003, Elsevier.

Crowley LV: *Introduction to human disease*, ed 4, Boston, MA, 1997, Bartlett.

Dalen J: The pulmonary artery catheter—friend, foe, or accomplice? *JAMA*, 286(3), 2001.

Deal D, Lambiase L, Li J: M2A capsule endoscopy, Jacksonville Medicine, June/July 2002: www.dcmsonline.org. Accessed November 2, 2006.

Dijkman AB, Mol BWJ, van der Veen F, et al: Can hysterosalpingocontrast-sonography replace hysterosalingography in the assessment of tubal subfertility? *EJR* 35:44–48, 2000.

Eisenberg R, Dennis CA: *Comprehensive radiographic pathology*, St. Louis, MO, 1995, Mosby.

Flanagan FL, Dehdashti F, Siegel BA: PET in breast cancer. *Semin Nucl Med* 28(4):290, 1998.

Gore RM, Levine MS: *Textbook of gastrointestinal radiology*, Philadelphia, PA, 1996, Saunders.

Gu P, Pan LL, Wu SQ, et al: CA 125, PET alone, PET-CT, CT and MRI in diagnosing recurrent ovarian carcinoma. A systematic review and meta-analysis. *EJR* 71:164–174, 2009.

Hoffman JR, Mower WR, Wolfson AB, et al, and the National Emergency X-Radiography Utilization Study Group: Validity of a set of clinical criteria to rule out injury to the cervical spine in patients with blunt trauma. *N Engl J Med* 343:94, 2000.

Hobbs C, Bilo R: Nonaccidental trauma: clinical and epidemiological aspects of child abuse. *Pediatr Radiol* 39:457–460, 2009.

Holmes JF, Akkinepalli R: Computed tomography versus plain radiography to screen for cervical spine injury: a meta-analysis. *J Trauma* 58(5):902, 2005.

Hubble W: Something old, something new: skeletal imaging with F18-sodium fluoride PET/CT. *Adv Med Imag Radiat Oncol*, 2011.

Jacobson HR, Striker GE, Klahr S: *The principles and practice of nephrology*, St. Louis, MO, 1995, Mosby.

Juranek J, Salmon M: Anomalous development of brain structure and function in spina bifida myleomeningocele. Developmental Disabilities Research Reviews [online]. 2010;16:23–30: http://onlinelibrary.wiley.com/doi/10.1002/ddrr.88/pdf. Accessed March 19, 2012.

Karavitka N, Cudlip S, Adams C, Wass J: Craniopharyngiomas. *Endocrine Rev [online]* 27(4):371–397, 2006: http://edrv.endojournals.org/content/27/4/371.full.pdf+html. Accessed March 19, 2012.

Karger S, Basel AG: European Stroke Initiative recommendations for stroke management. *Cerebrovasc Dis* 16:311, 2003.

Koopman WJ, Boulware DW, Heudebert GR: *Clinical primer of rheumatology*, Philadelphia, PA, 2003, Lippincott Williams & Wilkins.

Kumar V, Cotran R, Robbins S: *Basic pathology*, ed 7, Philadelphia, PA, 2003, Saunders.

Leyendecker J, Bllomfeld R, DiSantis D, et al: MR enterography in the management of patients with Crohn disease. *Radiographics* 29:1827–1846, 2009.

Lord SJ, Lei W, Craft P, et al: A systematic review of the effectiveness of MRI as an addition to mammography and ultrasound in screening young women at high risk of breast cancer. *EJC* 43:1905–1917, 2007.

Lovig KO, Ward BA: Benign breast diseases in elderly women and men. In Rosenthal RA, editor: *Principles and practice of geriatric surgery*, 2011, Springer Sciences + Business Media, LLC, pp 469–478.

Macari M, Bini EJ, Jacobs SL, et al: Significance of missed polyps at CT colonography. *Am J Roentgenol* 183(1):127, 2004.

Maier R: *Evaluation of abdominal trauma*, Chicago, IL, 2000, American College of Surgeons Trauma Committee.

McCance KL, Huether SE, Brashers VL, Rote, NS: *Pathophysiology: the biologic basis for disease in adults and children*, ed 6, St. Louis, MO, 2010, Mosby.

Mellors RC: *Congenital and hereditary bone disorders*, New York, 1999, Weill Medical College of Cornell University.

Merck manual of diagnosis and therapy, ed 19, Whitehouse Station, NJ, 2011, Merck & Co.

Minigh J: Traumatic injuries to the cervical spine. *Radiol Technol* 77(1):69, 2006.

Namasivayan S, Kalra MK, Torres WE, Small WC: Adverse reactions to intravenous iodinated contrast media: a primer for radiologists. *Emerg Radiol* 12(5):210–215, 2006.

National data archive on child abuse and neglect, Ithaca, NY, 2003, College of Human Ecology, Cornell University.

National Safety Council: Estimating the cost of unintentional injuries: http://www.nsc.org/news_resources/injury_and_death_statistics/Pages/EstimatingtheCostsofUnintentionalInjuries.aspx. Accessed.

Nursing Standard: Central venous lines quick reference guide 6, Nurs Stand 13(42), 1999: www.nursing-standard.co.uk/archives/ns/residentpdfs/quickrefPDFfiles/Quickref6.pdf. Accessed.

Old J, Colvert M: Vertebral compression fractures in the elderly. *Am Fam Phys* 69(1):111–116, 2004.

Overwalder PJ: Intraaortic balloon pump counterpulsation. *Internet J Thoracic Cardiovasc surg* 2(2), 1999: www.ispub.com/ostia/index.php?xmlFilePath=journals/ijtcvs/archives.xml. Accessed.

Payman S, Cox AJ, Ostendorf R: *Influence of airbags and restraining devices on the pattern of facial fractures in motor vehicle accidents*, Birmingham, AL, 2001, University of Alabama.

Pohost GM, O'Rourke RA, Berman DS, Pravin MS: *Imaging in cardiovascular disease*, Philadelphia, PA, 2000, Lippincott Williams & Wilkins.

Porth CM: *Essentials of pathophysiology*, ed 3, Philadelphia, PA, 2011, Lippincott Williams & Wilkins.

Rhoades R, Pflanzer R: *Human physiology*, ed 4, Pacific Grove, CA, 2003, Thomson Learning, Inc.

Saloner D, Uzelac A, Hetts S, et al. Modern meningioma imaging techniques. *J Neuro- Oncol [online]*, 2010. *DOI 10.1007/s11060-010-0367-6*: http://www.springerlink.com/content/71441438826w5m87/full-text.html. Accessed.

Sanders R: *Clinical sonography: a practical guide*, ed 3, Philadelphia, PA, 2011, Lippincott.

Saul T: *Management of head injury*, Chicago, 1998, American College of Surgeons Trauma Committee in conjunction with the Joint Section on Neurotrauma and Critical Care of the American Association of Neurological Surgeons and Congress of Neurological Surgeons.

Schilz A, Kornak U: CLCN7-related osteopetrosis, NIH October 14, 2010: www.ncbi.nlm.nih.gov/books/NBK1127. Accessed.

Schwartz HS, editor: *Orthopaedic knowledge update: musculoskeletal tumors 2*, Rosemont, IL, 2007, American Association of Orthopaedic Surgeons.

Smith R: *Netter's obstetrics, gynecology, and women's health*, Teterboro, NJ, 2003, Icon Learning Systems.

Society of Nuclear Medicine: SNM guidelines for sodium 18F-fluoride PET/CT bone scans, 2011: www.snm.org/docs/Practice%20Guideline%20NaF%20PET%20V1.pdf. Accessed.

Stiell IG, Wells GA, Vandemheen K, et al: The Canadian CT head rule for patients with minor head injury. *Lancet* 357(9266):1391, 2001.

Trancomano CA: Achondroplasia. In *Gene review*, 2006, National Institute of Health: www.genetests.org. Accessed April 23, 2006.

U.S. Department of Health and Human Services, Administration on Children, Youth and Families: Child maltreatment 2010: http://www.acf.hhs.gov/programs/cb/pubs/cm10/cm10.pdf#page=70. Accessed.

Van der A, Sherman J, Luciano D: *Human physiology*, ed 5, New York, 1990, McGraw-Hill Publishing.

WebMD LLC: Developmental dysplasia of the hip, 2011: Retrieved from emedicine.medscape.com/article/1248135. Accessed.

Wilson R, Alexander J: *Management of trauma—pitfalls and practice*, ed 2, Baltimore, MD, 1996, Williams & Wilkins.

Yochum TR, Rowe LJ: *Essentials of skeletal radiology*, ed 2, vols 1 and 2, Baltimore, MD, 1996, Williams & Wilkins.

Zuger J: *Positron emission tomography in lung imaging, PCCU Lesson 15*, vol 13, Northbrook, IL, 1999, American College of Chest Physicians.

Page numbers followed by "f" indicate figures, "t" indicate tables, and "b" indicate boxes.